The Emergence of International Health Policy in Southeast Asia, India, and Sri Lanka, 1937–1978

"Vivek Neelakantan has made a remarkable contribution to understanding the emergence, limits and obliteration of a progressive vision for international health and social reform in South and Southeast Asia during the 1930s. His book goes beyond Southeast Asia and is relevant to all scholars interested in two traditional perspectives on international health that are relevant to this day: a hegemonic perspective focused on technology; and a holistic perspective that emphasises the social determinants of disease. Neelakantan provides a novel examination of the complexity of the holistic Conference of Far-Eastern Nations on Rural Hygiene that took place in Bandoeng in 1937 – for many scholars, this was a crucial moment for the holistic perspective. Despite some important advances, like a call for a liaison between nutritionists and agriculturalists, there was no criticism at the event of the impact of colonial policies on nutrition, and rural change was overlooked. A naïve trust in the power of medical science prevailed, and the Cold War context of the post-Second World War period energised the hegemonic technocratic perspective. This is a crucial read for better understanding how to decolonize global health, and emphasising solidarity and equity as its organising principles."

—Marcos Cueto, Editor, *História, Ciências, Saúde-Manguinhos*, Casa de Oswaldo Cruz, Fiocruz, and President, Division of History of Science and Technology of the International Union of History and Philosophy of Science and Technology (IUHPST/DHST) for the period 2021–2025

"Vivek Neelakantan has offered a nuanced analysis of the history of medicine in interwar and post-war Southeast Asia. His monograph offers useful comparisons across the region and within South Asia, furthering our understanding of medicine within Asia, and globally. It is an excellent addition to the literature."

—Michitake Aso, Associate Professor, *Department of History and East Asian Studies, State University of New York at Albany*

"At a time when western concepts and institutions dominate the discourse on public health, this book brings sharp focus to Indigenous thinking within post-colonial Asia. Vivek Neelakantan's valuable research offers an inter-disciplinary perspective on public health, linking geographies, geopolitics and histories of the region."

—Rama Baru, Professor, *Jindal School of Public Health and Human Development, Jindal Global University*

"This pathbreaking book traces the history of international health endeavours in South and Southeast Asia during the critical middle decades of the twentieth century. Carefully researched and clearly written, the book exposes the tensions between technical approaches to health promotion – focusing on medicines, vaccinations and disease eradication – that were favoured before the war by colonial health departments, and after the war by the WHO, and a social approach that understood health in a broader sense. The proponents of the social approach – many of them based in international health organisations and missions – urged changes to the conditions in which Southeast Asians lived. Such changes often had the potential to undermine the colonial and post-colonial social orders. This book tells a fascinating story of ideological tension in the domain of public health. It is an important contribution to our understanding of modern South and Southeast Asian history."

—Robert Cribb, Emeritus Professor of Asian History, *Department of Political and Social Change, Australian National University*

Vivek Neelakantan

The Emergence of International Health Policy in Southeast Asia, India, and Sri Lanka, 1937–1978

palgrave
macmillan

Vivek Neelakantan
Southeast Asian Medical Historian
Mumbai, Maharashtra, India

ISBN 978-3-032-21232-0 ISBN 978-3-032-21233-7 (eBook)
https://doi.org/10.1007/978-3-032-21233-7

This Palgrave Macmillan imprint is published by the registered company Springer Nature Switzerland AG.
The registered company address is: Gewerbestrasse 11, 6330 Cham, Switzerland

Note on Orthography: Bahasa Indonesia

Place names follow Ejaan Yang Disempurnakan (1973). I retain the Dutch-era spelling (e.g., "Bandoeng" for the 1937 Rural Hygiene Conference) to reflect historical orthography. Post-independence names (e.g., "Bandung" for Bandung Plan and Asian-African Conference) reflect contemporary usage.

Note on Javanese Patronymics

Javanese are cited by their given name in subsequent mentions (e.g., Boentaran Martoatmodjo → Boentaran), conforming to regional naming conventions.

Note on Thai Patronymics

Thai individuals are likewise referred to by their given name in subsequent mentions (e.g., Sanguan Nitayarumphong → Sanguan).

Foreword

Epidemics do not respect national borders. Nor do health challenges such as obesity, diabetes, and cardiovascular disorders. The response to global challenges of ill-health and disability is therefore greatly facilitated by international cooperation. This conviction stimulated the founding of international health organizations including the World Health Organization. Yet the coordinated international response to health challenges requires relinquishing, to a certain extent, state sovereignty and state control. As Vivek Neelakantan's monograph analyses, most nations in Southeast Asia balked at that prospect. Despite the almost universal approval of coordination and cooperation, only a small number of modest initiatives have materialized.

During the 1950s, the World Health Organization (WHO) and UNICEF offered technical assistance and vertical solutions to health challenges. Neelakantan analyses the development of these efforts in Southeast Asia. The international malaria eradication campaign, which primarily focused on spraying DDT, is an example of a technocratic solution that ultimately failed. A second example is the smallpox eradication campaign, which was eventually successful. As Neelakantan trenchantly argues, these vertical approaches, which focus on specific diseases and consist of vaccination, antibiotics, and chemical substances to eradicate disease vectors—so-called magic bullets—might appear attractive but generally have limited effect in local contexts. Advocates of these technological and reductionistic approaches overlook the need for broader, holistic, and horizontal approaches to health and well-being, which emphasize local health infrastructures, public health programs, and public health education.

Yet health is more than just health—defined as those issues that physicians address in their everyday job. Addressing systemic issues including lack of sanitation and appropriate nutrition as well as absence of sewage systems lead to improvements in health. Similarly, poverty and disadvantage lead to adverse health outcomes. Research focusing on the social determinants of health has repeatedly and unequivocally demonstrated this. Unfortunately, finding solutions for broader issues is inherently complex, challenging, expensive, and often politically divisive. After World War II, developmental aid and community development programs focused issues, with mixed success.

At times, local and small-scale solutions, implemented by dedicated individuals, have proven to be successful. Neelakantan discusses programs like these in Indonesia, India, Sri Lanka, and Thailand. Small-scale local solutions have often functioned as inspiring examples in the publications of the World Health Organization, particularly those that appeared around the 1978 Alma-Ata conference and discussions about Primary Health Care. It has often been difficult to "scale up" successful local projects into global policies.

As Neelakantan concludes, formulating praiseworthy aspirations to improve health outcomes worldwide is relatively easy. To translate these ideals into tangible local policies and, ideally, local outcomes is far more difficult. This book highlights the ubiquitous tensions between global aspirations and local realities, national policies and ingrained practices, and the challenges of realizing high ideals into highly varied and ever-changing local contexts. In addition, pharmaceuticals, medical education, public health programs, and health care infrastructures are expensive. Even though most experts in international health policy emphasize that the limited financial strength of lower income countries are not the only obstacle in improving health outcomes worldwide, the lack of finance of health initiatives is one of the most serious obstacles.

Neelakantan analyses how international health experts, national politicians and powerbrokers, and local physicians and paramedical professionals have dealt with the various tensions in improving the health outcomes worldwide. He demonstrates how approaches and emphases have changed, have been changed back, and have been modified. At the same time, the health issues that confront us humans are changing as well. This book successfully analyses the interplay of evolving local and global responses to changing health challenges and the broader economic, social, political conditions in which they appear over almost two centuries.

Professor Hans Pols
The University of Sydney
Email: hans.pols@sydney.edu.au

Camperdown, NSW, Australia Hans Pols

Acknowledgments

I gratefully acknowledge financial support from the Rockefeller Archive Center (2016); Harry S. Truman and Dwight D. Eisenhower Presidential Libraries (2017); the Consortium for the History of Science, Technology and Medicine Research Fellowship (2018–2019), sponsored by the Wellcome Trust; and the Brocher Foundation (2023).

Conducting research for the monograph across four continents and nine countries was a formidable yet rewarding enterprise. I'm indebted to the staff of numerous institutions, including the Rockefeller Archive Center; the Truman and Eisenhower Presidential Museums and Libraries; the Archives of the WHO, ILO, the World Council of Churches, Geneva; the Perpustakaan Nasional Republik Indonesia Library, Jakarta; the Seeley Mudd Manuscripts and Rare Books at Princeton; the Yale Archives; the University of Auckland Special Collections; and the Tozzer and Arthur and Elizabeth Schlesinger Library on the History of Women at Harvard. Special thanks to Marie Villemin-Partow, Erard Reynald, Jacques Rodriguez, Remo Becci, Anne-Emanuelle Tankam, Ian Brailsford, Lee Hiltzik, and Monica Blanc.

This monograph draws its inspiration from the works of the late WHO scientist Socrates Litsios (1937–2021). Conversations with Shirish Kavadi and Marcos Cueto significantly shaped the evolution of the monograph's arguments, while Liping Bu, Patricia Rosenfield, Pierre-Yves Saunier, Terry Hull, and Omer Aloni offered invaluable perspectives. I thank Liat Kozma for inviting me to "Medicalizing the Pasts" workshop in 2023 at Haifa. The conference provided an opportunity to engage with emerging voices in global health histories. Special thanks go to Hans Pols and Eric

Tagliacozzo, whose support in my grant applications was instrumental. As my PhD mentor at the University of Sydney (2009–14), Hans encouraged me to present my preliminary findings on Southeast Asian medical history at HOMSEA conferences, which broadened my analytical lens beyond colonial and national frameworks.

I am grateful to the late Dutch mission doctor Arnoud H. Klokke (1920–2017) for sharing rare photographs, documenting the anti-yaws campaign in Borneo during the 1950s, from his personal collection. I am indebted to Rufino Macagba, Jon Rohde, Rolf Carrière, Henry Perry, Sharad Sapra, and Krisantha Weerasuriya for recounting their personal experiences related to the evolution of Primary and Selective Primary Health Care.

I thank Lucy Kidwell and her team at Palgrave Macmillan for being so supportive during the publication process.

Finally, this monograph would not have come to fruition but for the steadfast support of my parents. During one of the most difficult moments of my life, as I suffered from a debilitating illness, their quiet faith in my intellectual resilience strengthened me. This monograph is dedicated to Hans as a testament to his belief that principled academic labor must be sustained even when institutional scaffolding falters.

Competing Interests The author has no competing interests to declare that are relevant to the content of this manuscript.

Contents

About the Author

Vivek Neelakantan a Southeast Asian Medical Historian and a 2023 Brocher Foundation Visiting Fellow, interrogates the entanglements of public health, governance, and geopolitics across colonial and postcolonial Asia. His research agenda spans two major geographical and historical contexts. The first reconstructs cholera's history in nineteenth-century Bombay, tracing the interlocking of medical pluralism, imperial anxieties, Parsi philanthropy, and sanitary surveillance across urban and rural contexts. The second examines Indonesia's health policy under the Old and New Orders (1945–1998), mapping its incorporation into state-building and developmentalist rhetoric—and the ruptures therein.

Abbreviations

AIIHPH	All India Institute of Hygiene and Public Health
ANRI	Arsip Nasional Republik Indonesia, Jakarta [National Archives of Indonesia]
ANM	Auxiliary Nurse Midwife
ARO	UNICEF Regional Office for Asia
ASA	Association of Southeast Asia
ASEAN	Association of Southeast Asian Nations
BCG	Bacillus Calmette-Guérin
CDC	Centers for Disease Control and Prevention
CHD	Community Health Development
CHWs	Community Health Workers
CMC	Christian Medical Commission
CPT	Communist Party of Thailand
CRHP	Comprehensive Rural Health Project
DDT	dichloro diphenyl trichloroethane
DMK	Dravida Munnetra Kazhagam
DPT	diphtheria-pertussis-tetanus vaccination
DVG	Dienst der Volksgezondheid
EMRO	WHO Regional Office for the Eastern Mediterranean
FAO	Food and Agricultural Organization
FEATM	Far Eastern Association of Tropical Medicine
FOA	Foreign Operations Administration
GB	Gandhi Bhavan Collection, Bangalore
GH	Geneeskundige Hoogeschool
GOBI	Growth Monitoring, Oral Rehydration, Breastfeeding, and Immunization
ICA	International Cooperation Administration

IHB	International Health Board
IHC	International Health Commission
IHD	International Health Division
ILO	International Labor Organization
ILOA	ILO Archives
ILOL	ILO Library
ITC	International Tuberculosis Campaign
JMA	Japanese Military Administration
KB	Koninklijke Bibliotheek [National Library of the Netherlands]
LoN	League of Nations Archives
LNHO	League of Nations Health Organization
MCH	Maternal and Child Health
MSA	Mutual Security Agency
NAI	National Archives of India
NAM	Non-Aligned Movement
NARA	National Archives and Records Administration
NARIC	National Rice and Corn Corporation
NIAS	Nederlandsch-Indische Artsen School
NIEO	New International Economic Order
NLA	National Library of Australia
NLB	National Library Board, Singapore
NMP	Native Medical Practitioners
OIHP	Office International d'Hygiène Publique
PASB	Pan American Sanitary Bureau
PHC	Primary Health Care
PKI	Partai Komunis Indonesia
PMA	Philippine Medical Association
PNRI	Perpustakaan Nasional Republik Indonesia, Jakarta [National Library of Indonesia]
PRC	People's Republic of China
PUMC	Peking Union Medical College
RAC	Rockefeller Archive Center
RG	Record Group
SARS	severe acute respiratory syndrome
SEARO	WHO Regional Office for South-East Asia
SEAC	South-East Asia Command
SEATO	Southeast Asian Treaty Organization
SGMML	Seeley G. Mudd Manuscript Library, Princeton
SPHC	Selective Primary Health Care
SPI	State Pharmaceutical Corporation, Sri Lanka
STOVIA	School Tot Opleiding van Inlandsche Artsen
TAP	Technical Assistance Program

TCM	Traditional Chinese Medicine
TCPS	Treponematoses Control Program Simplified
TNSA	Tamil Nadu State Archives, Chennai
UHC	Universal Health Coverage
UMN	University of Minnesota Libraries
UN	United Nations
UNICEF	United Nations Children's Fund
UNRRA	United Nations Relief and Rehabilitation Administration
USAID	United States Agency for International Development
USPHS	United States Public Health Service
WEP	World Employment Program
WCC	World Council of Churches
WHA	World Health Assembly
WHO	World Health Organization
WHOA	World Health Organization Archives
WHOL	World Health Organization Library
WPHS	Western Pacific Health Services
WPRO	WHO Regional Office for the Western Pacific

List of Images

CHAPTER 1

Introduction

Conceptualizing Southeast Asia: A Microcosm of Global Health

While Southeast Asia is often defined in conventional terms—India to the west and China to the north—the introduction adopts a broader perspective.[1] This cartographic shorthand serves only as a foil, not the monograph's own definition of Southeast Asia. By adopting a wider remit, this chapter foregrounds Southeast Asia's coherence precisely through its entanglements with India, China, and international currents. Rather than treating Southeast Asia as a mere geographical expression, I approach the region as a historical arena shaped by the ebbs and flows of commerce, migration, European colonialism, decolonization, and the Cold War. Political boundaries alone cannot capture the region's socio-cultural, linguistic, or historical complexity. Since the early twentieth century, there has been a widespread tendency to focus on constituent parts of Southeast Asia rather than to develop a perception of the region as a whole.[2] This fragmentation has yielded valuable national histories but obscured the region's coherence as a historical sphere.

If Southeast Asia was an arena of historical entanglement, it was also on the ecological crossroads. The region's natural environment was central to its historical coherence:

V. Neelakantan, *The Emergence of International Health Policy in Southeast Asia, India, and Sri Lanka, 1937–1978*,
https://doi.org/10.1007/978-3-032-21233-7_1

> The Venetians monopolized it, then the Portuguese took control of it, and most European colonisers battled fiercely for nutmeg, mace, and cloves—once grown only in the Spice Islands of Indonesia, the world's largest tropical archipelago. Throughout its history, Southeast Asia has witnessed the rise and fall of cultures, empires, colonial powers and ideological regimes. Its natural environment mirrors its tumultuous past. Life-giving monsoons, so important for farming and sailing, also inundate and wreak destruction in local cities each year. Volcanic eruptions enrich and renew the topsoil, but also flatten scores of villages and bury vulnerable villagers. The wet and hot jungles between the Tropics of Cancer and Capricorn, friendly to infections and insurgents alike, also sustain animal and plant life unequalled in biodiversity.[3]

The environmental plenitude of the region—sustaining agriculture and biodiversity—nurtures prosperity yet exposes vulnerability to disasters and disease. Nature's precarious rhythms have tested the resilience of political institutions. In the sphere of public health, recurring disasters produce uneven outcomes, with some nations building resilient health systems, while others remain exposed to epidemics.

Although Southeast Asian nations share many elements of a common history and culture, the region is beset with socio-political contradictions. Agrarian economies, economic powerhouses, military, socialist, and democratic regimes are reachable within a short plane ride. Southeast Asia's teeming diversity also plays out in contemporary health achievements: in 2011, life expectancy ranged from 56 years in Myanmar to 81 years in Singapore.[4]

The region's teeming environment, however, also fosters zoonotic spillovers, as dense human-animal interactions have repeatedly generated Emerging Infectious Diseases—with the Nipah virus as a striking example. Nipah outbreaks exemplify how local ecological conditions can incubate pathogens that swiftly cross borders, testing both local responsiveness and international cooperation. First reported among swine farmers in northern Peninsular Malaysia in 1998, Nipah triggered outbreaks in Bangladesh, Singapore, India, and other countries between 2001 and 2005.[5]

Southeast Asia's experience with Emerging Infectious Diseases reveals tensions between national sovereignty and global health. Health systems across Southeast Asia have challenged existing global health regimes and precipitated debates over viral sovereignty and equitable access. For instance, Indonesia's refusal to share H5N1 avian influenza viral samples with the WHO in 2006 ignited a diplomatic inflection point over reconciling national interests with the global good.[6]

Between 1918 and 2020, Southeast Asia faced shared health challenges—pandemic influenza, beriberi, malaria, hookworm, and more recently, COVID-19. Yet, the region has lacked a mechanism for transnational health collaboration since the colonial period.[7] Between 1910 and 1938, the Far Eastern Association of Tropical Medicine (FEATM)—a short-lived regional body spanning colonial jurisdictions—convened congresses across monsoon Asia to address beriberi.[8] However, colonial states such as British India were unwilling to commit resources, precluding the operationalization of FEATM's regional strategy. Although the association dissolved before World War II, its fragmented posture resonated in geopolitical dilemmas that would later confront the WHO, including the partition of its Southeast Asia regional office—an indelible marker of state sovereignty.

Since its inception in 1948, the WHO implemented a policy of administrative decentralization or regionalization. Due to strategic compulsions, the organization partitioned the proposed regional office for Southeast Asia into the WHO Regional Office for South-East Asia (SEARO) and the Western Pacific (WPRO), along jurisdictional boundaries that remained fluid. This partition, in turn, reinscribed colonial fault lines in regional health governance.[9]

Ultimately, state sovereignty has eroded regional collaboration in health, from the FEATM initiatives to the WHO's partitioning of Southeast Asia and, more recently, the COVID-19 crisis. The Association of Southeast Asian Nations (ASEAN)—a regional grouping founded in 1967—recalibrated the WHO's International Health Regulations to Southeast Asia in the aftermath of the SARS (Severe Acute Respiratory Syndrome) outbreak in 2005. However, ASEAN's collective approach to strengthen emerging disease preparedness of member states contravened the regional grouping's cardinal principle of noninterference concerning the domestic affairs of sovereigns.[10] In Southeast Asia, individual nations' responses to COVID-19 were dictated by geopolitical equations with China. For instance, Cambodian premier Hun Sen visited Beijing at the height of the coronavirus panic in February 2020. He repeatedly claimed that fear of COVID-19 was more dangerous than the virus itself.[11] His rhetoric subordinated epidemiological caution to geopolitical posturing.

The fragmented response to COVID-19 across Southeast Asia underscored the tension between state sovereignty and regional health governance. On May 23, 2025—in the aftermath of the pandemic—Indonesia strategically shifted its alignment from SEARO to WPRO. The decision was finalized during the Seventy-Eighth World Health Assembly (WHA).[12] Indonesia's departure from SEARO forces a strategic reckoning: what constitutes a critical mass of states to sustain meaningful regional health cooperation?[13] The implications are immediate. Indonesia's transfer marks a departure from SEARO's traditional emphasis on equity, maternal health, and infectious disease control for lower- and middle-income countries to WPRO's focus on innovation, data governance, and pandemic preparedness.[14]

Indonesia's WPRO accession reflects shifting domestic health priorities. The country faces a dual burden—infectious diseases such as dengue and drug-resistant TB, and lifestyle diseases such as diabetes, hypertension, cardiovascular disease, and cancer. Mental disorders, climate shocks, and demographic aging compound systemic strain. In the context of planetary health—a framework that links the impacts of human disruptions on Earth's natural systems, including health—WPRO offers mechanisms to integrate climate resilience into health policy. This is critical for Indonesia, an archipelagic state exposed to rising sea levels, extreme weather, and transboundary haze.[15] Indonesia's niche within WPRO bridges regional concerns with global health diplomacy, advocating long-term environmental solutions that embed climate-linked determinants into health systems. This strategic reconfiguration—marked by Indonesia's WPRO membership—reaffirms that future resilience is contingent on cross-border epidemiological collaboration and addressing environmental determinants of health such as air pollution and climate change. In this context, Southeast Asia's diverse socioeconomic landscapes and unique health challenges position the region as a microcosm of global health, where resilience hinges on adaptation, innovation, and collaboration.

The Argument: The Nexus Between International Health and Geopolitics, Southeast Asia

This monograph traces the local antecedents of international health in Southeast Asia between 1937 and 1978. It delves into the non-Western critique of colonial medicine, the rapid transformations precipitated by political and economic decolonization in the aftermath of the Pacific War (1942–1945), and the incorporation of public health into postwar nation-building and Cold War geopolitics. Drawing on four case studies from Indonesia, India, Thailand, and Sri Lanka, this monograph argues that while Cold War ideological rivalries influenced the momentum toward PHC, the quest for PHC across Southeast Asia transcended geopolitical calculations alone. Local actors aligned PHC to suit national requirements. Context is central to understanding why the comprehensive approach—that linked public health to broader concerns of socioeconomic well-being—was eclipsed by a narrower technocentric approach, which prescribed the proverbial magic bullet to root out disease.

In sum, this monograph situates Southeast Asia's quest for PHC within a global framework, tracing the dynamic interaction between international health goals and regionally grounded interventions. It maps how regional health bodies such as SEARO and WPRO strategically aligned postcolonial aspirations with the normative prescriptions of international aid.

Extending the study of regional organizations, this monograph challenges extant international health historiography that privileges the centrality of the WHO and the Cold War, and instead advocates a decentering of Geneva from dominant global health narratives.[16] Furthermore, this monograph emphasizes the need to examine alternative international health frameworks pioneered by UNICEF (United Nations Children's Fund) and the International Labor Organization (ILO). UNICEF and the ILO articulated international health through fundamentally distinct paradigms—Selective Primary Healthcare (SPHC) and the Basic Needs Approach, respectively. SPHC and the Basic Needs Approach diverged in implementation logic. While SPHC pioneered technocratic cost-effective health interventions to address resource constraints in developing countries, the Basic Needs Approach advanced a rights-based structural orientation, rooted in social security.[17] In Southeast Asia, the PHC paradigm was not a WHO export but was reconfigured through regionally mediated health diplomacy.[18]

Region as a Geopolitical Construct

The crescent of land—that stretched from Bengal through Burma, the southern borderlands of Thailand, down the Malayan peninsula to Singapore island—was the hinterland of the Straits of Malacca, one of the world's prominent arteries of oceanic trade.[19] For centuries, the crescent drew millions seeking livelihood, especially from the ancient agrarian civilizations that bordered it. The advent of the colonial economy in the nineteenth century ushered in new opportunities. Waves of Chinese migrants, mainly from the hinterland of the southern seaboard, arrived in Nanyang or the Southern Seas as traders and artisans, pioneered the mines and plantations of Malaya, and provided the bulk of their workforce. South Asian communities populated numerous occupations: Muslim shopkeepers, Chettyar moneylenders, Sikh police, and Ceylonese lawyers. European rubber plantations in colonial Malaya attracted three-quarters of a million Tamils from the southern districts of Madras Presidency in British India. Many more Indians made the short journey from Bengal and Orissa to the rural economy of Burma. The main points of arrival for these migrants were Rangoon and Singapore, port cities with strong colonial underpinnings (Map 1.1).

Christopher Bayly and Tim Harper argue that during World War II, as retaining British India became a drain on the UK's domestic balance of payments, Southeast Asia emerged as the Empire's most prized asset. The region exported two-thirds of the world's tin, and British Malaya accounted for half the world's rubber production.[20] The economic resources of Southeast Asia were critical in ensuring the UK's postwar recovery. During the war, the Japanese sought to impose their worldview upon the crescent by incorporating it within the ambit of the Greater East Asia Co-Prosperity Sphere. However, Japan's military ascendancy was short-lived. The resurgence of the Allied naval power prevented the meaningful export of raw materials to Japan. When the rice exports from Burma and Thailand dried up in 1943 and 1944, the rest of the region faced dire food shortages, resulting in disease and malnutrition. The Pacific War (1942–1945) severed the region's old trade links with India and China.

At the end of the Pacific War, the crescent had to be forged anew. The instrument for this was the South-East Asia Command (SEAC), a brainchild of Admiral Lord Louis Mountbatten, a cousin of the British king-emperor, George VI. Created in 1943 at the zenith of the Pacific War, the SEAC was the first expression of Southeast Asia as a geopolitical entity.[21] Initially headquartered in New Delhi, capital of British India, the Command was transferred to Kandy, Ceylon in 1944. Ceylon's naval bases must have played a strategic role in the reconquest of Japanese-held territory in the World War II's eastern theater. Moreover, SEAC's inclusion of Ceylon (Sri Lanka since 1972) and the British Raj's northeastern frontiers—highlights the geopolitical importance of these areas, despite their exclusion from contemporary Southeast Asia. By contrast, the Netherlands Indies (now known as Indonesia), British Malaya, Singapore, and the

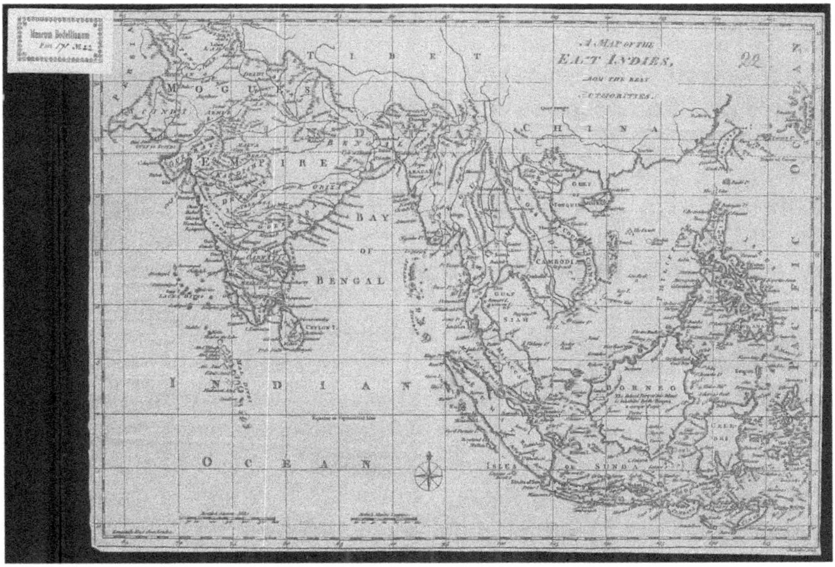

Map 1.1 A Map of the East Indies (Southeast Asia): From the Best Authorities, c. 1780. This 1780 map traces the arc of land from Bengal to Malaya—a littoral crescent that first served as an imperial maritime frontier, then as a colonial crucible of trade. During the nineteenth century, the crescent nurtured plantation economies, oceanic trade, and port-city formation, drawing Chinese and Indian migrants to Rangoon and Singapore, linchpins of colonial governance. Engraved by John Lodge. Shelfmark: COLLBN Port 175 N 22. Courtesy of Leiden University Libraries Digital Collection. Public domain. Persistent URL: http://hdl.handle.net/1887.1/item:3282488

Philippine Islands—under Japanese occupation between 1943 and 1945—were excluded from the jurisdiction of the Command. In this regard, the naming of Southeast Asia was a clear response to the historical fact that, by 1943, the Japanese Emperor's armies controlled the entire stretch between British Burma and the Philippine Islands.

The Pacific War catalyzed the ascendance of the notion of Southeast Asia as a geopolitical construct. Yet, the precise political boundaries of the region remained ambiguous until the creation of ASEAN in 1967. Benedict Anderson attributes the region's late unitary naming to three factors. First, the region lacked a historic hegemon such as the Ottomans for the Middle East or the Mughals of India. Second, the extraordinary religious diversity of the region—once Islam from the thirteenth century and Christianity from the sixteenth—broke up an essentially Hindu-Buddhistic syncretic civilization. Third, the region was imperially fragmented by the late nineteenth century, with the exception of Siam (Thailand since 1939), which served as a buffer state between British India and French Indochina. Unlike Africa, colonialism did not arrive in Southeast Asia in a late nineteenth-century rush but stretched across three centuries. For instance, the Portuguese and the Spaniards arrived in the late feudal sixteenth century, the Dutch in the mercantile seventeenth, the British in the industrialized eighteenth, the French in the industrialized nineteenth, and the Americans in the motorized twentieth. Each imperial power, jealous and rivalrous, sealed off its possessions so thoroughly that, by 1900, a young educated person in Batavia (Jakarta) knew more about Amsterdam than about Cambodia, with which their ancestors had close cultural affinity. Remote, heterogeneous, and imperially partitioned, it is therefore unsurprising that the region was late in its unitary naming.[22]

While the Pacific War marked the beginning of Southeast Asia's regional identity, the mottled nature of the region's colonial history offers an important context for its delayed unification. Regionalism is the act of forging a common platform. This includes constituting intergovernmental organizations and transnational civil society networks. The ultimate goal is to realize common objectives, and articulate a common identity.[23] Nationalist leaders, such as India's Jawaharlal Nehru, Burma's Aung San, and Soekarno of Indonesia, envisaged a balance between nationalism and international cooperation but were wary of subordinating national sovereignty to broader Asian ideals, delaying regional integration.[24]

Advancing decolonization was the underlying theme of the First Asian Relations Conference, convened in New Delhi in 1947. The Second Asian Relations Conference—hosted by Nehru in 1949—was directed toward supporting Indonesian nationalists after the Second Dutch Military Action in 1948. Despite talks of pan-Asian solidarity, proponents of the Asian Relations Conference were willing to offer verbal support rather than material assistance to advance the cause of the region's anti-colonial struggles. For example, India's aid to Indonesian freedom fighters did not extend to Ho Chi Minh.[25] The early stirrings of Pan-Asianism did not translate into enduring forms of regional cooperation.

At his inaugural address at the First Asian Relations Conference, Nehru asserted:

> It is fitting that India should play her part in this new phase of Asian development. Apart from the fact that India herself is emerging into freedom and independence, she is the natural centre and focal point of the many forces at work in Asia. Geography is a compelling factor, and geographically she is so situated as to be the meeting point of western and northern and eastern and southeast Asia. … Streams of culture have come into India from the west and the east and have been absorbed in India, producing the rich and variegated culture which is India today. At the same time, streams of culture have flowed from India to distant parts of Asia. If you would know India you would have to go to Afghanistan and western Asia, to Central Asia, to China and Japan and to the countries of southeast Asia. There you will find magnificent evidence of the vitality of Indian culture which spread out and influenced vast numbers of people.[26]

Delegates from Southeast Asia, particularly those from Burma, Indonesia, Thailand, Indochina, and Malaya, discerned in Nehru's inaugural address a strong Indian undercurrent, reading it as a bid for regional primacy under the guise of pan-Asian solidarity. As one Burmese delegate put it, "It was terrible to be ruled by a Western power, but it was even more so to be ruled by an Asian power."[27]

At New Delhi, Burmese leader Aung San espoused the formation of an Asian Commonwealth, which would constitute a united front against imperialistic rule. He argued, "While India should be one entity and China another, Southeast Asia as a whole should form an entity-then, finally, we should come together in a bigger union with the participation of other parts of Asia as well."[28] Building on his grand vision for a regional organization, Aung San proposed a more concrete Southeast Asian economic union. This regional framework included countries such as Burma, Indonesia, Thailand, Malaya, and Indochina (Vietnam, Laos, and Cambodia).[29] However, Burma's short-lived interest in regional cooperation evaporated with the tragic assassination of Aung San on July 19, 1947. Even more interested in regional relations during the late 1940s was Burma's neighbor to the east, Thailand.

On July 1, 1947, Thai Premier Thamrong Nawasawat proposed the creation of a Pan Southeast Asia Union, which would include, to begin with, Thailand, Vietnam, Cambodia, and Laos and would subsequently be expanded to include other states.[30] The proposed union would primarily concern itself with regional plans for the joint development of irrigation, fisheries, communications, and other resources of the area. However, the proposed association did not materialize. The Thai political opposition charged the Thamrong administration of colluding with French interests, leading the plan to be abandoned.[31] Marshal Phibun Songkhram—who usurped power following the November 1947 coup—revived the push for a regional dialog. He invited India, Burma, and the Philippines for talks in Bangkok in 1949 on political and economic matters but no conference was held due to a lack of enthusiasm from India and Burma.[32] During these years, Thailand also expressed interest in a Southeast Asian defense pact. Thailand's interest in a defense pact underscored Cold War tensions and the growing appeal of communism in Indochina.

The Philippines—a US colony that gained independence after the Pacific War—was genuinely concerned with the question of implementing an area accord during the early 1950s. Its status as a sovereign state, the enduring imprint of the colonial legacy, and lingering Cold War tensions in Indochina pivoted the Philippines toward Southeast Asia from its earlier orientation to the US. Following the Second Asian Relations Conference in 1949, Filipino diplomat General Carlos Romulo began working proactively towards an anti-Communist South and Southeast Asia regional bloc. The end of the Korean War in 1953 and escalating communist pressure on Vietnam—which led to the eventual partitioning of the country—changed Southeast Asia's geopolitical equation. In response, the US proposed a security cordon to contain communist advances beyond the northern portion of partitioned Vietnam, culminating in the establishment of SEATO (Southeast Asian Treaty Organization) in 1954.

SEATO's purview was expansive, encompassing the otherwise "unspecified general area of Southeast Asia," the equally "unspecified general area of the Southwest Pacific," and the member-state of Pakistan.[33] Although not geographically part of Southeast Asia, Pakistan joined the alliance due to geopolitical tensions with India. Notably, only two members of the military grouping—Thailand and the Philippines—were geographically situated in Southeast Asia. Between 1955 and 1970, neutral Cambodia and Laos declined to participate in the treaty—weakening its influence. Pakistan withdrew in 1972, and Vietnam's reunification in 1975 rendered the SEATO obsolete.

Donald K. Emmerson observes that SEAC and SEATO were Anglo-American initiatives—respectively anti-Japanese and anti-communist. Neither, however, was anti-colonial. SEAC facilitated the reassertion of the *status quo ante bellum*. SEATO, by contrast, was internally contradictory: its members pledged in Manila to "uphold equal rights and self-determination of peoples," while simultaneously opposing any effort in the treaty area to subvert sovereignty or territorial integrity.[34] Only after 1960 did indigenous forces in Southeast Asia begin spearheading the cause of a regional organization. In 1961, SEATO's Southeast Asian core—Thailand and the Philippines—joined Malaya in forming the Association of Southeast Asia (ASA), which lasted until 1967. The ASA dissolved in 1967, when the three states combined with Singapore and Indonesia to establish ASEAN. All five founding members of ASEAN suppressed communism as a political ideology and pursued a pro-Western orientation.

The destructive aspects of region formation in Southeast Asia should not be forgotten. What was once considered a culturally derivative borderland, roughly east of India and south of China, was reconstituted into a mosaic of specific states through the dynamic interplay between colonialism and nationalism. Colonial states imposed artificial political borders that disrupted pre-existing cultural networks. The redrawing of Southeast Asia's map since the nineteenth century has posed challenges to regional integration. The legacy of nationalism across Southeast Asia has subordinated global health goals to state sovereignty. For instance, in the case of Myanmar (Burma until 1989), the junta has drawn international criticism for its defiance of the concept of health as a human right, and the expectation that states should contribute to the collective security of the society of states through investment in and a commitment to public health domestically.[35] However, for nearly three decades, the military regime has allowed public health to deteriorate to such a degree that the country is now regarded as a disease reservoir, fanning disease outbreaks both within and outside Southeast Asia. Myanmar's lack of action to safeguard public health within its borders is crippling infectious disease control across neighboring states.

The shortcomings of public health leadership underscore the broader challenges posed by Southeast Asia's porous regional identity. Myanmar's historical positioning within South Asia—first, as a province of British India (1886–1935), separation from British India (1937), independence from the UK (1948), and eventual ASEAN accession (1997)—reveals the fluidity of Southeast Asia as a region.[36] Similarly, Afghanistan, though geographically situated in central Asia, joined SEARO in 1948, following the Asian Relations Conference (1947). At the conference, the Afghan delegate underscored the need for closer epidemiological coordination between his country and India.[37] However, by 1969, Afghanistan withdrew from SEARO to join the WHO Regional Office for the Eastern

Mediterranean (EMRO), citing socio-cultural and epidemiological affinity with the Middle East.[38] The shifting regional realignments across South, Southeast, East, and central Asia highlight incongruities between epidemiological coordination and geopolitical identity.

The selective focus on India and Ceylon—constituents of Mountbatten's SEAC—and ASEAN member states allows the monograph to delve deeply into the geopolitical dynamics that shaped Southeast Asia's fluid regional identity. In the epidemiological imagination of the nascent WHO, the central and South Eastern parts of Asia, together with Indonesia, represented the Monsoon Asia of Geographers.[39] The common denominator underlying health conditions of the area included endemic cholera and malaria, widespread food deficiencies of rice-eaters, and a high prevalence of TB. Furthermore, India and Ceylon—integrated into the activities of the FEATM, and the anti-hookworm campaigns of the Rockefeller Foundation's International Health Board (IHB) during the interwar period—shared close epidemiological ties with Southeast Asia. Despite being geopolitically positioned in South Asia, India, and Sri Lanka offer a compelling framework to investigate the dynamics between regional identity and international health collaboration. Conversely, this study excludes Pakistan, Bangladesh, Nepal, Bhutan, and the Maldives from South Asia, and Brunei from Southeast Asia.

The histories of Pakistan and Bangladesh (East Pakistan until 1971) are deeply entwined with the partition of the Subcontinent in 1947. Undivided Pakistan joined the EMRO in 1949, driven by geopolitical tensions with India over Kashmir. Bangladesh emerged as a newly independent country in 1971 after the nine-month liberation war and subsequently acceded to SEARO. In the case of Nepal and Bhutan, the mountainous topography and a strategic orientation toward India limited their geopolitical engagement in health with Southeast Asia.[40] Likewise, due to their islandness, the Maldives had closer epidemiological interactions with Sri Lanka and India rather than with Southeast Asia.[41] In Southeast Asia, the Sultanate of Brunei—a British protectorate during the period covered in this monograph (1937–1978)—was granted independence in 1984. However, health developments in Brunei fall beyond the scope of this study. Excluding these nations from the study prioritizes analytical depth over geographical breadth.

Conclusion

Southeast Asia's international health trajectory between 1937 and 1978 exemplifies the reconciliation of international health ideals and actionable goals at the local level. The monograph's central takeaway is the importance of a regional approach to international health history. Can meaningful progress be expected if international aid agencies continue to prescribe a one-size-fits-all? Such an approach risks not only inefficacy but also derailing technological advancements while failing to account for health systems shaped by local nuance.[42] If historians of international health lean toward global narratives, Southeast Asian medical historians have focused on national histories—overlooking the interconnectedness between local and global domains.[43] Bridging this divide requires a comprehensive framework integrating global, regional, and local perspectives to produce a layered analysis of health histories across scales.

My broad critique of the shortcomings of global and national historiographies of health is congruent with Sunil Amrith's *Decolonizing International Health: India and Southeast Asia, 1930–65*. Amrith argues that India played a central role in shaping the growing consensus on international health and formed the nodal point in a network of expertise and policies that spanned Southeast Asia, which touched some parts of the region more than others.[44] However, Amrith's line of argument overlooks the influence of Indonesia, the Philippines, or Ceylon in shaping the contours of international health in the aftermath of World War II. Additionally, while India's complex and diverse disease environment positioned it as the ideal laboratory for new medical technologies and policies, Amrith's generalization that solutions tested in India had universal applicability across the underdeveloped world risks flattening institutional textures underlying Southeast Asian health systems. The neglect of Southeast Asian actors, particularly the Philippines, underscores the need to situate India within a wider Southeast Asia framework, attentive to institutional diversity and regional nuances.

India's salience in this prominently Southeast Asia-focused monograph is a testament to its initiative in founding SEARO and as a source of influential health planning models. India's health planning prototypes included the Etawah community development model,

whose comparisons with postcolonial Philippines and Indonesia are highlighted in Chap. 6. Nehru's aspiration for regional leadership positioned India as the putative health hegemon. At the First Asian Relations

Conference (1947), by framing poverty as a "common problem" affecting Asia, Nehru cast India as the archetype for regional development.[45] Yet this very claim to representativeness risked obscuring the institutional diversity underpinning decolonizing Asia, where countries such as the Philippines and Ceylon pursued distinct trajectories of social policy.

The Bhore Committee Report (1946)—with its emphasis on integrating preventive and curative services, and prioritizing rural hygiene—became the cornerstone for asserting India's aspirational regional health hegemony in decolonizing Asia. The Bhore Committee principles were explicitly articulated at the First Asian Relations Conference (1947) and the ILO's Preparatory Asian Regional Conference in New Delhi (October–November 1947), bolstering India's claims to regional preeminence. Yet, the Committee's emphasis on integrated rural health services was ill-suited to Ceylon's plantation-dominated economy, where estate medicine—organized through employer-run dispensaries—remained the predominant framework.[46] Ceylon's plantation settings revealed that the Bhore Committee's rural hygiene principles were context-bound. By contrast, the implementation of Indonesia's rural health program—embodied in the Bandung Plan (1951), which likewise emphasized preventive-curative integration—was delayed by political instability and repeated military coups. The Plan echoed principles that paralleled those in the Bhore Report. Yet, there is no empirical evidence to suggest that Indonesian planners directly drew from the Report. What united the Bhore Report and the Bandung Plan was a shared emphasis on preventive hygiene, inspired by John B. Grant's Rockefeller-supported rural reconstruction in China, though refracted through distinct national and local priorities.

India's bid for regional health leadership was contested, as Pakistan and the Philippines advanced parallel claims that weakened India's positioning. Pakistan resisted Indian hegemony at forums such as the WHO, UNICEF, and ILO, while the Philippines implicitly contested India's authority to speak for Southeast Asian health problems at the Second World Health Assembly (1949).[47] At the Assembly, Philippine Health Secretary Antonio Villarama (1946–1948) asserted that no universal formula could address all health problems, and that local contexts should be given scope for devising their own solutions.[48] Villarama's insistence on local and regional specificity contrasted sharply with Indian attempts to generalize its own experience on rural hygiene, underscoring Southeast Asia's distinct international health trajectory.[49] This evidence complicates Amrith's argument that India functioned as the uncontested hub of international health expertise in Asia.[50] Far from enjoying unrivaled authority, India's interventions were persistently questioned and recalibrated, producing a regional health agenda that was shaped as much by local initiatives as by Indian models.

By situating India and Sri Lanka in the title, this monograph clarifies its remit. Southeast Asian and Sri Lankan health trajectories complicated India's role as putative health hegemon, producing a regional agenda that was forged through negotiation rather than domination.

The architecture of this monograph situates the histories of health in Southeast Asia, India, and Sri Lanka within a wider geopolitical framework, while following a chronological and thematic sequence. Each chapter integrates Southeast Asian case studies, with overlaps across chronology and themes. This convergence demonstrates how specific landmarks in international health histories intersected with regional dynamics.

Chapter 2 lays the groundwork for the monograph by situating the history of public health in Southeast Asia during the interwar period (1918–1939) within the broader context of colonialism, medical philanthropy, humanitarianism, and decolonization. Crucially, I argue that the discourse of rural hygiene articulated at the Intergovernmental Conference of Far-Eastern Nations in Bandoeng (1937)—which connected public health to broader social determinants of health—emerged from a series of fragmented public health experiments on the empire's periphery. The discourse reflected a spectrum of objectives, ranging from the holistic medical visions of nationalist leaders—particularly Abdoel Rasjid and Mahatma Gandhi—to the Rockefeller Foundation's efforts to reform hygienic practices in the Netherlands Indies and British India, respectively. Yet, at the commencement of the Pacific War, governments focused on quick-fix solutions to public health at the expense of rural hygiene initiatives. Chapter 3 traces the transformations propelled by wartime medical technologies, such as insecticide DDT trials, in British India and Ceylon. In turn, the chapter examines the circumstances that led to the reconfiguration of international health, i.e., from a loose network of technical experts during the interwar period to the notion that the state was responsible for guaranteeing the health of its citizens.

Chapter 4 discusses the postwar architecture of international health centered on the WHO. During the 1950s, amid Cold War tensions, the WHO steered away from its utopian vision of social medicine and adopted a pragmatic approach aimed at eradicating endemic diseases, such as malaria, which vitiated the population's productive capacity. In the

Southeast Asian context, the nascent organization had to tread cautiously between European powers—British, Dutch, Portuguese, and French—who jealously guarded their colonial territories. Meanwhile, leaders of newly independent states viewed public health as vital to their national reconstruction efforts. In this context, alongside the WHO, aid agencies such as UNICEF and the ILO incorporated a regionalization framework. This regional turn was mapped—albeit asymmetrically—by UNICEF and the ILO, reflecting both convergence on postwar state-building and institutional dissonance. Chapters 5 and 6 provide a parallel narrative to Chap. 4, highlighting the regional health activities of UNICEF and the ILO. UNICEF's regional program prioritized mass campaigns; the ILO's Universal Health Coverage (UHC) mandate, however, derailed amid Cold War geopolitics and institutional silos involving the WHO.

Set against the Cold War backdrop, Chapter 7 examines the local antecedents of PHC in Southeast Asia. Through case studies anchored in Indonesia, India, Thailand, and Sri Lanka, I argue that while Cold War rivalries influenced the early evolution of PHC, the normative momentum toward Alma-Ata transcended ideological binaries alone.

Note on Sources

The argument underpinning this monograph is shaped as much by the sources consulted as by the themes explored. Research was conducted across 30 repositories, ranging from the repositories of international organizations (The Rockefeller Archives, WHO, ILO, and UNICEF) to national and local archives and university special collections. Each source was scrutinized for its evidentiary strengths and potential pitfalls. The archives of international organizations—particularly those of the WHO and UNICEF—privilege technical solutions and institutional success. These narratives require interrogation and corroboration through biographies of international health diplomats and local physicians, private papers, official publications, and local archives that reveal administrative tensions beneath official claims.

Inspired by Ann-Laura Stoler's injunction to read along the archival grain, this study treats archival records both as a corpus of writing and as a force field: they channel knowledge toward particular institutional logics while minimizing alternative perspectives.[51] Official histories of international organizations—triangulated against national archives, private papers, and local repositories—reveal the stark asymmetries between institutional optimism and contestations that emerged at local levels over authority, the distribution of resources, and expertise. Attention is paid to the materiality of sources—handwritten diary notes, mimeographs, print sources (such as newspapers and magazines), and increasingly digitized files—since their format shaped both circulation and perceived authority. Equally important are the limits of access: restricted UNICEF files remind us that historical writing is contingent on archival access. While institutional archives, medical biographies, private collections, newspapers, and oral history collections dominate the study, I remain alert to the partial visibility of community voices. Their absence is historically conditioned—shaped by institutional priorities and archival logics.

These dynamics—involving materiality, authority, and access to sources—are not abstract. Both Indonesia's anti-yaws campaign and India's mass vaccination against tuberculosis reveal the collision between technocratic assurance and debates among local physicians and the wider community over the therapeutic efficiency of BCG and penicillin, respectively.

Indonesia's anti-yaws campaign provides a compelling case of how technocratic assurance was incorporated into official narratives while overlooking local medical debates. The campaign was overseen by Spurgeon Milton Keeny, then director of the UNICEF Regional Office for Asia (ARO). Keeny's 1953 report—his first major account of the campaign—depicted it as a cooperative endeavor.[52] The report foregrounded logistical challenges: shortage of personnel, erratic penicillin supplies, and difficulties in coordinating polyclinics across the Indonesian archipelago. Keeny's account—unlike unpublished UNICEF documents—circulated as a printed source, reflecting the agency's official narrative. Yet UNICEF's administrative rationality—evident in Keeny's report—privileges technical expertise and minimizes local debates between Indonesian physicians M. Soetopo and Raden Kodijat over penicillin's therapeutic efficacy. By contrast, Soetopo and Wasito's study in the *Bulletin of the World Health Organization* highlights disagreements over penicillin's administration and uneven diagnostic precision.[53] Their account illustrates how local epidemiological perspectives were subordinated to international technical expertise.

Echoing the pattern of post-World War II technological optimism encountering local skepticism observed in Indonesia, India's mass vaccination campaign against tuberculosis was inaugurated in 1948. It reveals the same asymmetry: WHO and UNICEF's administrative rationality emphasized institutional success, while local contestations questioned the safety, efficacy, and prophylactic value of the Bacillus Calmette Guérin (BCG) vaccine. In his report, Keeny acknowledged these bottlenecks but emphasized Delhi's BCG success, reflecting trust in international technical authority.[54] In contrast, Tamil newspapers—such as *Dina Thanthi*, sourced from the Tamil Nadu State Archives in Chennai—documented local resistance to BCG.

The two cases expose a broader methodological challenge: the evidentiary imbalance created by the dominance of WHO records and the limited accessibility of UNICEF unpublished reports. Niels Brimnes' monograph—while illuminating the logical challenges associated with tuberculosis control in twentieth-century India—exemplifies the tendency of historical scholarship to privilege WHO, UNICEF, and state repositories.[55] Crucially, biographies of international health diplomats such as Keeny—who crafted UNICEF's regional approach in Asia—remain absent in the historiography. Such exclusive reliance on the repositories of international aid agencies and state archives entrenches institutional perspectives, while simultaneously overlooking local contestations of disease—both from the scientific community and the general population.[56] This obscures the very dynamics that explain why the proverbial magic bullet approach—anchored in technical fixes such as penicillin or BCG—often tended to overshadow holistic perspectives rooted in the social determinants of health.

The monograph's historiographical intervention consists in the recovery of neglected biographies of international health diplomats, systematically juxtaposing international records with non-English sources, and reframing archival silences as evidence in their own right. By emphasizing the politics of archives—the materiality of sources and the asymmetry of institutional authority—this study shows how narratives of international health were curated through selective visibility and erasure. In doing so, this monograph pivots the history of international health away from institutional histories and toward contested terrains where technical expertise collided with local skepticism, resistance, and alternative epistemologies.

Notes

1. For a conventional definition of Southeast Asia as a bounded terrain, see D.G.E. Hall, *A History of South-East Asia* (New York: St. Martin's Press, 1955).

2. J.D. Legge, "The Writing of Southeast Asian History," in *The Cambridge History of Southeast Asia: Volume 1, From Early Times to 1800*, Nicholas Tarling edited (Cambridge: Cambridge University Press), 1–50, 5.
3. Jose Acuin, Rebecca Firestone, Thein Thein Htay, et al., "Southeast Asia: An Emerging Focus for Global Health," *The Lancet* 377, no. 9765 (February 2011): 534–35, 534.
4. Ibid., 534.
5. Ziqi Cui, Jing Li, Ling Meng, et al., "Nipah Virus: a Re-emerging Public Health Concern," *Lancet Microbe* 5, no. 3 (March 2024): e212.
6. Celia Lowe, "Viral Sovereignty: Security and Mistrust as Measures of Future Health in the Indonesian H5N1 Outbreak," *Medical Anthropology Quarterly* 6, no. 3 (2019): 109–32, 115–16.
7. Vivek Neelakantan, "History of Pandemics in Southeast Asia: A Return of National Anxieties?" *ISIS* 114, S1 (2023): S419–46, S440.
8. David Arnold, "Tropical Governance: Managing Health in Monsoon Asia, 1908–1938," Asia *Research Institute Working Paper* Series 116 (2009). Accessed April 10, 2025.https://papers.ssrn.com/sol3/papers.cfm?abstract_id=1645149.
9. Vivek Neelakantan, "Introduction," *The Geopolitics of Health in South and Southeast Asia: Perspectives from the Cold War to COVID-19*, Vivek Neelakantan edited (Abingdon, Oxon: Routledge, 2023), 1–26, 7.
10. Sara Davies, *Containing Contagion: The Politics of Disease Outbreaks in Southeast Asia* (Baltimore, MD: Johns Hopkins University Press, 2019), 4.
11. Carl Grundy-Warr and Shaun Linn, "COVID-19 Geopolitics: Silence and Erasure in Cambodia and Myanmar in Times of Pandemic," *Eurasian Geography and Economics* 61, nos. 4 and 5 (2020): 493–510.
12. WHO, "Reassignment of Indonesia from the South-East Asia Region to the Western Pacific Region: Report by the Secretariat," *WHO: Seventy-Eighth World Health Assembly: Report by the Secretariat*, Provisional Agenda Item 25, May 12, 2025, Doc. A78/31 (Geneva: WHO, 2025), WHO website. Accessed May 28, 2025. https://apps.who.int/gb/ebwha/pdf_files/WHA78/A78_31-en.pdf.
13. Habib Benzian, and Manu Raj Mathur, "Indonesia Leaves SEARO: What it Means for Regional Health and WHO," *The Lancet Regional Health–Southeast Asia* 43 (2025): 10031, https://doi.org/10.1016/j.lansea.2025.100660.
14. Ilham A. Ridlo, "Indonesia Just Left WHO's Southeast Asia Region: Here's Why It Matters for Global Health," *Science Watchdog.id,* May 25, 2025. Accessed May 28, 2025. https://sciencewatchdog.id/2025/05/26/indonesia-just-left-whos-southeast-asia-region-heres-why-that-matters-for-global-health/.
15. Ibid.

16. Randall Packard, *A History of Global Health: Interventions into the Lives of Other Peoples* (Baltimore, MD: Johns Hopkins University Press, 2016); Marcos Cueto, Theodore Brown, and Elizabeth Fee, *The World Health Organization; A History* (Cambridge: Cambridge University Press, 2019). For the wider Cold War context, see Erez Manela, "Smallpox and the Globalization of Development," *The Development Century: A Global Perspective*, Stephen Macekura and Erez Manela edited (Cambridge: Cambridge University Press, 2018), 83–104; See also Anne-Emanuelle Birn, and Nikolai Krementsov, "'Socialising' Primary Care? The Soviet Union, WHO and the 1978 Alma-Ata Conference," *BMJ Global Health* 3 (2018): e000992. Doi: 10.1136/ bmjgh-2018-000992.
17. World Bank, *World Development Report 1993: Investing in Health* (New York: Oxford University Press, 1993).
18. For a contrast with Africa, see Guillaume Lachenal, "A Genealogy of Treatment as Prevention (TasP): Prevention Therapy and the Tensions of Public Health in African History," *Global Health in Africa: Historical Perspectives on Disease Control*, Tamara Giles-Vernick and James L.A. Webb Jr edited (Athens: Ohio University Press, 2013), 70–91; See also Jennifer Tappan, "The True Fiasco: The Treatment and Prevention of Severe Acute Malnutrition in Uganda, 1950–74," in the same volume, 92–116. While Tanzania and Ethiopia incorporated elements of the Barefoot Doctor model, PHC across much of Sub-Saharan Africa was externally driven—emphasizing "Treatment as Prevention" strategies for yaws, sleeping sickness, and malnutrition, displacing community-based care.
19. Christopher Bayly and Tim Harper, *Forgotten Wars: The End of Britain's Asian Empire* (London: Penguin, 2007).
20. Ibid.
21. Ibid.
22. Benedict Anderson, *The Spectre of Comparisons: Nationalism, Southeast Asia and the World* (London: Verso, 1998), 3–6.
23. Amitav Acharya, "Asia is Not One," *The Journal of Asian Studies* 69, no. 4 (2010): 1001–13, 1002.
24. Acharya, "Asia is Not One," 1005.
25. Acharya, "Asia is Not One," 1006.
26. Jawaharlal Nehru, "Inaugural Address," in *Asian Relations: Being Report of the Proceedings of the First Asian Relations Conference New Delhi, March to April 1947* (New Delhi: Asian Relations Organization, 1948), 23–24.
27. William Henderson, "The Development of Regionalism in Southeast Asia," *International Organization* 9, no. 4 (1955): 463–76, 466.
28. Amry Vandenbosch and Richard Butwell, *The Changing Face of Southeast Asia* (Lexington, Kentucky: Kentucky University Press, 1966), 343.
29. Ibid., 343.

30. Vandenbosch and Butwell, *The Changing Face*, 341.
31. Ibid., 341.
32. Vandenbosch and Butwell, *The Changing Face*, 342.
33. Donald K. Emmerson, "Southeast Asia: What is in a Name," *Journal of Southeast Asian Studies* 15, no. 1 (1984): 1–21, 9.
34. Emmerson, "Southeast Asia," 10. SEATO's jurisdiction also included the British colonial territories of Malaya, Singapore, Brunei, Sarawak, and North Borneo.
35. Michael A. Stevenson and Andrew F. Cooper, "Overcoming Constraints of State Sovereignty: Global Health Governance in Asia," *Third World Quarterly* 30, no. 7 (2009): 1379–94, 1381.
36. Neelakantan, "Introduction," 4.
37. Abdul Majid, *Public Health Activities in Afghanistan: Asian Relations Conference, March to April 1947* (New Delhi: Indian Council of World Affairs, 1947), 3.
38. World Health Assembly 22, "Inclusion of Afghanistan in the Eastern Mediterranean Region. World Health Organization," *Twelfth Plenary Meeting: Committee on Administration, Finance and Legal Matters, Fourth Report*, Doc. WHA 22.19, The World Health Organization Library and Historical Collections, Geneva (hereafter WHOL).
39. WHO Interim Commission, "Delimitation of Regional Health Areas on an Epidemiological Basis," March 31, 1947, Doc. WHO IC//61 (Rev.1), Subject 452, Series 1, File 5, *WHO First Generation Files* (*WHO.1*), Archives of the World Health Organization, Geneva (hereafter WHOA).
40. Susan Heydon examines the intersections between foreign aid and public health in the context of Nepal. See Susan Heydon, *Modern Medicine and International Aid: Khunde Hospital, Nepal, 1966–1998* (Hyderabad: Orient BlackSwan, 2009). In the case of the smallpox eradication program in Bhutan, for example, the WHO wielded limited influence. The agency had to navigate the interests of powerful neighbors such as India and China. See Sanjoy Bhattacharya, "International Health and the Limits of its Global Influence: Bhutan and the Worldwide Smallpox Eradication Programme," *Medical History* 57, no. 4 (2013): 461–86.
41. Eva-Maria Knoll, "Malaria Eradication and Modernization in Maldives and Sri Lanka," *The Geopolitics of Health in South and Southeast Asia: Perspectives from the Cold War to COVID-19*, Vivek Neelakantan edited (Abingdon, Oxon: Routledge, 2023), 77–98.
42. To understand the realignment of the Global Smallpox Eradication program to local conditions, see Sanjoy Bhattacharya and Carlos Eduardo D' Avila Pereira Campani, "Re-assessing the Foundations: Worldwide Smallpox Eradication, 1957–67," *Medical History* 64, no. 1 (2020): 71–93.

43. To analyze global health narratives overshadowing local particularities, see Javed Siddiqui, *World Health and World Politics: The World Health Organization and the UN System* (London: Hurst and Company, 1995). To understand the continuities and changes in international health, see Anne-Emanuelle Birn, "The Stages of International (Global) Health: Histories of Success or Successes of History?" *Global Public Health* 4, no. 1 (2009): 50–68. On the social and political ramifications of global health initiatives, see Packard, *Global Health.* For individual case studies on Southeast Asia, see, for example, *Southern Medicine for Southern People: Vietnamese Medicine in the Making*, Laurence Monnais, C. Michele Thompson, and Ayo Wahlberg edited (Newcastle-upon-Tyne: Cambridge Scholars, 2012); Davisakd Puaksom, "A Promise of Desire: On the Politics of Health and Moral Discourse in Thailand, 1950–2010," *Public Health and National Reconstruction in Post-War Asia: International Influences, Local Transformations*, Liping Bu and Ka-che Yip edited (London: Routledge, 2015), 175–96.
44. Sunil Amrith, *Decolonizing International Health: India and Southeast Asia, 1930–65* (Basingstoke: Palgrave Macmillan, 2006), 12.
45. Jawaharlal Nehru, "Speech at the Closing Plenary Session of the Asian Relations Conference: Asian Relations Organization," April 2, 1947, in *Selected Works of Jawaharlal Nehru* volume 2 (New Delhi: Jawaharlal Nehru Memorial Fund, 1984), 247–51.
46. See, for example, "Preparatory Asiatic Regional Conference of the International Labour Organisation, New Delhi 1947," *Problems of Social Security: First Item on the Agenda*, Report I (New Delhi: ILO, 1947), 111, ILOL.
47. WHO, "Speech by Dr. Antonio Villarama, Philippines," June 15, 1949, *Official Records of the World Health Organization: Second World Health Assembly*, no. 21, June 13–July 2, 1949 (Geneva: WHO, 1949). WHOL.
48. Ibid.
49. See, for example, WHO, "Speech by Rajkumari Amrit Kaur, India at Fourth Plenary Meeting," June 14, 1949, *Official Records of the World Health Organization: Second World Health Assembly*, no. 21, June 13–July 2, 1949 (Geneva: WHO, 1949). WHOL.
50. Amrith, *Decolonizing International Health*, 12.
51. Ann-Laura Stoler, *Along the Archival Grain: Epistemic Anxieties and Common Sense* (Princeton: Princeton University Press, 2009), 22.
52. S.M. Keeny, "Two Cooperative Projects of the WHO and UNICEF," *Public Health Reports* 68, no. 6 (1953): 606–608.
53. M. Soetopo, and Wasito, "Experience with Yaws Control in Indonesia: Preliminary Results with a Simplified Approach," *Bulletin of the World Health Organization* 8 (1953): 273–91.

54. Keeny, "Two Comparative Projects," 607–608.
55. Niels Brimnes, *Languished Hopes: Tuberculosis, the State and International Assistance in Twentieth Century India* (Hyderabad: Orient Blackswan, 2015), 17.
56. See, for example, Bhattacharya, "Introduction," *Expunging Variola*, 1–12.

CHAPTER 2

Beyond Medicine: International Health in Southeast Asia During the Interwar Period, 1918–1941

Introduction

Historical studies have examined the period between 1851 and 1945 to investigate how international health was intertwined with concerns of imperialism, philanthropy, humanitarianism, and decolonization.[1] Such scholarship foregrounds the uneven trajectory from the ineffectual implementation of International Sanitary Conventions to the institutionalization of permanent health bodies. By the 1930s, two versions of international health ran parallel to each other: (1) the hegemonic perspective that was based on an excessive reliance on medical technology and validated health as an accelerator to economic growth; and (2) the holistic perspective that emphasized social reforms to improve public welfare and solidarity between countries.[2]

In this chapter, I argue that the discourse of rural hygiene, articulated at the Intergovernmental Conference of Far-Eastern Nations on Rural Hygiene, Bandoeng (1937), emerged from a series of Rockefeller Foundation-initiated, fragmented public health experiments in Ceylon, the Philippine Islands, the Netherlands Indies, and British India on the periphery of the colonial empire.[3] Furthermore, the discourse embodied a range of aspirations, from Abdul Rasjid and M.K. Gandhi's quest for holistic medicine to the Rockefeller Foundation's attempts to transform hygienic practices in the Netherlands Indies and British India, respectively.

V. Neelakantan, *The Emergence of International Health Policy in Southeast Asia, India, and Sri Lanka, 1937–1978*,
https://doi.org/10.1007/978-3-032-21233-7_2

But at the start of the Pacific War in 1942, the holistic vision of rural hygiene was eclipsed by a narrower technocentric approach to public health.

Regional Health Initiatives in the Far East: Contributions of the Rockefeller Foundation, Far Eastern Association of Tropical Medicine, and the League of Nations Health Organization

The genesis of international health is conventionally traced to the First Sanitary Conference held in Paris in 1851. It took a further 56 years and 11 conferences to set up a full-time agency, the Office International d' Hygiène Publique (OIHP) in Paris (1907). Institutional progress notwithstanding, political and economic rivalries between imperial powers delayed the signing of international health accords, limited their enforcement, and resulted in an England versus France and everybody else rhetoric. [4] As England and France remained imbricated in diplomatic asymmetry, the US and Mexico developed their own system of epidemic surveillance. In 1902, the Pan American Sanitary Bureau (PASB) was founded with initiative from the United States Public Health Service (USPHS). Concurrently, the Red Cross (founded in 1861) provided war relief, establishing a second axis of humanitarian intervention—distinct from epidemiological surveillance.

Just as the OIHP was created, a new player in international health emerged. The Rockefeller Foundation was established by the oil mogul John D. Rockefeller in 1913 to "promote the well-being of mankind throughout the world."[5] The Foundation oversaw a global enterprise of health organized through field offices in Paris, Cali, and New Delhi. The Foundation's International Health Division (IHD, founded in 1927) spearheaded campaigns against hookworm and malaria. The LNHO—provisionally founded in 1921 and formally established in 1923—occasionally challenged the IHD's biomedical model.[6] Despite the LNHO's epistemic divergence, its operational viability—especially its capacity to fund study tours and gather epidemiological intelligence—was predicated on Rockefeller funding.

Influenced by the Progressive Movement that swept the US during the early twentieth century, Rockefeller used public philanthropy to apply scientific knowledge to further the social good. In 1910, he established the

Sanitary Commission for the Eradication of Hookworm Disease with assistance from his philanthropic advisers, namely Frederick Gates, Charles Stiles, and Wickliffe Rose. Gates, Stiles, and Rose attributed anemia-provoking hookworm disease to the economic backwardness of the Southern States.[7] The Rockefeller Foundation created the International Health Commission (IHC) in 1913 to eradicate hookworm in other countries.[8] Rose was appointed Director General of the IHC and visited the British West Indies, Egypt, Ceylon, and the Malay States to inaugurate the IHC's anti-hookworm campaign in collaboration with local governments.[9]

The IHC, renamed the International Health Board (IHB, 1916–1927), launched a hookworm treatment program in Ceylon's plantations beginning in 1915. From the outset, planters resisted Rockefeller intervention, fearing disruption to their operations.[10] Victor Heiser, Director of the IHB Operations in the Far East (1915–1934), had to navigate resistance from tea planters while conducting the campaign under the colonial health service.[11] In 1914, there was a plague scare in Ceylon soon after the harvest season, causing thousands of estate workers—recruited from the Madras Presidency in British India—to flee.[12] The colonial health authorities coerced workers into taking the plague vaccine. The exodus threatened plantation productivity, exposing the fragility underpinning colonial labor regimes.

Heiser persuaded planters by offering to have the IHB bear nearly half the cost of the hookworm control project—an incentive neither they nor the colonial government could refuse.[13] In 1916, the IHB in Ceylon drafted a plan of operations, placing select plantation estates under the supervision of American medical personnel.[14] The government pledged support to improve estate sanitation. A pilot demonstration area in the Matale district was selected, followed by others.[15] The campaign integrated chenopodium oil trials, latrine experimentation, and worker education, treating at least 40,000 people, with 78 percent cured on microscopic re-examination.[16]

Despite clear health gains among workers treated with the wonder-drug chenopodium, estate managers remained unconvinced about undertaking sanitary improvements, particularly latrine construction, previously recommended by the IHB. Colonial authorities—acting under IHB pressure—mandated latrine construction on estates. However, compliance remained limited, sustaining continued infection rates.

Health education was a weak component of the hookworm elimination campaign in Ceylon. In his letter to Heiser, Wilbur Sawyer—who was Assistant Director of the IHB in the East between 1923 and 1924—conveyed a sense of pessimism with respect to the results of the campaign:

> An educational failure of the present is the inability of the Anchylostomiasis [*sic*] Campaign to treat villagers in the vicinity of Colombo, and the excuse given is that nothing can be done with them [schoolchildren] because they have Western ideas and are not under complete control of the headmen. Isn't it time that a program is invented that will appeal to such people with more modern ideas. If this is not done it can be predicted that the permanent control will have diminishing effect.[17]

Soma Hewa notes that Rockefeller philanthropic medicine that assisted British authorities in Ceylon served the long-term economic and political interests of US industrial capitalism.[18] The intervention did not materialize because estate owners were unable to grasp the symbiotic relationship between labor health and their own interests.

In 1923—following a survey determining major health problems and their underlying causes—Rockefeller officer William P. Jacocks realized that treatment alone was not a panacea for hookworm. Rural communities demanded attention to immediate health problems. The rationale of treating hookworm—an insidious infection—at the expense of debilitating diseases such as typhoid, smallpox, dysentery, or malaria—revealed a dissonance between the Rockefeller-supported biomedical model and everyday experience. Ceylon's anti-hookworm campaign (1916–1922) recalibrated the role of community participation within IHB strategy. During the 1920s, Western-educated Ceylonese intelligentsia impelled the colonial state to intervene in rural health—a shared IHB concern.[19] In collaboration with colonial authorities, the IHB developed the Kalutara rural health unit in Ceylon by 1926. Under Jacocks' stewardship, Kalutara evolved into a prototype for decentralized health delivery (Image 2.1).

The Rockefeller Foundation's policy of working "with and through governments" was apparent not only in Ceylon but also in the Philippine Islands, then an American colony. In 1914, Heiser—Director of Public Health in the Philippines (1905–1915)—endorsed Rose's proposal to appoint a commission to assess the deleterious effects of hookworm, but the colonial government lacked funding.[20] At the time, the United Missionary Campaign for New England led a hookworm survey in the

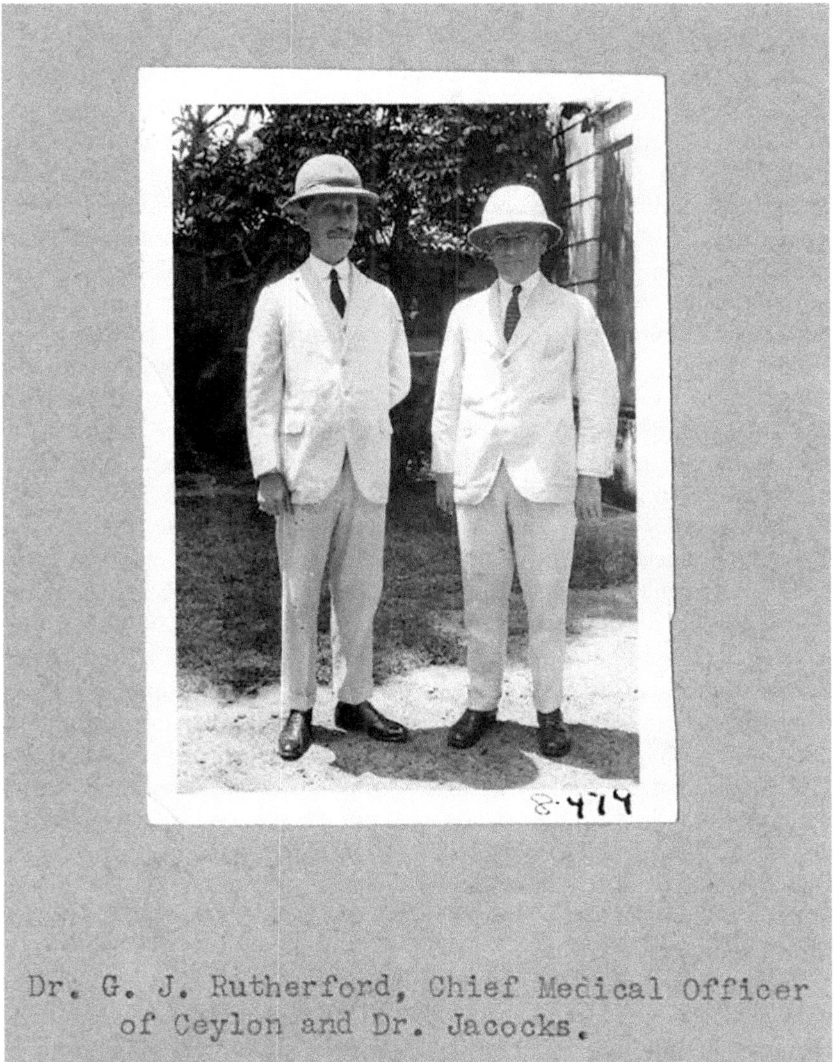

Image 2.1 Where Colonial Medicine Intersects with Rockefeller Philanthropy: Ceylon, 1920s. Dr G.J. Rutherford, Medical Officer of Ceylon (left), with Dr William P. Jacocks of the International Health Division (right). Photograph of Dr G.J. Rutherford, Chief Medical Officer of Ceylon, with Dr Jacocks, William P. Jacocks Series 1055, Photographs, Jacocks, William Pickard. With Permission from the Rockefeller Archive Center

Philippine Islands and established an ecumenical hospital for the treatment of more severe cases.[21]

In the annual report of the Philippine Health Service compiled for 1915, Heiser's successor, J.D. Long, included a lengthy discussion on soil pollution in the archipelago.[22] American health administrators in the Philippines were apprehensive that "Filipino promiscuous defecation" might spread cholera or typhoid germs.[23] Hookworm apparently figured in the list of public health concerns, but authorities did not explicitly mention it in the annual report. Instead, they focused on installing a pail system of toilets. The plan never gained traction due to difficulties in securing personnel for the repulsive tasks of collecting, dumping, and cleaning. Health authorities subsequently experimented with simple pit latrines, where bodily wastes were covered with earth or lime, but the pit bred flies.[24] The failures of colonial sanitary interventions set the stage for the emergence of 1920s Rockefeller-sponsored demonstration centers in Cavite and Laguna.

During the 1920s, American officials—amid volatile debates on Philippine independence—invited the IHB to support reconstruction efforts.[25] Disease control became a site of institutional experimentation and symbolic reform. In 1928, the Rockefeller Foundation—learning from earlier anti-hookworm treatment failures—launched a rural health demonstration in Cavite province, offering potable water, sanitary excreta disposal, malaria control methods, dispensaries, immunization programs, education, and propaganda. A primary healthcare initiative in Laguna (1929) emphasized sanitary latrines, school health programs, and maternal and child care.[26] These achievements, however, were not replicated elsewhere. Nurses opposed regulations regarding the use of latrines, since they felt that these regulations contravened "local sensitivities."[27] These initiatives unfolded amid Heiser's imagination of the Filipino body as a site of bodily reform.

Heiser hoped to transform the Filipino from what he perceived as a weak and feeble race into a strong and enduring people. His methods required modification of sanitary habits to make the Filipino well-disciplined and attentive to environmental nuisances.[28] Yet, by the 1920s—principally shaped by his conversations with Filipino physicians, particularly Jacobo Fajardo and José Fabella—Heiser recalibrated his approach to hygiene education. He shifted the focus from racial typologies to the broader populace as subjects of expansive health interventions.[29]

Heiser, a health advisor to the Philippine colonial government, founded the Far Eastern Association of Tropical Medicine (FEATM) in 1908. A multilateral cooperative initiative, the FEATM aimed to advance the knowledge of tropical medicine and foster international collaboration among physicians.[30] At its inaugural meeting in Manila in April 1910, Heiser shaped the association's regionwide anti-beriberi campaign, though the proposal encountered resistance from a few delegates. The FEATM also promoted the regionalization of quarantine practices.[31]

The FEATM incorporated beriberi (vitamin B1 deficiency) into its regional health agenda from the outset for two reasons. First, beriberi was endemic in the region encompassed by the FEATM, i.e., the "Far East," a zone virtually coterminous with the world's principal rice-producing and rice-consuming societies. Second, as the FEATM was being established, a breakthrough in beriberi research coincided with intensified investigations by colonial regimes across the region.[32] At its inaugural meeting, the association shared preliminary research findings of Hans Aron (the Philippine Islands), Ambrose Thomas Stanton, and Henry Fraser (British Malaya).[33]

Following the pioneering contributions of Aron, Stanton, and Fraser, delegates to the Second FEATM Congress in Hong Kong in 1912 discussed the problem of beriberi. Indochina delegates shared M.R.L. Montel's proposals for establishing small maternity centers staffed by local midwives in French Indochina with their colleagues from the Netherlands Indies at the Third Congress in Saigon in 1913.[34] The Netherlands Indies colonial health authorities subsequently implemented Montel's ideas.

Between 1913 and 1921—a hiatus of eight years—the FEATM was left almost moribund due to World War I. The Fourth Congress of the FEATM—held at Batavia (now Jakarta) in 1921—marked its revival. Heiser, chairing the beriberi committee, cited Fraser and Stanton's research and urged delegates to press their governments on the need to legislate against milled rice.[35]

Despite Heiser's appeal, early efforts to regulate rice milling—such as those piloted in the Philippines—faced economic and logistical challenges. In the words of Sawyer:

> No one Far Eastern country seems to be in a favourable position for discouraging the over-milling of rice, as it would put the millers at a disadvantage in international competition. The plantation manager hesitates to feed his coolies with brown rice because it might give his competitor who feeds with white rice an advantage in securing labor.[36]

Beriberi appeared as a pathological symptom wherever highly milled rice entered consumption.

Amidst a divergence of views on the etiology of beriberi, the FEATM convened the Fifth Congress in Singapore in 1923. The Filipino delegate proposed that imported rice be graded based on its phosphorous pentoxide content and suggested taxing over-milled rice.[37] However, Dr F.H. Guérin (French Indochina) and Dr Cornelius de Langen (Netherlands Indies) questioned whether these measures would effectively prevent beriberi.[38]

While scientific uncertainty persisted regarding the causation of beriberi, the Japanese delegate Dr S. Kanai argued that substituting undermilled for polished rice would control beriberi. However, he warned that such a measure would encounter cultural resistance, as a "change of taste of a nation" was a serious concern.[39] Kanai instead recommended correcting nutritional deficiencies caused by over-milled rice through the incorporation of complementary foods in cooking.

The Fifth FEATM Congress concluded that an international convention on beriberi was impractical due to conflicting perspectives.[40] Instead, it recommended that governments tailor anti-beriberi campaigns to suit local conditions and devise strategies to reduce reliance on milled rice. The Singapore resolution reflected the inherent complexity of implementing a uniform regional health agenda across colonial territories.

The FEATM shaped international health in interwar Asia in two key ways. First, the association recognized colonial governments of Asia as de facto national units and fostered an intercolonial expert network. The LNHO had incorporated FEATM's practices into its Asian operations by the mid-1920s.[41] Second, FEATM's schemes enabled national experts from colonial Asia to present research at international venues. Yet, as David Arnold notes, the association's effectiveness was constrained by the absence of a permanent headquarters, the insecure funding, and lack of an executive body.[42] These limitations were exacerbated by FEATM's recognition of colonial sovereignty, which impeded coordinated anti-beriberi efforts. At the Fifth Congress, for instance, while the Government of India endorsed international action against beriberi, it declined to provide financial support.[43]

By the time the LNHO was founded in 1921, the FEATM had already been advancing regional health-governance agendas for over a decade. Directed by Polish bacteriologist Ludwik Rajchman (1921–1939), the LNHO sought to define international health priorities.[44]

The LNHO faced two existential problems: should international health be philanthropic or League-accountable, and would a supranational authority erode state sovereignty in health.[45] To allay these concerns, Rockefeller authorities contended that the IHB should complement— not duplicate— the LNHO, focusing on laboratory research, experimental local health stations, and fieldwork in epidemic control. In 1922, Rajchman partnered with the IHB to establish an international service for medical intelligence and statistics.[46]

Edgar Sydenstricker, chief of the LNHO's division of Epidemiological Intelligence and Public Health Statistics, worked primarily in Europe.[47] To extend its reach, the LNHO needed to adapt its epidemiological strategy for the Far East, given the region's colonial dynamics.[48] Rajchman appointed a Far Eastern Committee—Sir George Buchanan, Professor Albert Calmette, and Masatsugu Miyajima— to assess the feasibility of a Far East regional epidemic intelligence center.[49]

Between November 1922 and July 1923, Norman White—a LNHO staff and former Sanitary Commissioner with the Government of India—undertook a study tour to examine epidemic diseases in the Far East and assess preventive strategies. White's expedition exposed the limits of LNHO's engagement with colonial governments. Medical authorities in British India resisted sharing epidemiological data.[50] They pointed out that White's proposal to substitute ports for ships contravened the revised draft of the International Sanitary Convention (1912), which left the authority to classify ports to the discretion of individual governments. The Government of India feared that supranational port classification would disrupt commerce—underscoring the tensions between international governance and the sovereignty of the colonial state.

Upon the completion of his trip to Asia, White authored a three-part report. To quote White:

> It is obvious that no discussion can be profitable without a comprehensive and detailed study of the behaviour of these diseases both in the ports and territories adjacent. A study of these matters necessitates an appreciation of public health and medical organisation and activities of the countries concerned. This in itself, constitutes a very large subject of enquiry, as the countries in all stages of public health and sanitary development are included in the Far Eastern arena.[51]

The above quote illustrates the geopolitical ambiguity of the term "Far East," which initially referred to North Asia (China, Manchuria, and Japan) and later encompassed Southeast and South Asia, parts of Australia and the Southwest Pacific, East Africa, and parts of Northeast Africa—any country of the Pacific and Indian Ocean rims connected by maritime activity.[52] While the "Eastern Bureau" was the accepted designation for the regional epidemic center, White's use of "Far Eastern arena" was disputed by the LNHO for its military overtones. The League instead recommended "eastern seas" as a more appropriate nomenclature.[53]

Singapore was chosen as the Eastern Bureau's headquarters due to its strategic location as a maritime gateway to the Far East. The Eastern Bureau collected information about infectious diseases—plague, cholera, and smallpox—via telegraph, compiled vital statistics from Far Eastern ports and hinterlands, and tracked sanitary regulations.[54] The Rockefeller Foundation committed US$ 125,000 in funding to establish the bureau.[55] This support facilitated the bureau's establishment during the Singapore Conference in February 1925, attended by delegates from the Straits Settlements, the Federated Malay States, India, the Dutch Indies, Indochina, Siam, Japan, China, Hong Kong, Ceylon, British Borneo, and the Philippines. [56] The French Indochina delegate to the conference, Dr L' Herminier, cautioned against publishing epidemiological data but affirmed public health as a long-term investment.[57] Until the Japanese occupation of Singapore (1942) forced its closure, the Eastern Bureau disseminated epidemiological information to 137 ports across the Indian Ocean and the Western Pacific, spanning Asia, Africa, and Australasia.[58]

The Bureau's expansive reach, however, raised questions about regional representation and epidemiological coverage—particularly from Australia—whose expanding commercial ties with Asia prompted a parallel initiative. During the 1920s, as commercial contacts between Asia and Australia intensified, Australian medical authorities grew concerned about the potential spread of diseases. To address these concerns, Australia convened the International Pacific Health Conference in Melbourne in 1926. The conference highlighted the need for improved epidemiological data for the Melanesia and Polynesia Island groups in the Austral-Pacific Regional Zone.[59] At the Melbourne conference, Australia expressed its interest in hosting an epidemiological bureau modeled after the Singapore Bureau but calibrated to the region's specific needs. Yet concerns emerged that such a bureau might eclipse the Eastern Bureau by severing its links with the Pacific islands.[60]

The activities of the IHD impeded Australia's quest for medical dominance in the Pacific region. While the British Empire utilized the Western Pacific Health Services (WPHS)— a centralized disease control institution, funded in part by the Rockefeller Foundation—to manage healthcare for colonial subjects, Australia elected a different alternative. [61] By declining to participate in WPHS activities, it prioritized training Papuan students in first aid instead.[62] The WPHS operated under the authority of the Chief Medical Officer of Fiji and was overseen by the Western Pacific High Commission.

Between 1928 and 1931, the WPHS implemented campaigns against hookworm and yaws in the British Solomon Islands, New Hebrides, Ellice Islands, and Fiji.[63] Rockefeller-trained Native Medical Practitioners (NMPs)—graduates from the Central Medical School at Suva—provided mass treatments for hookworm using carbon tetrachloride and ethylene tetrachloride. By 1931, NMPs treated 106,029 hookworm-afflicted individuals with no adverse effects.[64] For yaws, NMPs administered 222,000 salvarsan injections to children aged two to seventeen and adults with symptoms, suggesting eradication potential among dispersed island groups.[65]

Despite these successes, WPHS efforts in the field of rural sanitation were less effective across the Pacific islands. In 1931, following a dysentery outbreak in rural Suva, Fiji, the WPHS installed 1250 bored-hole latrines under the successful supervision of NMPs.[66] However, in New Hebrides, the program had to be abandoned due to the shortage of NMPs and financial constraints.

While the IHD, LNHO, Eastern Bureau, and WPHS professed to engage local communities, their interventions were driven more by governance imperatives and geopolitical considerations rather than by a commitment to the right to health. Eliminating endemic diseases such as malaria, yaws, and hookworm—associated with vitiated labor productivity—was central to the Rockefeller international health model, which fused tropical medicine with geoeconomic strategy. However, the foundation took great care to avoid infantile diarrhea or tuberculosis, as these diseases demanded socially sensitive, long-term solutions that clashed with its technical focus.[67] After World War II, aid agencies—especially the WHO and UNICEF—modeled their regional architecture on the Rockefeller Foundation's field offices, calibrated to local contexts.

Public Health Experiments on the Empire's Periphery

In Asia, debates on rural hygiene unfolded on the colonial periphery, reflecting a kaleidoscope of aims. These ranged from Abdul Rasjid and M.K. Gandhi's pursuit of holistic healthcare in the Netherlands Indies and British India to John Lee Hydrick's Rockefeller-backed sanitary outreach in Java. These initiatives wove local health experiments into a transnational health tapestry.

The Netherlands Indies

Between 1924 and 1939, the IHD led a hygiene program in Java that connected with Indonesian nationalism. The project—directed by Rockefeller Foundation field officer Hydrick—shifted from the hospital-based medicine of the *Dienst der Volksgezondheid* (Netherlands Indies Public Health Service or DVG) to rural hygiene. The project established a Hygiene Mantri School in Banjumas (Central Java), training local elites as hygiene educators who would teach disease prevention and sanitation to Javanese villagers through home visits and outdoor cinema.[68] Heiser laid the foundation for this program in 1915, adapting the IHC's successful model of fighting hookworm in the American South to the Dutch East Indies.[69]

On March 29, 1915, Heiser met with H.M. Neeb, a faculty at STOVIA (School tot Opleiding van Inlandsche Artsen or the School for Training Native Physicians, established in 1902). He sought to convince Neeb of the necessity of starting a Java hookworm control program. Heiser noted:

> My task in the Orient is indeed a delicate one and my one hope to accomplish something seems to consist in going slow. It has become more and more apparent by the results which have been achieved that the Philippines are doing us a good service, and without the officials of other countries openly admitting it, it is evident there is much emulation of what has been done there.[70]

Although STOVIA faculty were appreciative of Heiser's public health initiatives in the Philippines, they cautioned Heiser that comparable measures were not scalable in Java due to the limited authority of the local police to enforce the population's adherence to sanitary standards. To address these bottlenecks, Heiser informed W. Frederick Indenburg,

Governor General of the Netherlands Indies, about the IHC's intent to collaborate with governments on health initiatives, emphasizing that hookworm eradication was significant "for the lever which it gave to other health reforms."[71]

The Netherlands Indies Governor General expressed strong interest in the work of the IHC in tropical disease control and introduced Heiser to the chief medical officer. On the officer's recommendation, the Governor General agreed to assign a government physician to support any commission the Rockefeller Foundation required to investigate hookworm in the Netherlands Indies.[72] Although plans were underway to launch an anti-hookworm campaign in Java in 1915, Heiser noted that fierce competition between the Rockefeller-owned Standard Oil Company and the Dutch-owned petroleum industry led colonial authorities to view the motives of the Rockefeller Foundation with suspicion.[73] In 1916, Heiser returned to Java, traveling from Soerabaja to Batavia (now known as Jakarta), where he documented widespread hookworm infestation.[74] By the end of his itinerary, an agreement was reached for Dr Samuel Darling of the Rockefeller Foundation to return later that year to conduct a formal survey of the hookworm situation in Java.

The Darling Commission investigated the impact of hookworm infection on health and efficiency in Malaya, Java, and Fiji.[75] They found that 90 percent of Java's inhabitants had hookworm, with the heaviest cases in mid-Java.[76] Following the Darling Commission's Report, prospects emerged for collaborative anti-hookworm efforts between the Rockefeller Foundation and the Netherlands Indies authorities, though implementation remained uncertain. However, a photograph published in the report depicting a Javanese laborer with the caption, "In the great struggle for subsistence in the beautiful island of Java, men and women become beasts of burden but are not brutalized in the process"—offended colonial sensibilities.[77] This led to an eight-year delay (1916–1924) in collaboration between the Rockefeller Foundation and the Netherlands Indies Public Health Service (Image 2.2).

In order to iron out misunderstandings with Dutch authorities, the Rockefeller Foundation hired Hydrick, an American citizen of Dutch heritage, in April 1924 to handle hookworm control in Java. In November 1924, Hydrick wrote a letter to Heiser noting that circumstances varied across west, central, and east Java. Colonial authorities recommended that the Netherlands Indies Health Service concentrate efforts on east and central Java, while the foundation focused on controlling hookworm in west

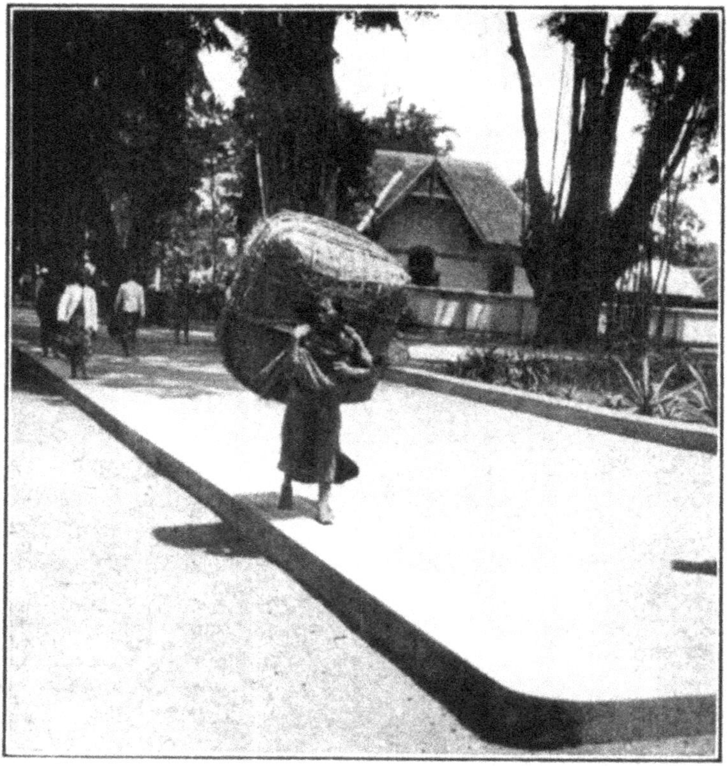

Image 2.2 Tension between Human Dignity and Structural Exploitation (1920). S.T. Darling, M.A. Barber and H.P. Hacker, "Hookworm and Malaria Research in Malaya, Java and the Fiji Islands: Report of Uncinariasis Commission to the Orient, 1915–17," *International Health Board Publication*, No. 4 (New York City: Rockefeller Foundation International Health Board, 1920), 9. With permission from the Rockefeller Archive Center

Java.[78] The Dutch strategy—centered on chenopodium treatment and mandatory latrine construction—stood in stark contrast to Hydrick's educational strategy.[79] The district of Serang in west Java—noted for anti-government unrest—was assigned to the foundation, while the Netherlands Indies Health Service worked in Kroja, central Java, where ethnic Javanese residents were recognized for their compliance.[80] The foundation organized its health demonstration unit in Serang in 1925.

In early 1926, Heiser steamed into Batavia and was received by Hydrick and Dr van Lonkhuijzen, Head of the DVG. Heiser—accompanied by Dr Tutyer of the sub-district and Dr Mollinger, head of the health services for west Java—proceeded to the IHB health demonstration unit in Serang.[81] The *mandoers* [Javanese: overseers on plantations] led hygiene education efforts, and villagers responded in large numbers for treatment. Hydrick set about proving to the Dutch that, despite the virtues of treating hookworm-infected villagers with chenopodium, the most important task before the DVG and the IHB was to prevent reinfection. Accordingly, he began a campaign against soil pollution, paired with latrine construction and treatment.[82]

But Dr van Lonkhuijzen remained skeptical of the results in rural sanitation achieved by the IHB. At Kroja, Heiser and Hydrick noted that 150,000 latrines had been constructed and 115,000 villagers had received hookworm treatment. Yet Lonkhuijzen observed that latrine use lagged behind treatment— and, in many cases, was absent.[83] Convinced of the need to develop hygiene education, he enlisted Heiser and Hydrick to help develop pedagogical models adaptable across Java. [84]

From 1926 until 1939, Hydrick served as the director of the DVG's newly established Department of Health Education. He played a key role in recruiting *mantri* [Malay: health technicians], who underwent extensive training in sanitation and public health. House visits by *mantri* were used to educate the *kampoeng* [Malay: village] about soil pollution. The educational component of rural sanitation in Java experienced a marked transformation by 1927. Informal discussions on hygiene were held at schools by mobile demonstration cars, accompanied by a health demonstrator equipped with charts, models, lantern slides, and moving graphics.[85] Rising demand for hygiene education outpaced the department's capacity.[86] In response, the department began offering basic hygiene classes in Malay and Sundanese in the residency of Banjumas, with government officials and teachers participating (Image 2.3).

From 1925 to 1936, Poerwokerto in Banjumas Regency provided the backdrop for Hydrick's rural hygiene experiments, which he subsequently reflected in his treatise *Intensive Rural Hygiene Work in the Netherlands East Indies*. Hydrick's vision was to awaken lasting public interest and promote habits conducive to sustained health.[87] Throughout the 1930s, Hydrick followed Heiser's 1915 strategy and moved steadily from hookworm eradication to a broader spectrum of diseases linked to poor sanitation and nutrition.[88] Experience at Poerwokerto revealed the limits of

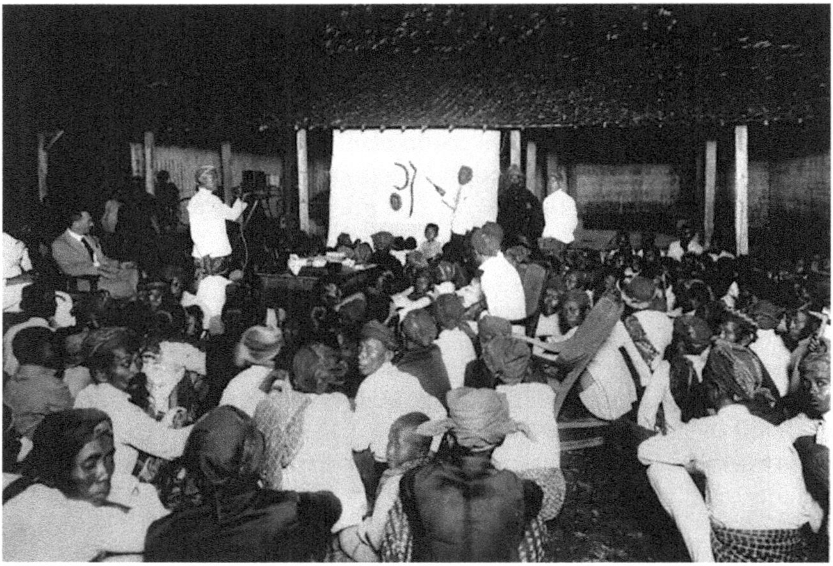

Image 2.3 Hookworm Visual Pedagogy in the *Kampoeng* (c. 1929). Staged by the Dienst der Volksgezondheid as a part of the rural hygiene campaign in Java. Image no: TM-ALB-0116-10. Source: The Dutch Museum of World Cultures. URL: https://collectie.wereldmuseum.nl/#/query/ded4f184-6451-45e8-9b1e-13802f4b818e. Public Domain

education alone, prompting Hydrick and his Dutch Indies colleagues to advocate for locally funded health services.[89] Decentralized health units were expected to meet this demand. By 1936, these efforts culminated in the Hygiene Mantri School at Poerwokerto—an institutional hub for training preventive health cadres destined for deployment across the Indies archipelago.

In certain respects, the coming of the Rockefeller Foundation's rural hygiene projects on Java in the 1920s enabled Indies physicians to break with the orthodoxy of Dutch clinical practice and engage directly with rural publics.[90] Rasjid was one such physician who was inspired by Hydrick's rural hygiene projects in Java. A 1914 STOVIA alumnus, Rasjid was a descendant of one of the former sultans of the Batak highlands, known as South Tapanoeli on the island of Sumatra.[91] He was an elected member of the Dutch East Indies' Volksraad (Legislative Assembly) from

1931 until the Japanese annexation of the Indies in 1942.[92] Rasjid's political career coincided with the Depression decade (1929–1939).

In collaboration with Dr ten Haaf and Abdul Wahab, school overseers in Medan, northern Sumatra, Rasjid began implementing student-led health brigades in October 1931. Boy Scout leaders from the top two secondary grades instructed students in first aid and basic hygiene.[93] The DVG provided bilingual Dutch and Malay instructional materials to assist the brigades, while the Rockefeller Foundation provided a subvention to underwrite their publication. Between 1929 and 1931, health brigades mobilized 8000 Javanese schoolchildren to reach underserved communities.[94]

During the Depression years, the colonial administration launched an ambitious decentralization program to acquaint Indonesians with democratic institutions. Hendrikus Colijn and other colonial administrators believed that the Indies archipelago's ethnic groups were best governed locally, citing the codification of *adat* [Malay: customary law] as evidence.[95] In his 1930s Volksraad speeches, Rasjid endorsed these policies, arguing that only traditional leaders possessed intuitive knowledge of their ethnic group. Deploying biological metaphors, Rasjid described traditional communities as organisms whose internal dynamics required a medical approach—one that positioned physicians as their natural leaders.[96]

During the early 1930s, Rasjid prioritized extending modern medicine to his people. Given the severe shortage of doctors in the Netherlands Indies, Rasjid proposed a dual system that would include both doctors, nurses, and midwives trained in modern medicine alongside native medical men of the villages (Malay: *doekoens*). Rasjid's innovation lay in deploying *doekoens* as first aid providers and informants for physicians.[97] He envisioned a regency health service for South Tapanoeli, staffed by four doctors, sixteen nurses, eight midwives, and one *doekoen* for each village. The community would fund the activities of the health service, with each member paying a tax of 0.25 guilders annually for curative care.[98] To support this, Rasjid established a private foundation for the promotion of hygiene in South Tapanoeli, named after the Dutch resident Fagginger Auer, to support this effort.[99]

Rasjid established a rapport with Dr Offringa, head of the DVG, and accompanied him on his medical tours. In 1931, Rasjid arrived in Batavia with proposals to reorganize the health service in Tapanoeli regency.[100] He argued that health funds already allocated for South Tapanoeli could be better utilized through decentralization of services.

In 1933, Rasjid approached the DVG with a proposal to entrust the curative mandate of public health to the Fagginger Auer Foundation. He was subsequently successful in transferring the management of the government hospital in Penjaboengan, South Tapanoeli, to his foundation.[101] However, this act of reconfiguration provoked resistance from seven village heads, who—fearing an affront to their traditional authority—objected to community-directed self-help.[102]

Like most Indies doctors, Rasjid greeted the Poerwokerto Health Demonstration Unit enthusiastically. After visiting Poerwokerto in 1935, he reported having seen his long-cherished principles of hygiene operationalized with structural clarity.[103] He particularly appreciated the Rockefeller leadership's attunement to local socio-cultural rhythms and needs. He continuously promoted the health demonstration projects of the Rockefeller Foundation and called for their institutional scalability across the Indies archipelago.[104]

Rasjid noted that Western medicine was expensive to implement in the Indies archipelago. In his Volksraad speech, he brought up the paradox that while the Netherlands Indies had an excess of doctors in its cities, there was a persistent shortfall in the countryside.[105] Rasjid made a distinction between medicine and hygiene. He maintained that while hygiene improved communities' physical and mental resilience, medicine in its more limited sense, especially infectious disease containment, had a defensive nature. Investments in hygiene yielded compound returns—measurable in taxation, economic resilience, and physical health.[106] Hygiene measures constituted the foundational axis of infectious disease control. In a diagnostic rebuttal to colonial medicine, he excoriated the DVG for its incapacity to collaborate with local communities and its refusal to acknowledge the embedded social and economic dimensions of illness. Rasjid supported Indonesian traditional medicine and urged the DVG to utilize *doekoens* to provide community health services based on local initiative.[107] Rasjid incorporated the core ideas of Hydrick's Poerwokerto project into his medical nationalism: public health programs were the most effective means of enhancing Indonesians' resilience both physically and mentally.[108]

Aided by the IHD, the ideas of Hydrick and Rasjid eventually coalesced into the body of technical expertise known as public health. Their efforts gained visibility within the LNHO, which endorsed the social transformation catalyzed by the rural health experiments. The League's approval to host the Intergovernmental Conference of Far-Eastern Nations on Rural Hygiene in Bandoeng (1937) was a testament to the enduring imprint of the Poerwokerto Regency Health Service on rural hygiene.

British India

Between 1920 and 1928, the Rockefeller Foundation launched an anti-hookworm campaign in Madras Presidency, marking the beginning of the foundation's public health activities in British India. The foundation suspected indentured labor from Madras, exported to British colonies, particularly Ceylon, as potential disease carriers.[109] The campaign transpired during a moment of administrative recalibration, when public health was framed as a provincial subject. Following World War I, the Government of India devolved public health to the provinces to alleviate the central government's growing administrative burden. Yet this structural shift, while enabling IHB entry, exposed deeper fault lines: underfunded provincial health services. Despite transnational linkages, the Madras hookworm campaign did not translate into effective organization due to colonial prejudices and widespread poverty.[110]

In 1916, the IHB conducted an initial enquiry into hookworm prevalence in Madras Presidency.[111] Although presidency authorities dismissed hookworm as a minor concern—relegated to mineworkers and plantation laborers—Rockefeller delegations prompted detailed investigations. From 1916 to 1919, the Indian Research Fund Association undertook hookworm investigations in the presidency under the supervision of Dr K.S. Mhaskar of the King Institute of Preventive Medicine. In 1921, John F. Kendrick—who had earlier conducted a hookworm survey for the IHB in Mauritius—was deputed to Madras.[112] Between 1921 and 1928, Kendrick and Mhaskar jointly undertook surveys of hookworm incidence, conducted awareness programs, experimented with latrine types, and launched experimental trials of vermifuges.

IHB officials, particularly Sawyer and Kendrick, warned that without adequate sanitary measures to prevent reinfection, the hookworm program would yield limited value. Yet Madras authorities supported mass treatments, as poverty made household privies unfeasible. In his 1924 letter to Heiser—exposing weaknesses in the educational aspects of the campaign—Sawyer observed:

> Certain things were taught over and over again without regard to the fact that no results were being produced, and no one seemed to be worried about it. Success was measured by the number of people who swallowed their one dose of medicine and not by the complete failure of the sanitary phase of the program. People are being told, as a part of the routine, to come back for second and third treatments, and almost no one ever comes.

> This does not seem to suggest to the medical officers that this ineffective advice cheapens all the instruction and should be omitted or else altered so as to become effective.[113]

Effectiveness of the sanitary aspects of the anti-hookworm campaign in Madras Presidency hinged on local initiative. In 1926, the Madura district board—led by an Englishman—sanctioned rupees 20,000 for latrine work, expecting a matching government grant.[114] The government declined. Undeterred, board authorities went ahead and constructed latrines in Usilampatti and neighboring villages. Kendrick, funded by the board, experimented with various latrine types, including the pit model from Java, which villagers approved as suitable to local conditions.[115] Kendrick noted that latrine use increased when educational campaigns accompanied installation.[116]

In the 1927 provincial budget, although the Madras government had allocated funds to treat hookworm on the plantations and in schools, no funds were provided to assist district boards with latrine construction.[117]

The Madura experiment, which prioritized health education and rural sanitation over the mass treatment of afflicted individuals, ran counter to the Madras Presidency's broader anti-hookworm effort. After the Rockefeller Foundation withdrew in 1928, the Madras government took over the campaign, nominally emphasizing rural sanitation and the prevention of soil pollution.[118] Yet, in 1938–1939—when hookworm work was undertaken in six presidency districts—the hookworm infection was still at 90 percent.[119] The persistent reliance on mass treatment—contrary to the foundation's stated emphasis on health education—contributed to the program's failure in Madras Presidency.

The 1918–1919 influenza pandemic precipitated nationalist mobilization around health in British India.[120] Arnold notes that while the plague epidemic of the 1890s and 1900s generated extensive photographic and statistical documentation, pandemic influenza—despite claiming 12 million lives—left a negligible archival imprint. One reason, he suggests, is that British India was an unmodern society ruled over by an unmodern state: indifferent to mass mortality and desensitized by decades of pestilence and famine.[121] Hunger, poverty, and soaring prices defined the material stakes.[122]

Local newspapers criticized the colonial government's inaction.[123] As influenza unfolded alongside political unrest, nationalist leaders capitalized on the colonial state's weakness amid public hardships to extract political concessions. Within months, Gandhi shifted from recruiting soldiers for the Raj to leveraging anti-colonial discontent.[124]

Gandhi's quest for health evolved from his broader critique of modern civilization. Since the West was considered as the birthplace of modern civilization—the system of allopathic medicine being a part of it—Gandhi's critique was a symbolic defiance of Western modernity.[125] Although doctors and hospitals signified progress, Gandhi viewed them as signs of decadence for two reasons: (1) they undermined self-control; and (2) fostered dependency on cure over prevention.[126]

Sunil Amrith notes that health and nutritive food marked the beginnings of Gandhi's envisioned transformation. Bodily discipline, in Gandhi's vision, would awaken national consciousness and strengthen the Indian race.[127] Gandhi linked polished rice to national debility, citing contemporary nutritional research—particularly Robert McCarrison's "Rice in Relation to Beri-Beri in India."[128] In "Polished vs Unpolished," Gandhi contended, "If public opinion was strong, it will make rice-mills an impossibility by simply insisting on unpolished rice and appealing to the owners of rice mills to stop a traffic that undermines the health of a whole nation and robs the poor people of an honest means of livelihood."[129]

In quest for dietary reform and national vitality, Gandhi turned to the League of Nations Health Committee's groundbreaking research on the Physiological Basis of Human Nutrition, prominently featured in *Harijan*.[130] Gandhi drew on League research to lend scientific credibility in framing nutrition as a sovereign domain.[131]

In his article "Green Leaves," Gandhi asserted, "Since the economic reorganization of villages has been commenced with food reform, it is necessary to find the simplest and cheapest foods that would enable villagers regain lost health."[132] His village restructuring culminated in the revised Constructive Program by 1940, where sanitation and health education were key pivots.[133] Gandhi argued, "If rural reconstruction were not to include rural sanitation, our [India's] villages would remain the muck-heaps that they are today."[134] Rural reconstruction—premised on economic equality—ensured every villager a proper house, balanced food, and *khadi* [Hindi: handspun cloth] for clothing.[135]

Gandhi's health vision—steeped in the material realities of rural poverty and the symbolic urgency of national regeneration—ideationally resonated with Bandoeng (1937). The final report of the Bandoeng Conference emphasized rural reconstruction, land reform, nutrition, and public health as foundational to economic growth. Theodore Brown and Elizabeth Fee argue that these elements not only reflected the progressive ethos of the LNHO but also embodied the values of nationalist movements such as Gandhi's in India.[136]

The Bandoeng Ambiguities

Divergent views exist among historians about the significance of the 1937 Bandoeng Conference. According to Brown and Fee, the conference was a "milestone event" marking the culmination of a wave of interwar interest in rural hygiene. Unlike the European Conference on Rural Hygiene convened in Geneva (1931), which featured sovereign states, the Bandoeng meeting brought together colonial states negotiating various phases of decolonization.[137] The Bandoeng agenda—training native medical personnel attuned to local environments—differed markedly from Geneva.[138] Alternatively, Omer Aloni notes that topics such as sanitation were also raised at Geneva, challenging Bandoeng's distinctiveness.[139] This further calls into question whether the Conference represented a distinct international health intervention or merely an extension of European medical governance in colonial Asia. Laurence Monnais and Hans Pols emphasize that the Bandoeng meeting functioned less as a turning point in international health and instead reinforced colonial medical governance. [140] All public health initiatives were implemented under colonial medical authority, occasionally assisted by local physicians.

Debates over the significance of Bandoeng (1937) reflect not only its strong colonial underpinnings but also international deliberations that underscored the Conference agenda. In 1932, Chinese and Indian delegates to the LNHO were the first to propose the idea of convening a conference on rural hygiene in the Far-East. This proposal initiated a complex decision-making process within the LNHO in Geneva and the Eastern Bureau in Singapore, reflecting the need to incorporate rural hygiene within the contours of colonial health governance. The conference architecture emerged from a dynamic interplay between international health administrators and colonial authorities.

Emerging from this layered decision-making process, the LNHO accepted the Dutch government's invitation to host a conference in Bandoeng (1937). Dr de Langen, Dr E.J. Pampana from the LNHO, and the ex-Colonial Secretary of the Malay States, A.S. Haynes, constituted a Preparatory Committee.[141] Their mandate involved comparative assessments of regional health conditions and thematic evaluations of rural reconstruction, medical assistance, nutrition, and agriculture.

On April 9, 1936, Haynes arrived in Bombay and subsequently sailed to Burma, Siam, Malaya, Indochina, the Philippines, the Netherlands Indies, and Ceylon.[142] On April 11, 1936, Haynes and Dr de Langen visited Gordhandas Sunderdas Medical College in Bombay, exploring a potential visit to Wardha to observe Gandhi's rural reconstruction initiatives.[143] While the attempt to link the conference with Gandhi's program underscored its utopian aspirations, the proposal was abandoned due to scheduling constraints.

The tour of the Preparatory Committee benefited from favorable timing. Haynes observed:

> The countries which we have visited are almost entirely agricultural; their 'backbone' is the peasantry. In each country Rural Reconstruction' is prominent in the newspapers, and is on everyone's lips. It is perhaps somewhat strange that this should occur simultaneously in all the countries concerned and that it should he so recent and so comparatively sudden.[144]

During the tour, the committee confined its scope to evaluating key challenges linked to health and rural reconstruction in the Far East. In correspondence with Rajchman, members noted that hygiene in Eastern countries constituted only one dimension of a broader rural reconstruction agenda.[145] Other components included nutrition, agriculture, education, and cooperative movements.

Selskar N. Gunn—vice president of the Rockefeller Foundation in 1932— jointly led a rural reconstruction project in China with John B. Grant of the Peking Union Medical College (PUMC).[146] Grant viewed public health as integral to socioeconomic development and advocated integrating preventive and curative medicine within community health services.[147] In China, he bridged public health and medical education in ways that deviated from the biomedical model espoused by the Rockefeller Foundation.[148] Gunn authored the introduction to the Bandoeng report.[149]

Based on the Preparatory Committee's recommendations, five main topics guided the conference agenda:

1. Health and medical services: Weighing the merits of training assistant doctors versus deploying auxiliary medical staff under physician supervision;
2. Rural reconstruction and collaboration of the population;
3. Sanitation and housing: Addressing water supply, waste disposal, and fly control;
4. Nutrition: Investigation of disorders and strategies for remediation;
5. Disease control in rural districts: Targeting malaria, plague, ancylostomiasis (hookworm), tuberculosis, pneumonia, yaws, leprosy and mental diseases, and drug addiction.[150]

Held from August 3 to 13, 1937, the Bandoeng conference drew delegates from North Borneo, Burma, Ceylon, China, Gilbert and Ellice Islands, New Hebrides, Hong Kong, British India, four Indian princely states, the Netherlands East Indies, French Indochina, the Philippines, British Malaya, Siam, Japan, the British Solomon Islands, and Tonga. Participants represented veterinary science, education, sanitary engineering, agriculture, and health disciplines. Conscious of their historic mission, Bandoeng delegates engaged with broader stakes. Sir Mirza Ismael, the Diwan (Chief Minister) of Mysore and head of the Indian delegation, declared, "It is no light task to advise one half of the human race as to the measures necessary to ensure them a fuller, happier and a healthier life."[151] Caught between revolutionary unrest in British India and conservative authority, Ismael emphasized that debility and poverty stunted a country's social and economic progress, and that enduring reform required raising living standards.[152]

In his speech, W.R. Aykroyd, Director of the Nutrition Research Laboratory at Coonoor, noted that half of the human race—as referenced by Ismael—was not a homogeneous group.[153] He challenged Ismael's view that improving Asian diets was futile due to poverty and population pressures.[154] Aykroyd argued that the gravest effects of nutritional disorders in Asia were not deficiency diseases but a broader impairment of health and vitality.

The report of the Preparatory Committee urged medical students to engage with traditional wisdom—a prerequisite for adapting to their social environment.[155] While confident in its merits, Offringa acknowledged the challenges in implementing Western medicine in non-Western settings. He argued:

> It seems to me that I am not going too far, if I speak of a victory, which Western medicine in the fields of curative and of preventive care has made in the Orient. Over the whole area a rapid progress in the activities for public health is manifest. The interest in Western medicine comes as a flood over these countries of the Far East, inevitable consequence as it is of increasing knowledge and development. Western capability also as regards medicine proves to be of enormous significance.[156]

Yet later in his speech, Offringa admitted difficulties in organizing medical activities in the Far East. He cautioned that imitating the West—however appealing—could hinder progress.[157] The Bandoeng conference established a complex narrative around the diffusion of Western medicine in Asia.

Hydrick—rapporteur to the commission on Health and Medical Services—drew extensively from the Rockefeller Foundation's Poerwokerto experiment. On organizing rural health services, Hydrick recommended:

> Emphasis should be laid not so much on centres from which the people are reached, but upon securing of the co-operation of the village people who will come to the centres. Intensive activities by house-visits of the personnel in the villages must create confidence in the people and win their support to make the centres efficient, and the place to secure the confidence of the people, especially in the beginning of a service, is in the village home, and not in centres and hospitals. Although the work is very intensive in the beginning and reaches only a small number of people, readjustments for extension can be made later, so that it becomes less intensive in those areas in which the people give their co-operation, but intensive in the newly added areas.[158]

In organizing rural health services, Hydrick emphasized self-help.

Extending Hydrick's community-based model— Henri Morin, head of the Pasteur Institute of Indochina—drew on 1930s anti-malarial work in Indochina's rubber plantations, emphasizing the need to localize disease control efforts.[159] Invoking a military metaphor, he wrote, "The peasantry of Asia represent an army of workers," to emphasize the urgency and scale of anti-malarial activities.[160] He cautioned that relying exclusively on synthetic remedies to alleviate rural malaria was "a mere drop in the ocean," alluding to the centrality of community mobilization.[161]

Building on Bandoeng's advocacy for community-centered approaches, the LNHO sought collaboration with British India and the Netherlands Indies to address the domestic fly issue in the Far East—linking public health with composting practices using waste and animal dung. Rajchman noted that securing specialists to work on this problem required patience and persistence, often unfulfilled.[162]

While the Conference devoted considerable attention to describing various health problems entrenched in local conditions, actionable solutions remained scarce despite extensive deliberations. A definite tone of conservatism permeated rural health discussions, exemplified by Ismael's call to cultivate a sanitary conscience among villagers and allocate limited government resources with restraint.[163] To this end, Ismael suggested that administrators improve existing arrangements and avoid introducing comparatively new and expensive arrangements from outside.[164]

At the same time, scientists and experts were called upon to innovate rural diets, provide clean drinking water, and control insects and other vectors of disease.[165] The conference report emphasized the need for affordable malaria control methods rooted in coordination between public health, agriculture, engineering, and housing.[166] The foremost priority at Bandoeng included leveraging public health as the entering wedge for a broader program of rural reconstruction—encompassing education, economics, sociology, engineering, and agriculture.

Conclusion

As Iris Borowy contends, "For all practical purposes, the Bandoeng Conference was both the high point and the end of significant LNHO work in Asia. It was also a demonstration of an increasing LNHO commitment to a concept of health as a global and social good."[167] Specific conference recommendations included safe water provision, disposal of waste, and the study of flies. However, the influence of economic constraints and local specificities rendered the conference conclusions ambiguous and subject to interpretation.

For example, the conference acknowledged that responsibilities associated with rural reconstruction were heavy. Yet, it cautioned against the drastic introduction of rural reconstruction programs that overlooked economic circumstances and local customs.[168]

This chapter does not regard the Bandoeng conference as a milestone event in international health. Rather, it compares the proposed agenda of the conference with the actual report produced. Socrates Litsios notes that during the conference, issues were discussed in a fragmented manner.[169] Discussion of diseases was separated from environmental sanitation. Diseases such as malaria, leprosy, or yaws were left hanging with little linkage to environmental sanitation or health and medical services. In discussing nutrition, for example, the Bandoeng conference report acknowledged that nutrition was correlated with economic conditions. Additionally, it called for liaison between nutritionists and agriculturalists. There was no critique of colonial policies on nutrition.

The interwar period opened new avenues for addressing international health concerns in Southeast Asia. Initially, the Rockefeller Foundation and the LNHO focused on a technocentric approach to public health, emphasizing benchmarks in nutrition and housing. By the 1930s, international health organizations and colonial governments began to acknowledge the underlying social and economic determinants of disease. Rockefeller-supported public health experiments undertaken in Ceylon, the Philippines, the Netherlands Indies, and British India departed from earlier colonial medical initiatives in the degree to which they acknowledged participation of local communities in health improvement. Across the chapter's four cases, the co-option of local authorities in implementing public health programs contributed to a bottom-up view of technical assistance rather than a top-down view that characterized the early work of the IHB, the LNHO, and the colonial state.

But there were limits to progressive approaches. Continued belief in the power of medical science to redress health problems and inability of rural reconstruction programs across Asia to redress questions related to inequitable land distribution meant that the progressive approaches of Gunn, Grant, or Gandhi remained unfulfilled.[170] Colonial authorities half-heartedly devolved decision-making to local populations who, for many administrators, were seen as needing external assistance. Nonetheless, the 1930s should be regarded as a decade of great optimism for international health in Southeast Asia—the beginnings of a utopian vision that sought to tackle the social and economic roots of disease.

The Pacific War (1942–1945) disrupted attempts to implement the alternative vision of health and created a humanitarian crisis. The war also transformed international organizations. The LNHO was disbanded in 1946. Between 1943 and 1948, new international organizations such as the United Nations, the United Nations Relief and Rehabilitation Administration (UNRRA), and a new World Health Organization (WHO) were established to deal with the postwar world order. America's Cold War politics greatly augmented malaria control. It was believed that control of the disease would augment agricultural productivity and win the hearts and minds of rural populations in newly decolonized Asia threatened by communism.[171] The discovery of the insecticide DDT during World War II provided optimism for the American authorities and the newly established WHO that malaria eradication was possible, while overlooking underlying causes such as poverty. Rural hygiene was a casualty of the Cold War.

Notes

1. For a nuanced understanding of the colonial origins of international health, see Mark Harrison, "A Global Perspective: Reframing the History of Health, Medicine, and Disease," *Bulletin of the History of Medicine* 89, no. 4 (2015): 639–89. For an exploratory study of the humanitarian imprint on international health, see Mark Anderson, Kristin Becknell and Joanna Taliano, "History of Humanitarian Emergencies," *Health in Humanitarian Emergencies: Principles and Practices for Public Health and Healthcare Practitioners,* David Townes edited (Cambridge: Cambridge University Press, 2018), 9–24. To understand the philanthropic origins of international health, see Anne-Emanuelle Birn, "Philanthrocapitalism, Past and Present: The Rockefeller Foundation, the Gates Foundation, and the Setting(s) of the International/Global Health Agenda," *Hypothesis* 12, no. 1 (2014): e8, doi:10.5779/hypothesis.v12i1.229. To discern continuities and changes between colonial and postcolonial health in Southeast Asia, see Sunil Amrith, *Decolonizing International Health: India and Southeast Asia, 1930–65* (Basingstoke, Oxon: Palgrave Macmillan, 2006).
2. See, for example, Marcos Cueto, "The History of International Health: Medicine, Health and Two Socio-Medical Perspectives, 1851–2000," in *The Oxford Handbook of Global Health Politics*, Colin McInnes, Kelley Lee and Jeremy Youde edited (New York: Oxford University Press, 2020).
3. For nuanced colony-level studies, see Soma Hewa, "The Hookworm Epidemic on the Plantations in Sri Lanka," *Medical History* 38, no.1 (1994): 73–90; Warwick Anderson, *Colonial Pathologies: American Tropical Medicine, Race and Hygiene in the Philippines* (Durham, NC: Duke University Press); Eric Stein, "Colonial Theatres of Proof: Representation and Laughter in 1930s Rockefeller Foundation Hygiene Cinema in Java," *Health and History* 8, no. 2 (2006): 14–44; Shirish Kavadi, " ' Parasites Lost and Parasites Regained': Rockefeller

Foundation's Anti-Hookworm Campaign in Madras Presidency," *Economic and Political Weekly* 42, no. 2 (2007): 130–37.

4. Norman Howard Jones, *The Scientific Background of the International Sanitary Conferences* (Geneva: WHO, 1975). For details on the English system of quarantine, see, for example, Krista Magden, K, "'The First Line of Defense': British Quarantine and the Port Sanitary Authorities in the Nineteenth Century," *Social History of Medicine* 15, no. 3 (2002): 413–28, 424; See also Birn, "Philanthrocapitalism. Past and Present." The internationalization of health in Southeast Asia dates back to the mid-nineteenth century. The transmission of cholera along transnational oceanic routes rendered the Hajj a dangerous pilgrimage. Legislations were passed in various colonial empires to try and rationalize shipping, maintain clean water supplies and a modicum of space for individual Hajj pilgrims. See Eric Tagliacozzo, "Pilgrim Ships and the Frontiers of Contagion: Quarantine Regimes from Southeast Asia to the Red Sea," in *Histories of Health in Southeast Asia: Perspectives on the Long Twentieth Century*, Tim Harper and Sunil Amrith edited (Bloomington, Indiana: Indiana University Press, 2014), 47–60.
5. See Rockefeller Foundation, *The Rockefeller Foundation Annual Report, 1913–14* (New York: Rockefeller Foundation, 1915), 7.
6. Tomoko Akami, "The League of Nations Health Organization," *Oxford Biographies in the History of Medicine* (Oxford: Oxford University Press, 2025), Tomoko Akami, "The League of Nations Health Organization," *Oxford Biographies in the History of Medicine*, Jacalyn Duffin edited (Oxford: Oxford University Press, 2025), DOI 10.1093/obo/9780197768723-0039.
7. Anne-Emanuelle Birn and Elizabeth Fee, "The Art of Medicine: The Rockefeller Foundation and the International Health Agenda," *The Lancet* 381, no. 9878 (September 2013): 1618–19.
8. Rockefeller Foundation, *Annual Report, 1913–14*, 12.
9. Rockefeller Foundation, *Annual Report, 1913–14*, 13–14.
10. Soma Hewa, "Tropical Disease and Imperial Medicine in Colonial Sri Lanka," *Galle Medical Journal* 24, no. 2 (2019): 25–32, 28.
11. Doctor Victor Heiser, *An American Doctor's Odyssey: Adventures in Forty-Five Countries* (New York: W.W. Norton, 1936), 329.
12. Heiser, *An American Doctor's Odyssey*, 330.
13. Hewa, " Tropical Disease and Imperial Medicine," 28.
14. Ibid., 28.
15. Ibid., 28.
16. Ibid., 28.
17. "Letter from Wilbur A. Sawyer to Victor Heiser," March 21, 1924, Report on Ceylon Part III, Rockefeller Foundation Records: Officers'

Diaries, Record Group (RG) 12, S-Z; Sawyer, Wilbur A., Rockefeller Archive Center (RAC).

18. Hewa, "Tropical Medicine and Imperial Medicine," 26.
19. Soma Hewa, "The Alma-Ata Declaration, Rockefeller Foundation and the Development of Primary Health Care in Sri Lanka: A Model for Health Prevention," in *Science, Public Health and the State in Modern Asia*, Liping Bu, Darwin Stapleton and Ka-che Yip edited (Abingdon, Oxon: Routledge, 2012), 71–92, 79.
20. Rockefeller Foundation, *The Rockefeller Foundation Annual Report, 1922* (New York: Rockefeller Foundation, 1922), 130.
21. "Letter from the United Missionary Campaign to Wickliffe Rose," July 28, 1913, Folder 160. Philippine Islands (1911–14), Rockefeller Sanitary Commission for the Eradication of Hookworm Disease Records; Field Offices Series 2, Philippines, RAC.
22. Warwick Anderson, "Going through the Motions: American Public Health and Colonial 'Mimicry,'" *American Literary History* 14, no. 4 (2002): 686–719, 702.
23. Anderson, "Going Through the Motions," 703.
24. Ibid., 703.
25. For the wider political context, see "Independence Stand Vigorously Defended," *The Michigan Daily*, March 22, 1924, The University of Michigan Library, Michigan Daily Digital Archives. Available at: https://digital.bentley.umich.edu/midaily/mdp.39015071755743/323.
26. Anderson, " Going through the Motions," 705.
27. Anderson, " Going Through the Motions," 706.
28. Anderson, *Colonial Pathologies*, 69.
29. Anderson, *Colonial Pathologies*, 70.
30. "Far Eastern Association of Tropical Medicine," *The British Medical Journal* 1, no. 2470 (May 2, 1908): 1061–62.
31. Tomoko Akami, "Imperial Polities, Intercolonialism, and the Shaping of Global Governing Norms: Public Health Expert Networks in Asia and the League of Nations Health Organization, 1908–37," *Journal of Global History* 12, no.1 (2017): 4–25, 10.
32. See David Arnold, "Tropical Governance: Managing Health in Tropical Asia, 1908–38," *Asia Research Institute Working Paper* 116 (May 2009), https://doi.org/10.2139/ssrn.1645149.
33. See, for example, Victor Heiser, "Practical Experiences with Beriberi and Unpolished Rice in the Philippines," *Journal of the American Medical Association* LVI, no. 17 (1911): 1237–38, 38.
34. A.L. Hoops, *The Prevention of Disease in the Tropics: An Address Delivered before the Fifth Congress of the Far Eastern Association of Tropical Medicine* (Singapore: Government Printing Office, 1923), Dossier Concerning

the Fifth Congress of the Far Eastern Association of Tropical Medicine, Singapore, Doc. R19/12B/32210, League of Nations Archives Geneva (henceforth LoN). For a comprehensive understanding of the application of French ideas of infant care to local communities in Indochina, see Thuy Linh Nguyen, "French Educated Midwives and the Medicalization of Childbirth in Colonial Vietnam," *Journal of Vietnamese Studies* 5, no. 2 (2010): 133–82.

35. Arnold, "Tropical Governance."
36. Wilbur A. Sawyer, *Advantages of Nation-Wide and International Organization of Disease Control, with Special Reference to Hookworm Disease and Beri-Beri* (Singapore: Government Printing Office), 8.
37. *Statements Laid Before the Committee on Beri-Beri Control and the Resolution Recommended by the Committee and Passed at the General Council of the Fifth Congress of the Far Eastern Association of Tropical Medicine, 1923* (Singapore: Government Printing Office, 1923), Dossier Concerning the Fifth Congress of the Far Eastern Association of Tropical Medicine, Singapore, Doc. R19/12B/32210, LoN.
38. "Statement: Dr F.H. Guèrin on Behalf of the Delegation of Indochina," *Statements Laid Before the Committee on Beri-Beri Control and the Resolution Recommended by the Committee and Passed at the General Council of the Fifth Congress of the Far Eastern Association of Tropical Medicine, 1923* (Singapore: Government Printing Office, 1923), Dossier Concerning the Fifth Congress of the Far Eastern Association of Tropical Medicine, Singapore, Doc. R19/12B/32210, LoN; "Statement by C.D. de Langen of the Netherlands East Indies Delegation," *Statements Laid Before the Committee on Beri-Beri Control and the Resolution Recommended by the Committee and Passed at the General Council of the Fifth Congress of the Far Eastern Association of Tropical Medicine, 1923* (Singapore: Government Printing Office, 1923), Dossier Concerning the Fifth Congress of the Far Eastern Association of Tropical Medicine, Singapore, Doc. R19/12B/32210, LoN.
39. "Statements by Dr S. Kanai and Dr Honna on Behalf of the Delegations of Japan and Formosa," *Statements Laid Before the Committee on Beri-Beri Control and the Resolution Recommended by the Committee and Passed at the General Council of the Fifth Congress of the Far Eastern Association of Tropical Medicine, 1923* (Singapore: Government Printing Office, 1923), Dossier Concerning the Fifth Congress of the Far Eastern Association of Tropical Medicine, Singapore, Doc. R19/12B/32210, LoN.
40. " The Resolution Recommended by the Committee as Amended by the Council and Passed at the General Meeting of the Fifth Congress of the FEATM," *Statements Laid Before the Committee on Beri-Beri Control and*

the Resolution Recommended by the Committee and Passed at the General Council of the Fifth Congress of the Far Eastern Association of Tropical Medicine, 1923 (Singapore: Government Printing Office, 1923), Dossier Concerning the Fifth Congress of the Far Eastern Association of Tropical Medicine, Singapore, Doc. R19/12B/32210, LoN.

41. Akami, "Imperial Polities," 6.
42. David Arnold, "British India and the Beriberi Problem, 1798–1942," *Medical History* 54, no. 3 (2010): 295–314.
43. "Possibility of International Action for Control of Beriberi: From Governor of the Straits Settlements dated April 19, 1923," Deputation of Medical Officers from the Provinces of India to the Fifth Congress of the Far Eastern Association of Tropical Medicine to be Held at Singapore, Department of Education and Health (1923), Identifier PR_000003001391, File No Education and Health_Sanitary_B_1923_Jun_102–125, National Archives of India (NAI). Accessed April 24, 2024. https://indianculture.gov.in/archives/deputation-medical-officers-provinces-india-5th-congress-far-eastern-association-tropical.
44. Akami, "Imperial Polities," 11.
45. Paul Weindling, "Philanthropy and World Health: The Rockefeller Foundation and the League of Nations Health Organization," *Minerva* 35 (1997): 269–81.
46. "Letter from Wickliffe Rose to Rajchman," September 2, 1922, Collaboration between the Health Organization of the League of Nations and the International Health Board of the Rockefeller Foundation, Doc. R839/12B/21836, Jacket 1, LoN.
47. See, for example, Philip Clarke and Guido Erreygers, "Edgar Sydenstricker: A Pioneer of Health Economics," The *European Journal of the History of Economic Thought* 29, no. 6 (2022): 1066–88.
48. Yi-Tang Lin, *Statistics and the Language of Global Health: Institutions and Experts in China, Taiwan and the World, 1917–60* (Cambridge: Cambridge University Press, 2022), 96.
49. League of Nations, "Health Committee: Report on the Far Eastern Commission of Enquiry," January 8, 1923, Commission d' Enquête en Extrême Orient, Doc. R843/12B/23230/25592, LoN.
50. "Letter Signed by E.J. Turner to Secretary General, League of Nations," Far Eastern Sanitary Convention: August 15, 1925, Doc. R903/12B/30818/35026, LoN.
51. Norman White, "The Prevalence of Epidemic Disease and Port Health: Organizations and Procedures in the Far East," Report Presented to the Health Committee of the League of Nations, Geneva (1923), Doc. C/167M/43/1924/III, LoN.

52. See Lenore Manderson, "Wireless Wars in the Eastern Arena: Epidemiological Surveillance, Disease Prevention and the Work of the Eastern Bureau of the League of Nations Health Organisation, 1925–1942," in *International Health Organisations and Movements*, Paul Weindling edited (Cambridge: Cambridge University Press, 1995), 109–33, 117.
53. "Letter Addressed to Gilbert Brooke, Director of the Eastern Bureau," May 7, 1925, Far East Epidemiological Intelligence Bureau: Organisation of the Work of the Bureau, Doc. R925/12B/34275/45102, LoN.
54. League of Nations Health Organisation, "Minutes of a Conference held in Singapore Regarding the Establishment of an Epidemiological Intelligence Bureau for the Far East," Doc. R925/12B/34275/42212, LoN.
55. Norman White, "Morning Session," February 4. 1925, Epidemiological Intelligence Bureau in the Far East: Proceedings of the Singapore Conference, February 1925, Doc. R925/12B/34275/42212, LoN.
56. "Telegram from Norman White to Ludwik Rajchman," Received in the Health Section of the League of Nations on February 5, 1925, Epidemiological Intelligence Bureau in the Far East: Proceedings of the Singapore Conference, February 1925, Doc. R925/12B/34275/42212, LoN.
57. "First Session," February 4, 1925, Epidemiological Intelligence Bureau in the Far East: Proceedings of the Singapore Conference, February 1925, Doc. R925/12B/34275/42212, LoN.
58. Lin, *Statistics and the Language of Global Health*, 100.
59. Alexander Cameron Smith, "Australian Imperialism and International Health in the Pacific Islands," *Australian Historical Studies* 41, no. 1 (2010): 57–74, 64.
60. Commonwealth of Australia, *Report of the International Pacific Health Conference held at Melbourne, 11th to 25 December 1926*, Conference on Health Problems in the Pacific Islands, Melbourne (December 1926), Doc. R983/12B/52362, LoN.
61. See, for example, Ho Hee Cho, *Imperial Health: Centralisation of Medical Institutions in the South Pacific* (PhD diss., Oxford University, 2022).
62. Smith, "Australian Imperialism," 72.
63. Western Pacific Health Services, *Fourth Annual Report 1931*, MSS & Archives 2003/1, NHBS 1/I, Vol 3 Series I., File 146/1932, Special Collections, University of Auckland Libraries and Learning Services.
64. Ibid.
65. Ibid.
66. Ibid.

67. Birn, "Philanthrocapitalism."
68. See, for example, Eric A. Stein, "Hygiene and Decolonization: The Rockefeller Foundation and Indonesian Nationalism, 1933–58," *Science, Public Health and the State in Modern Asia*, Liping Bu, Darwin Stapleton and Ka-che Yip edited (Abingdon, Oxon: Routledge, 2012), 51–70, 52.
69. Terence Hull, "Conflict and Collaboration in Public Health: The Rockefeller Foundation and the Dutch Colonial Government in Indonesia," *Public Health in Asia and the Pacific: Historical and Comparative Perspectives*, Milton J. Lewis and Kerrie L. Macpherson edited (Abingdon, Oxon: Routledge, 2008), 139–52, 140.
70. Victor Heiser, "Buitenzorg, March 29, 1915," Notes on the 1915 Trip, Rockefeller Foundation Records, Officers' Diaries, RG 12, F–L; Heiser, Victor G., RAC.
71. Victor Heiser, "Buitenzorg, March 30, 1915," Notes on the 1915 Trip, Rockefeller Foundation Records, Officers' Diaries, RG 12, F–L; Heiser, Victor G., RAC.
72. Hull, "Conflict and Collaboration in Public Health," 141.
73. Victor Heiser, "Steamship Oranje, April 2, 1915," Notes on the 1915 Trip, Rockefeller Foundation Records, Officers' Diaries, RG 12, F–L; Heiser, Victor G., RAC.
74. Rockefeller Foundation International Health Board, "Itinerary of Doctor Victor G. Heiser, Director for the East," Notes on the 1916 Trip (vol. 1), Rockefeller Foundation Records, Officers' Diaries, RG 12, F–L; Heiser, Victor G., RAC.
75. A.T. Darling, M.A. Barber and H.P. Hacker, *Hookworm and Malaria Research in Malaya, Java and the Fiji Islands: Report of the Uncinariasis Commission to the Orient, 1915–17* (New York: The Rockefeller Foundation International Health Board, 1920), 15.
76. Hull, "Conflict and Collaboration in Public Health," 142.
77. Darling, Barber and Hacker, *Hookworm and Malaria Research*, 9.
78. Hull, "Conflict and Collaboration in Public Health," 143.
79. Ibid., 143.
80. Ibid., 143.
81. Victor Heiser, "Hotel des Indies, Weltevreden, January 10, 1926," Diary of Heiser: World Trip, September 17, 1925 to June 8, 1926, Rockefeller Foundation Records, Officers Diaries, RG 12, F–L; Heiser, Victor G., RAC.
82. Heiser, *An American Doctor's Odyssey*, 476.
83. Victor Heiser, "Hotel Tram, Poerwakarta, January 12, 1926," Diary of Heiser: World Trip, September 17, 1925 to June 8, 1926, Rockefeller Foundation Records, Officers Diaries, RG 12, F–L; Heiser, Victor G., RAC.

84. Ibid.
85. Rockefeller Foundation, *The Rockefeller Foundation Annual Report, 1927* (New York: Rockefeller Foundation, 1927), 120.
86. Rockefeller Foundation, *Annual Report, 1927*, 121.
87. John Lee Hydrick, *Intensive Hygiene Work in the Netherlands East Indies* (New York City: Rockefeller Foundation, Netherlands Information Bureau, 1944), 12.
88. Hull, "Conflict and Collaboration in Public Health," 146.
89. Hull, "Conflict and Collaboration in Public Health," 147.
90. Stein, "Hygiene and Decolonization," 52.
91. "S.t.o.v.i.a.," *Het Nieuws van den Dag voor Nederlandsch-Indië*, July 11, 1914, Koninklijke Bibliotheek or KB [Dutch].
92. Hans Pols, *Nurturing Indonesia: Medicine and Decolonisation in the Dutch East Indies* (Cambridge: Cambridge University Press, 2018), 149.
93. "Gezondheidbrigades ter Oostkust: Goed Werk van den Dienst der Volksgezondheid," *De Sumatera Post*, March 8, 1932, KB [Dutch].
94. Ibid.
95. Pols, Nurturing Indonesia, 149.
96. Pols, *Nurturing Indonesia*, 151.
97. "J.L. Hydrick: Trip to Batavia and Sumatra, 1932," RG 2 General Correspondence Indonesia HYD-2, Box 558, Folder 3773, RAC.
98. Ibid.
99. Vivek Neelakantan, *Science, Public Health and Nation-Building in Soekarno-Era Indonesia* (Newcastle-upon-Tyne: Cambridge Scholars, 2017), 37.
100. "Zeikenverzorging in Z. Tapanoeli," *De Sumatera Post*, November 3, 1932, KB [Dutch].
101. "Dr Offfringa te Medan Conferentie met Dr Rasjid," *Het Nieuws van den Dag voor Nederlandsch-Indië*, December 28, 1934 [Dutch].
102. "Veel Besproken Kwestie en Tapanoeli: Zeven Hoofden Tegen Plannen van Dr Rasjid," *De Sumatra Post*, January 17, 1935, KB [Dutch].
103. Susan Abeyasekare, "Health as a Nationalist Issue in Colonial Indonesia," in *Nineteenth and Twentieth Century Indonesia: Essays in Honour of Professor J.D. Legge*, C.D. Cowan, and O.W. Wolters edited (Clayton, Victoria: Monash University Press, 1986), 1–9.
104. Pols, *Nurturing Indonesia*, 152.
105. *Redevoeringen van de Leden van den Volksraad: Abdul Firman Gelar Maharadja Soangkoepon en Abdul Rasjid Gelar Maharadja Mahkota Soangkoepon over het Zittingsjaar, 1936–37* (Buitenzorg: Buitenzorgsche Drukkerij, 1938), 155–61, KB.
106. Ibid.
107. Ibid.

108. Pols, Nurturing Indonesia, 152.
109. Heiser, *An American Doctor's Odyssey*, 340.
110. Shirish Kavadi, "'Wolves Come to Take Care of the Lamb': The Rockefeller Foundation's Hookworm Campaign in Madras Presidency," in *The Politics of the Healthy Life: An International Perspective*, Esteban Rodrìguez-Ocaña edited (Sheffield: European Society for the History of Medicine, 2002), 89–111.
111. Kavadi, 'Wolves Come to Take Care of the Lamb,' 91.
112. Kavadi, 'Wolves Come to Take Care of the Lamb,' 92.
113. "Letter from Wilbur Sawyer to Victor Heiser: Report on Trip to Madras Presidency," April 28, 1924, Rockefeller Foundation Records, Officers Diaries RG 12, S-Z; Sawyer, Wilbur A., RAC.
114. Kavadi, 'Parasites Lost and Parasites Regained,' 135.
115. "Letter from Kendrick to Heiser," April 7, 1927, Rockefeller Foundation Records, International Health Board/Division Records RG 5, Correspondence Series 1_02 Project Correspondence, Sub Group 1926; India Subseries 1926_464; Kendrick, J.F., RAC.
116. Ibid.
117. Ibid.
118. Kavadi, 'Parasites Lost and Parasites Regained,' 136.
119. Ibid., 136.
120. David Arnold, "Death and the Modern Empire: The 1918–19 Influenza Epidemic in India," *Transactions of the Royal Historical Society* 29 (2019): 181–200, 185–86.
121. Arnold, "Death and the Modern Empire," 186.
122. Arnold, "Death and the Modern Empire," 195.
123. For details see Mridula Ramanna, *Bombay Presidency, 1850–1920: Disease, Sanitation and Public Health Personalities* (New Delhi: Primus, 2024), 317.
124. Arnold, "Death and Modern Empire," 198.
125. Shamshad Khan, "Systems of Medicine and Nationalist Discourse in India: Towards 'New Horizons' in Medical Anthropology and History," *Social Science and Medicine* 62 no.11 (2006): 2786–97, 2793.
126. Ibid., 2793.
127. Amrith, *Decolonizing International Health*, 32.
128. Robert McCarrison, "Rice in Relation to Beri-Beri in India," *The British Medical Journal* 1, no. 3297 (1924): 414–20.
129. M.K. Gandhi, "Polished vs Unpolished," *Harijan,* October 26, 1934, Gandhi Bhavan Collection, Bangalore (hereafter GB).
130. M.K. Gandhi, "Physiological Basis of Human Nutrition," *Harijan*, April 25, 1936, GB.
131. Amrith, *Decolonizing International Health*, 33–34.

132. M.K. Gandhi, "Green Leaves," *Harijan*, February 15, 1935, GB.
133. M.K. Gandhi, "Implications of Constructive Programme," *Harijan*, August 18, 1940, GB.
134. Ibid.
135. Ibid.
136. Theodore Brown and Elizabeth Fee, "The Bandoeng Conference of 1937: A Milestone in Health and Development," *American Journal of Public Health* 98, no. 1 (2008): 42–43, 43.
137. Brown and Fee, "The Bandoeng Conference," 42.
138. Iris Borowy, *Coming to Terms with World Health: The League of Nations Health Organisation, 1921–46* (Frankfurt: Peter Lang, 2009), 347.
139. Omer Aloni, *The League of Nations and the Protection of the Environment* (Cambridge: Cambridge University Press, 2022), 218.
140. Laurence Monnais and Hans Pols, "Imperial Social Medicine in Southeast Asia: The Bandung Intergovernmental Conference on Rural Hygiene," *Medicine on a Larger Scale: Global Histories of Social Medicine*, in Ann Kveim Lie, Jeremy Alan Greene and Warwick Anderson edited (Cambridge: Cambridge University Press, 2025), 81–105, 103.
141. "Undated Statement," Rural Hygiene Conference in the Far East: Correspondence Exchanged during Dr Pampana's Mission, April to August 1936, Doc. R6093/8A/25509/8855, LoN.
142. "Letter from A.S. Haynes, Chairman of the LNHO Committee on Rural Hygiene to Private Secretary, His Excellency, the Viceroy of India," August 22, 1936, Rural Hygiene Conference in the Far East: Correspondence Exchanged during Dr Pampana's Mission, April to August 1936, Doc. R6093/8A/25509/8855, LoN.
143. "Letter from Haynes to Jivraj Mehta," June 11, 1936, Rural Hygiene Conference in the Far East: Correspondence Exchanged during Dr Pampana's Mission, April to August 1936, Doc. R6093/8A/25509/8855, LoN.
144. "Letter from A.S. Haynes to Private Secretary to His Excellency the Viceroy," August 22, 1936, Rural Hygiene Conference in the Far East Preparatory Measures: Correspondence Exchanged During Dr Pampana's Mission, April to August 1936, Doc. R6093/8A/25509/8855, LoN.
145. "Confidential Letter to Dr Rajchman," April 14, 1936, Rural Hygiene Conference in the Far East Preparatory Measures: Correspondence Exchanged During Dr Pampana's Mission, April to August 1936, Doc. R6093/8A/25509/8855, LoN.
146. Socrates Litsios, "Bandoeng Conference of 1937," *American Journal of Public Health* 98, no. 5 (2008): 777.
147. Liping Bu, "Beijing First Health Station: Innovative Public Health Education and Influence on China's Health Profession," in *Science,*

Public Health and the State in Modern Asia, Liping Bu, Darwin H. Stapleton and Ka-che Yip edited (Abingdon, Oxon: Routledge, 2012), 129–43, 129.

148. Litsios, "Bandoeng Conference," 777.
149. Ibid., 777.
150. League of Nations Health Organisation, *Report of the Intergovernmental Conference of Far-Eastern Nations on Rural Hygiene Held at Bandoeng (Java), August 3rd–13th, 1937* (Geneva: League of Nations Health Organisation, 1937), 7.
151. "Speech by Sir Mirza Ismael, Dewan of Mysore," Rural Hygiene Conference in the Far East, August 1937: Speeches by Delegates, Rapporteurs, etc., Doc. R6017/8A/37715/8855, LoN.
152. Ibid.
153. "Speech by W.R. Aykroyd, Director of Nutrition Research Laboratory, Coonoor," August 4, 1937, Rural Hygiene: Conference in the Far East, August 1937: Speeches by Delegates, Rapporteurs, etc., Doc. R6107/37715/8855, LoN.
154. Ibid.
155. "Far Eastern Rural Hygiene Conference," *Current Science* 6, no. 2 (1937): 70–72.
156. "Speech of Dr Offringa," Rural Hygiene Conference in the Far East, August 1937: Speeches by Delegates, Rapporteurs, etc., Doc. R6017/8A/37715/8855, LoN.
157. Ibid.
158. "Report to the Plenary Meeting of the Conference by Dr J.L. Hydrick: Commission I, Health and Medical Services," Rural Government Conference in the Far East, August 1937: Reports of Commissions, Doc. R6107/8A/37714/8855, LoN.
159. For details see Michitake Aso, "Patriotic Hygiene: Tracing New Places of Knowledge Production about Malaria in Vietnam, 1919–75" *Journal of Southeast Asian Studies* 44, no. 3 (2013): 423–43.
160. Morin, "On the Prevention of Malaria in the Far East," July 21, 1937, Intergovernmental Conference of Far-Eastern Countries on Rural Hygiene, Item V, Hygiène Rural Conférence en Extrême-Orient: Rapports des Gouvernements, Doc. R6096/8A/26763/8855, LoN.
161. Ibid.
162. "Letter from Ludwik Rajchman to Dr Park, Director of the Eastern Bureau," December 10, 1937, Rural Hygiene: Study of the Fly Problem in the Far East, Doc. R 6094/8A/26055/8855, LoN.
163. "Report to the Plenary Meeting of the Conference by Dr J.L. Hydrick."

164. "Commission II: Introductory Remarks by Sir Mirza M. Ismael," Rural Hygiene Conference in the Far East, August 1937: Speeches by Delegates, Rapporteurs, etc, Doc. R6017/8A/37715/8855, LoN.
165. See also Annick Guénel, "The 1937 Bandung Conference on Hygiene: Towards a New Vision of Healthcare?", *Global Movements, Local Concerns: Medicine and Health in Southeast Asia*, Laurence Monnais and Harold Cook edited (Singapore: NUS Press, 2012), 62–80, 73.
166. League of Nations Health Organisation, *Report of the Intergovernmental Conference*, 30.
167. Borowy, *Coming to Terms with World Health*, 356.
168. See, for example, League of Nations Health Organisation, *Report of the Intergovernmental Conference*, 26.
169. Socrates Litsios, "Revisiting Bandoeng," *Social Medicine* 8, no. 3 (2014): 113–19.
170. Packard, *A History of Global Health*, 87.
171. See also Socrates Litsios, "Rural Hygiene in the Early Years of the World Health Organization: Another Casualty of the Cold War?" *Anais do Instituto de Higiene e Medicina Tropical* 15 (August 2016): 125–32, 32.

CHAPTER 3

"Healthy People, Strong Nation": Mobilizing Public Health During the Pacific War and Its Aftermath, 1942–1947

Introduction

Historians have depicted the Pacific War (1942–1945) as a period of transition or continuity.[1] This chapter addresses the Pacific War in Southeast Asia from a public health perspective, emphasizing change. It details the wartime trials of insecticide DDT in Ceylon, British India, and Malaya, illustrating the intersection between public health and wartime exigencies. In order to ensure their success in the Pacific War, the Japanese instrumentalized public health as a tool for political mobilization. Speaking of a New Java and a New Society (Malay: *Masjarakat Barœ*), Indonesian doctors reclaimed public health as a terrain of medical decolonization.[2] Yet postwar health governance in Southeast Asia remained tethered to prewar legacies. For example, Dutch doctors could no longer claim responsibility for rural hygiene in Java after the Japanese surrendered in 1945; instead, 1930s Rockefeller-trained Indonesian physicians did.

This chapter interrogates the historical events that contributed to the recognition of health as a "right" in the aftermath of the Pacific War. Additionally, it traces the epistemic and institutional shifts in international health governance—from an interwar period of loose expert networks to a postwar environment grounded in state responsibility for population health.

V. Neelakantan, *The Emergence of International Health Policy in Southeast Asia, India, and Sri Lanka, 1937–1978*,
https://doi.org/10.1007/978-3-032-21233-7_3

Public Health in the Greater East Asia Co-Prosperity Sphere

At the close of World War I, the legitimacy of colonialism came under attack from Gandhi and Russian revolutionary Vladimir Lenin. The war's end catalyzed national self-determination and complicated the justification for imperialism. Peter Duus contends that the acquisition of partial sovereignty over "backward peoples" or territories— a practice normalized by Western powers—required rhetorical reframing to align with liberal constructions of nationhood.[3]

The principal Japanese response to the intellectual dilemmas of interwar imperialism was the vision of a Greater East Asia Co-Prosperity Sphere, coined by Foreign Minister Arita Hachiro on June 29, 1940. The Sphere sought to reconcile the Asian aspirations for independence with Japan's ambitions for regional hegemony.[4] It ensured resources and markets for Japanese industries while strategically excluding Western rivals from Southeast Asia. During the Pacific War, Japan launched total mobilization campaigns under slogans such as "Greater East Asia War" and "Construction of New Java."[5] Health was central to wartime mobilization, particularly in Java.

On March 1, 1942, the Japanese attacked Java. Eight days later, the Dutch Commander-In-Chief of the Allied Forces, Ter Poorten, capitulated without consulting British and American allies. Indonesians viewed this as Dutch capitulation—akin to Vichy's Indochina—and welcomed the Japanese.[6] The lifting of the Dutch bans on the red-and-white flag and the singing of Indonesia Raya signaled a rupture in colonial authority.[7] Believing Indonesian nationalist leaders posed no significant threat, Japan sought to exploit Indonesia's natural resources, launching the *Pergerakan Tiga A* [Malay: Three A Movement] in April 1942. The Three As stood for slogans such as "Japan, the Leader, Protector, and Light of Asia."[8] Only a few nationalists, notably Soetan Sjahrir—who openly criticized the occupation—gained traction among medical students.[9]

Soon after Japan invaded Java, education at the Batavia Medical School (Geneeskundige Hoogeschool or GH) and the Surabaya Medical School (NIAS) was suspended. In August 1942, a small group of medical students from Surabaya traveled with Indies physician Abdul Rasjid to Jakarta and implored the military administration to restart medical education. On April 29, 1943, commemorating the birthday of the Japanese emperor, the Ika Daigaku [Japanese: Medical College] was inaugurated.[10] Malay replaced Dutch as the lingua franca. Like other professional organizations, the Association of Indies Physicians was dissolved and reconstituted in 1943 as the Java Medical Service Association (Japanese: Djawa Izi Hōkōkai).[11] *Berita Ketabiban,* the association's journal—saturated with pro-Japanese rhetoric—pledged loyalty to building a new Indonesia under the aegis of the Greater East Asia Co-Prosperity Sphere.[12]

In his 1943 speech, nationalist leader Soekarno emphasized that a doctor not only treated the sick but also prevented disease and educated the population on hygiene. This, he argued, would lead to a strong and healthy nation (Malay: *ra'jat sangat sehat dan koeat*).[13] Soekarno urged members of Djawa Izi Hōkōkai to not only dedicate themselves to their patients but to all layers of society.[14]

Leiden-educated Indonesian physician Boentaran Martoatmodjo, vice president of Djawa Izi Hōkōkai, was acting director of Semarang Central Hospital in 1941 and had joined an underground organization preparing for the Japanese occupation of Java. He headed the Semarang division of the Organization to Aid Victims of War (Malay: Penolong Korban Perang), a Java-wide network that sought to undermine Dutch defenses.[15] When the Japanese arrived, he transformed the group into the Local Committee for Indonesian Independence (Malay: Komiti Indonesia Merdeka) to welcome the victors.[16] In August 1943, Boentaran was appointed to the Central Advisory Committee, a quasi-parliamentary body that replaced the Volksraad. Concurrently, the military administration deputed him to Japan to study the organization of preventive and curative health systems.[17] On his return to Java, he described Japanese initiatives, such as: improving population quality and quantity, focusing on maternal and child health, enhancing physical well-being, promoting industrial hygiene, and preventing epidemics.[18] Boentaran concluded that preventive measures outweighed curative efforts in significance.

Boentaran's observations were enthusiastically received by colleagues in Djawa Izi Hōkōkai who recommended that Indonesian physicians broaden their understanding of preventive medicine to nurture a strong and healthy citizenry. Inspired by his visit to Japan, Indonesian physicians proposed several initiatives in *Berita Ketabiban.* One physician emphasized the importance of exercise in the realization of New Java, while another advocated for the physical and mental well-being of Indonesians, describing public health as a pillar of society (Malay: *tiang masjarakat*).[19] During the Japanese occupation, three days each month were designated as health days (Malay: *hari kesehatan rakjat*), featuring hygiene education and street cleaning (Images 3.1 and 3.2).

The emphasis on civic hygiene and population discipline was echoed in the broader propaganda apparatus, most notably in the Malay-language daily, *Asia Raya*. This flagship of the Java Propaganda Squad (Japanese: *Bunkeyin*) was published from April 29, 1942, to September 7, 1945. *Asia Raya* emphasized Japan's vision for a united and prosperous Asia and downplayed coverage related to wartime medical shortages or war crimes that might provoke Indonesian resentment.

Ethan Mark argues that *Asia Raya* had to walk a tightrope between Indonesian nationalism and Japanese schemes for the Greater East Asia Co-Prosperity Sphere. Indonesian journalists recruited by *Asia Raya* evoked expectations Japan had raised in promising to lead Indonesia's development on modern lines, recognize Indonesia as an equal member of the Greater East Asia Co-Prosperity Sphere, and deliver results swiftly.[20]

Articles in *Asia Raya* contrasted health conditions during the final years of Dutch colonialism (1939–1940) with the first year of Japanese occupation (1942–1943). One report claimed over a tenfold decline in protein-energy malnutrition—from 4000 cases in 1940 to fewer than 300 by 1943.[21] To address malnutrition, the article emphasized cross-sectoral coordination linking health, agriculture, and industry under the Japanese Military Administration as part of broader efforts to inculcate civic hygiene and augment productivity.[22]

The military administration promoted campaigns for the eradication of mass diseases, particularly yaws, that debilitated the productive capacity of the Javanese. Yaws—a bacterial infection caused by the spirochete treponema pertenue, which spreads through open wounds—afflicted nearly 5 percent of the Javanese population during the Pacific War.[23] Incidence was particularly high among rural children. Insanitary conditions facilitated transmission. The disease destroys the nasal cartilage and toes, and the rural Javanese euphemistically referred to yaws as the "beautiful flowering disease" (Javanese: *kembang ayau boenga patèk*).[24] The disease was treated with salvarsan injections from the late colonial period in the Netherlands Indies, but supplies dwindled during the Pacific War. In his article, Raden Kodijat—medical graduate from STOVIA (1914) and regency physician in East Java (1930–1942)—recommended distancing from infected individuals and maintenance of personal hygiene as preventive measures.[25] The military administration dispensed mass yaws treatments in Java between March and May 1944 through mobile clinics. The treated

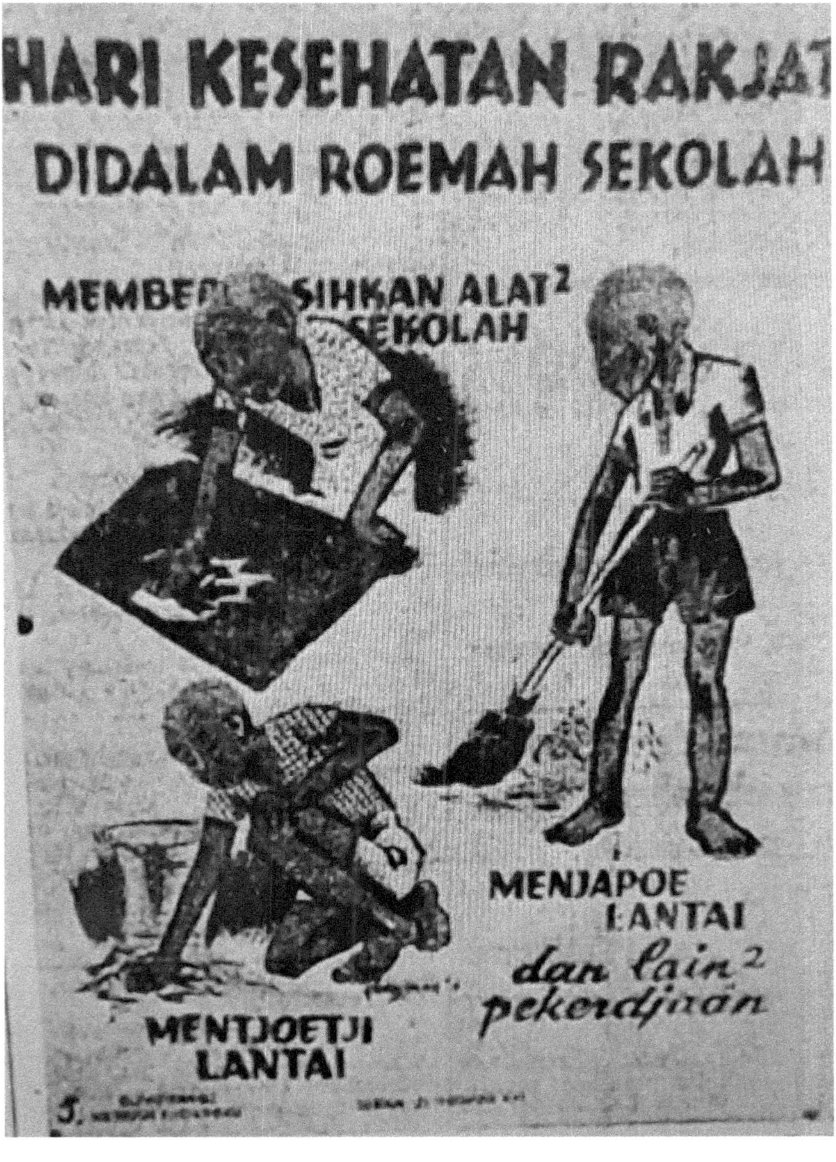
HARI KESEHATAN RAKJAT
DIDALAM ROEMAH SEKOLAH
MEMBE SIHKAN ALAT2
SEKOLAH
MENJAPOE
LANTAI
dan lain2
pekerdjaan
MENTJOETJI
LANTAI

Image 3.1 Mobilizing Public Health in Wartime Java: School Hygiene as a Civic Ritual, 1943. Source: *Asia Raya*, October 11, 1943, p. 2. Leiden University Libraries Digital Collections. Public Domain. Persistent URL: http://hdl.handle.net/1887.1/item:3206099

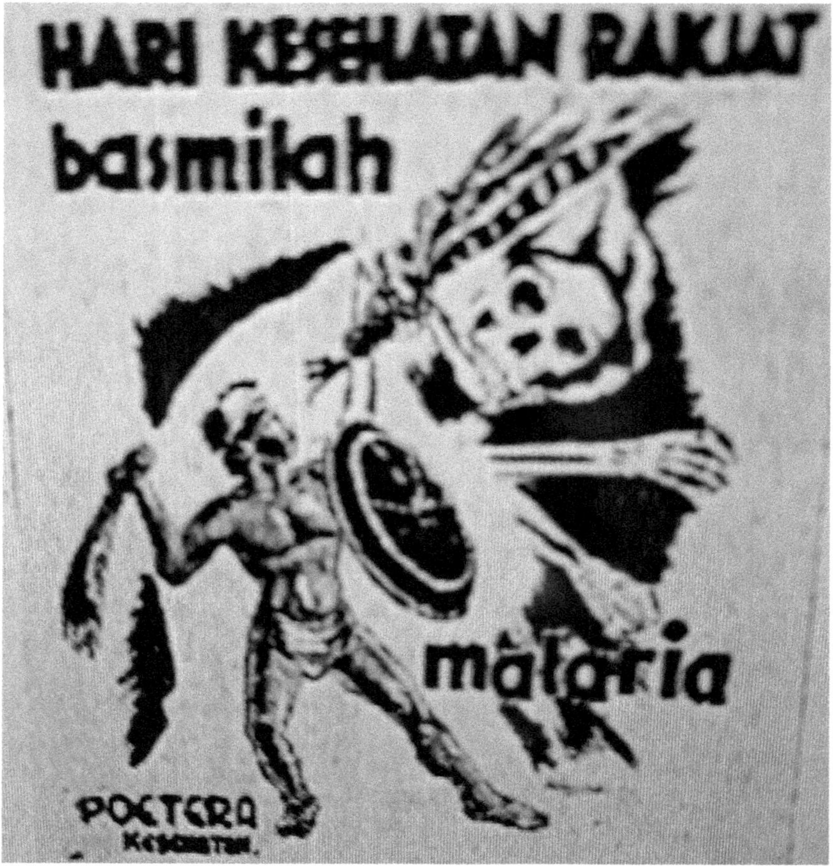

Image 3.2 Java, 1943: Militarized Metaphors in the War Against Malaria. Malaria—cast as a skeletal figure—evokes the visual imagery of death. Public Health is enacted through embodied civic rituals on People's Health Day, emphasizing eradication as a sacrament. Source: "Hari Kesehatan Rakjat, Bulan XI (2603)," *Asia Raya*, November 6, 1943, p.4. Courtesy: Leiden University Libraries. Persistent URL: http://hdl.handle.net/1887.1/item:3216029. Public Domain

individual became a symbol of national vitality in Japanese wartime propaganda (Image 3.3).

Prominent Indonesian physicians showcased their medical nationalism in theatrical pageantries staged by the Japanese.[26] However, the masses suffered from poverty, malnutrition, and infectious disease. The lack of

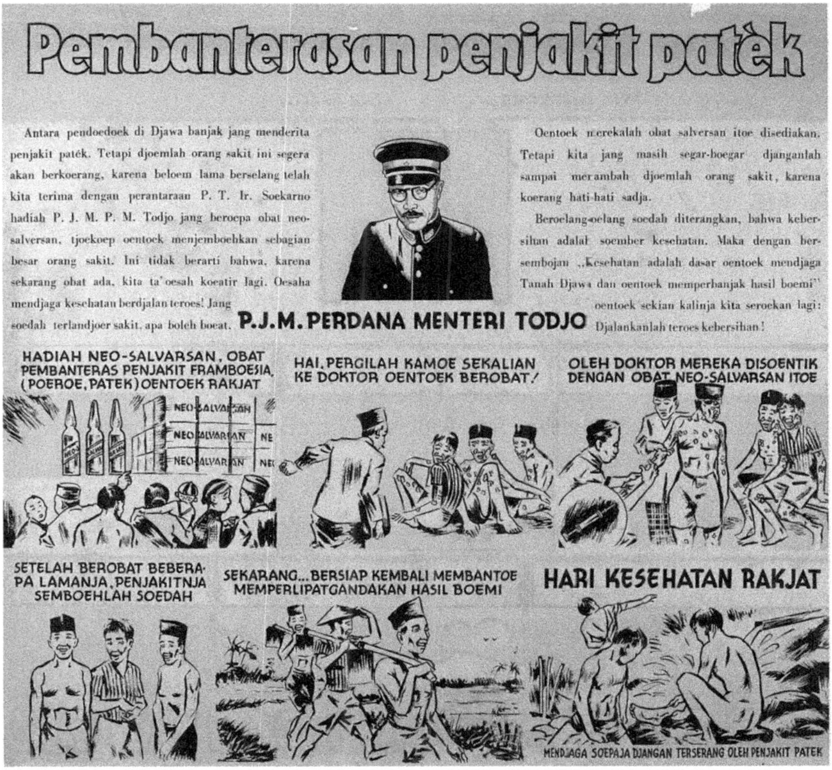

Image 3.3 Visual Pedagogy Aligned with Patriotic Hygiene: Yaws Eradication in Java (1943). An educational poster in Malay published by Varia (1943) during the Japanese occupation, promoting yaws prevention among the Javanese—issued jointly by Eiseikyoku [Japanese: Department of Public Health] and Djawa Izi Hōkōkai [Japanese: Medical Service Association]. The comic-style panels transformed healing into a spectacle. Citation: Author Unknown. *Pemberantasan Penjakit Patèk*. Djakarta: Varia. With permission from Perpustakaan Nasional Republik Indonesia

effective medications and the total collapse of health facilities further aggravated their suffering.

Dutch estates on Java closed following the Japanese occupation, rendering their workforce unemployed. Japanese authorities responded by reviving Dutch-era transmigration from densely populated Java to resource-rich Sumatra.[27] They also initiated relief works for the unemployed. In 1943, the military administration proposed a Java-wide network of recruitment agencies. Yet the scale of mobilization proved counterproductive: mass conscriptions led to rural labor shortages, and fields were left uncultivated. Over 2.6 million *romushas* (corvée laborers) were employed by the Japanese. Alongside them, 200,085 individuals were conscripted (Japanese: *kinro hoshi*)—a symbolic enactment of civic duty, intended to promote the spirit of Dai Nippon [Japanese: Great Japan], and reinforce Japan's vision for a unified Asia.[28]

As the Pacific War progressed, workers' wages became inadequate to sustain themselves and their families due to high inflation. The Japanese struggled to procure adequate rations and were eventually forced to reduce supplies to *romushas*. Disease was a major problem in South Sumatra. Large-scale movement of *romushas* into swampy areas led to outbreaks of malaria, while unsanitary living conditions triggered dysentery and yaws.[29] As malnutrition was widespread, work efficiency registered a conspicuous decline.

Benedict Anderson notes that toward the close of the Pacific War (1944–1945), a sense of impending catastrophe gripped Java. Socioeconomic conditions deteriorated under a combination of natural calamities, administrative chaos, and dislocations. The 1944 harvest was devastated by drought. To quote Anderson:

> The close of the Japanese occupation was a time of growing darkness and desolation. For the first time in living memory, people were falling dead in the streets from starvation and disease, mendicancy spread silently but horrifyingly through the cities, and the sense of being precipitated out of a stable order increased with every month that passed.[30]

Neither 1940 nor 1941 were good years for the rice harvest in Java, but both 1942 and 1943 were, which helped alleviate supply shortages.[31] Gregg Huff argues that although the 1944 famine in Java could be attributed to a decline in the availability of rice, its incidence was uneven and discriminate. In each residency of Java, nearly 50–60 percent of estate workers and landless families were at risk due to entitlement failure.[32] This failure—both in endowment and exchange—was foreseeable amid the wartime collapse of Java's estate economy. High inflation pushed unemployed estate workers and landless families—even those with occasional work—to the brink of starvation, as wages were not able to keep up with living costs. For Javanese villagers, migration to cities offered an opportunity to work or access rations. But by 1944, the Japanese had introduced a population registration system to determine rice rationing after the 1943–1944 harvest.[33] Those left out of the public distribution system formed a large destitute group and accounted for a substantial share of the famine's victims.

Huff argues that in wartime famine zones, while decisions for war and erratic weather are exogenous factors, human agency is not.[34] Voluntary action may avert a potentially avoidable famine— or fail to do so due to misguided policy. Despite extremely unfavorable weather and wartime bombing, the Vietnam famine (1944) could have been averted if one or more of the three main political actors intervened to supply food to the famine-affected Tonkin delta and North Annam. Those whose decisions might have prevented the famine included the French administrative machinery (the Vichy regime, indirectly under Japanese control), the Japanese military, who occupied Vietnam (March 9, 1945 coup), and the Americans who bombed Vietnam. Estimates of Vietnam's famine-induced mortality varied from a lower bound of 700,000 to an upper one of 2 million, the latter enshrined in Vietnamese communist mythology.[35] By 1943, famine signs were evident due to a typhoon in September and year-end output declines, but the severity escalated only in late 1944.[36] Between August and October 1944, coastal areas in Vietnam witnessed three successive typhoons and a tidal wave, rupturing dikes and damaging standing paddy. The November harvest was almost entirely lost, leaving 558,383 individuals destitute.[37]

When food was scarce, rural Tonkinese would turn to nontraditional nutritional sources: paddy husks, banana tree roots, and clover. According to Huff, the amount of paddy produced in northern Tonkin and Annam was 12.5 percent less in 1944 than in 1942 (1.64 million tons), highlighting fragile subsistence margins among peasants.[38] Rice stocks were further depleted in autumn 1943, as Vietnamese peasants were compelled to sell surplus rice to the Vichy regime. To compound the situation, the cold winter of 1944–1945 devastated a large proportion of non-rice crops. With Japan sending little to no textiles to Vietnam to make up for prewar imports, many people were left without adequate clothing or food.[39] Sheer desperation pushed countless individuals to trek along "starvation roads" in search of relief in provincial towns and cities.

During the Pacific War, the food situation in the Philippines paralleled that of Java and Vietnam. The Japanese occupied Manila on January 2, 1942, and established the Japanese Military Administration (JMA). A Philippine Executive Commission, composed of prewar Filipino leaders, assisted the Japanese in enforcing policies. Concerned about food shortages, the JMA liaised with NARIC (National Rice and Corn Administration, established in 1936) to regulate rice prices. Japan granted nominal independence to the Philippines on October 14, 1943, appointing José Laurel as president. In Luzon's rice bowl, Laurel faced the left-leaning and peasant-based Hukbalahap rebellion. The Huks obstructed rice procurement and viewed NARIC as a Japanese instrument. Guerrillas loyal to the US cause likewise opposed the Laurel government.[40] Key rice-producing districts in Luzon remained under anti-Japanese guerrilla control, prompting Laurel to consider martial law in Nueva Ecija, the country's rice granary.

Food scarcity had reached crisis proportions when Laurel assumed office. He continued the 1942 food production campaign and boosted vegetable and tuber output. To court farmer support, Laurel declared November 19 as Farmers' Day.[41] But rice distribution was hampered by transportation issues. Laurel's plan for a controlled economy crumbled under logistical and incentive failures, as NARIC fixed procurement prices, discouraging rice cultivation. Manila faced a rice shortage in November 1943. Hopes for harvest recovery dimmed as a typhoon devastated neighboring provinces, disrupted transport, and caused prices to quintuple.[42]

While the Laurel government discouraged exodus of the rural population to Manila, the Japanese were eager to recruit laborers for airfield construction and military cargo transportation. To make matters worse, the war turned against Japan by 1944. Japanese reinforcements arrived in the Philippines—intensifying competition with civilians for scarce rice supplies, particularly in Manila.[43]

Even though they were hungry, people joked about the Japanese occupation by saying that the Philippines was no longer "Pilipinas," but was now "Pilapinas" [Tagalog: queue]. The Japanese had brought only *rasyon* [Tagalog: rations], prices of foodstuffs were controlled only on paper; when buyers showed price lists from the *Tribune,* sellers sarcastically told them to buy them at the newspaper office.[44] But people had to buy rice regardless of government plans. Many resorted to smuggling, stealing, and bribery; some Filipinos framed these acts as patriotic, arguing they undermined the Japanese and their Filipino collaborators.[45] People traveled to the rural areas, often bartering furniture or jewelry to purchase rice as inflation debased the Japanese-issued currency. As Laurel found no solution to the rice crisis, the Japanese forced him to abdicate. Meanwhile, the Americans made a comeback on the island of Leyte (October 1944) and Luzon (January 1945)—freeing towns and reinstating food rationing.

Malaya did not suffer from food shortages to the same extent as Indonesia, Vietnam, or the Philippines due to higher living standards at the onset of the Pacific War. Many smallholders cultivated rice and other food crops alongside rubber.[46] Malaya benefited from its insular geography and proximity to Thailand, from where rice could be more readily sourced. Overall nutrition levels were minimal—barely sufficient to sustain basic functionality.[47]

Among the population, Indians suffered the most nutritionally, while Chinese adapted more successfully due to access to the black market and subsistence farming.[48] Indian estate laborers and their families faced dire subsistence hardship, with some conscripted by the Indian National Army or forced into Japanese labor, leaving dependents to starve.[49] *Kampong* Malays (village Malays), despite small landholdings, often sold foods such as eggs and coconuts in the market, where they fetched high prices, paradoxically worsening their own dietary intake.[50]

As the Japanese military imposed excessive demands on Malay cultivators and instituted wartime rationing in urban centers, food production declined precipitously.

British Orientalist J.M. Gullick, who served in the British Military Administration at the close of the Pacific War (1945), noted in his memoirs:

> Sickness had taken its toll. In the Lenggeng Valley a footpath ran between the houses or hamlets on the slightly higher ground above the ricefields. Coconut trees grew around or near the houses. Here and there one found the houses standing empty—all the household had died or moved away. The people who remained were dispirited and half-starved. As I have said, the occupation period was remembered for years afterwards as the time when people perforce ate tapioca (Malay: *ubi kayu*) which was fairly abundant but reported to be slightly poisonous, and always very unpalatable.[51]

Throughout Malaysia, the mid-1940s were remembered as *zaman ubi kayu* [Malay: era of tapioca] due to rice scarcity and subsistence collapse.[52]

By Southeast Asian standards, food shortages in Thailand were modest during the war. The country specialized in rice rather than estate crops such as rubber. Unlike Malaya or the Philippines, Thailand lacked significant anti-Japanese resistance. Thailand's birth rate fell from 35 per 1000 during the 1930s to 25.7 by 1945.[53] Despite stable death rates during the Pacific War, a quinine shortage drove malaria-related deaths from 213.6 per 100,000 in 1940 to a peak of 341.0 in 1943, followed by marginal decline.[54] Infant mortality surged late in the war, fueled by malaria escalation and tinned milk scarcity. The Thai government shielded local workers from Japanese excesses, often at the expense of Chinese laborers conscripted for the Thai-Burma Railway.[55]

Burma, similar to Thailand, was rice-surplus during the Pacific War, though regional disparities persisted. By 1943, half of Burma's transport system had been damaged, and Japan controlled the rest—making food deficits inevitable.[56] Sharp price variations across regions signaled local rice shortages.[57] Japan lacked transport to move rice north from Lower Burma, where surpluses accumulated, while central and northern regions faced acute scarcity. Rangoon witnessed high malnutrition rates, and by mid-1944, Mandalay's rice situation was deemed serious.[58]

In 1942—following Burma's capitulation to the Japanese—all rice imports from that quarter to Bengal, an overpopulous rice-deficit province in British India since the 1930s, ceased. In mid-October, a cyclone ripped through the coastal districts of Midnapur and 24 Parganas, major paddy-producing areas. More than 14,400 persons and 180,000 cattle perished during or after the cyclone.[59] Elsewhere, plant diseases whittled away paddy yields. In coastal Midnapur, the cyclone was followed by brutal repression of the Congress-led rebellion: the Tamluk Jatiya Sarkar, a parallel government that challenged the Raj (December 1942). Both episodes directly triggered starvation. In Chittagong, situated in the eastern part of Bengal province, famine surfaced in early 1943. The famine coincided with Allied troop build-up, mass refugee influx from Burma, a sudden scarcity of consumer goods, and the near-collapse of British credibility.

The political threat posed by the Japanese proximity to Bengal eroded public faith in the British ability to maintain order or defend Calcutta.[60] The Japanese bombed Calcutta on December 12, 23, 24, and 28, 1942, followed by sporadic attacks on the city in early 1943. Under these circumstances, the Bengal provincial government took a strong stance against organized grain traders—sealed grain stocks across Calcutta and its environs and remunerated traders below market rates. Relations between traders and the government cooled. Clinging to New Delhi's assurances of external procurement, Bengal ministers downplayed scarcity to deflect blame and avert public panic.[61] Rationing, implemented elsewhere in British India, was haphazardly set up in Bengal in 1944.

In 1943, despite claiming that grain stocks were adequate, the Bengal government made large purchases from the Calcutta market to supply its own employees and army. Furthermore, the government encouraged large industrial concerns around Calcutta to pay industrial workforces in grain to oil the war machinery while avoiding inflationary wage increases. In May 1943, as the price of grain reached rupees 30 per maund in the Calcutta wholesale market, buying agents of the Bengal government, big merchants, and speculators fanned out into rural Bengal.[62]

As Paul Greenough points out:

> In effect the superior purchasing capacity of a great city moved like a vacuum cleaner through the hinterland, buying up large and small quantities of grain. Rice which ordinarily flowed in non-commercial exchanges between cultivators and their dependents began to veer into the commercial channel, and a much larger proportion than usual of the stored rice supply fell into the hands. of outsiders. In some areas payments in kind gave way to payments in cash as cultivators responded to prices that reached a plateau level of more than Rs 30/ per maund wholesale all over Bengal.[63]

Starving villagers were aware that food was available at urban relief centers, and a large exodus began from rural Bengal to the cities. Between 80,000 and 150,000 villagers migrated to Calcutta by July 1943 and took refuge in air raid shelters before being repatriated.[64] Relief failure and mass starvation drove excess deaths sharply upward.

By winter 1943, outright starvation was averted as the rice harvest reached markets, prices fell, and the army initiated rural relief. But by the summer of 1944, outbreaks of smallpox, cholera, and malaria sustained excess deaths among an already emaciated population. Greenough notes that famine mortality was strictly rural.[65] In March 1943, the Bengal government scrapped price controls and urged New Delhi to declare eastern British India—Bengal, Bihar, Orissa, and Assam—as a free trade zone. The policy that succeeded in supplying rice to Bengal's cities did so by stripping stocks from Bihar and Orissa.[66] Ironically, more rice flooded Calcutta during the famine's peak than the urban population could consume.

The famines in Java, Vietnam, the Philippines, and Bengal were contemporaneous. Beyond natural disaster and loss of Southeast Asian rice as a consequence of Japanese victories, the four famines were boom famines—driven by inflationary pressures attributed to the Pacific War. Grain prices soared, and vulnerable groups in each of the four famine-affected regions lost exchange entitlements to food. Yet the gravest hardship during the Japanese occupation stemmed from food availability. Southeast Asia, once a net food exporter, saw its infrastructure devastated, disrupting distribution and triggering localized food shortages. With trade at a standstill, Japanese administrations urged local territories—especially Java—to pursue self-sufficiency in food. Though necessary under wartime exigency, this policy was antithetical to the notion of a Greater East Asia Co-Prosperity Sphere.

"Bombing Malarial Mosquitoes"

Since the late 1930s, the political landscape upon which malaria control was debated in the US and Western Europe gravitated to the right.[67] This shift was evident in US Surgeon General Hugh Cummings' vehement opposition to League of Nations Health Organization (LNHO) director Ludwik Rajchman's proposal to convene a conference on rural hygiene in Latin America—modeled on the LNHO Intergovernmental Conference of Far-Eastern Countries, Bandoeng (1937). Conference delegates championed a holistic approach to malaria control that evolved during the interwar period as part of a broader public health movement. But by the onset of World War II, the idealism that underpinned Bandoeng fractured, and malaria control contracted to insecticide use, sidelining comprehensive public health strategies.

Malaria devastated Allied troops, particularly in the Pacific theater, where traditional vector control methods consisted of draining swamps, spraying larvicides, and sanitation. However, the Japanese occupation of Java in 1942 cut off quinine supplies. In August 1942, the US representative of the Swiss firm J.R. Geigy introduced Gesarol, an insecticide containing Dichloro Diphenyl Tricholoroethane (DDT). Once DDT was sprayed on house walls, mosquitoes contacting treated surfaces suffered nervous damage and died instantly.

The career of Ceylonese Tamil malaria assistant Wilfred Chellapah is illustrative of the hubris and horrors associated with the earliest trials of the insecticide DDT in Southeast Asia. Chellapah's trajectory also coincided with the Allies' establishment of the South-East Asia Command (1943), coordinating operations from Ceylon and India against Japan.[68]

After graduating from the Royal Sanitary Institute, London, in 1939, Chellapah was deputed on a three-year contract to Ceylon as a malaria assistant. The control methods that he and his team pioneered in Ceylon were illustrative of the environmental engineering approach introduced during the interwar years: draining marshy areas, systematic oiling, and targeting stagnant pools.[69] On estates reporting malaria outbreaks, Chellapah conducted preliminary surveys: marking pools where drainage was required and conducting spleen examination on estate children under ten to determine whether malaria cases were local or imported. As children rarely left the estates, spleen data enabled him to gauge the true incidence of malaria in each locality.[70]

In 1943, soon after Chellapah's contract with the Royal Sanitary Institute ended, J.W. Sharpe, chief medical officer of the South-East Asia Command, enlisted him as a personal assistant on an experimental DDT project in eastern India. His deputation coincided with a cholera outbreak in Calcutta and the onset of the Bengal famine.[71] He was flown to the Royal Air Force camp in Charbatia, Orissa, where military scientists secretly tested aerial DDT spraying. Chellapah observed scientists collecting mosquitoes and insects affected by the insecticide.[72] His daily reports helped them hypothesize DDT's effectiveness.

DDT was introduced in Southeast Asia due to wartime exigencies. Before its arrival, the Allied Forces used another insecticide pyrethrum. But with the Japanese occupation of Java—then a major pyrethrum supplier—the British were left defenseless against malaria. In Chellapah's words, "At that moment they just wanted to get rid of mosquitoes and save the people."[73] Faced with a shortage of pyrethrum, the British urgently sought an alternative pesticide and abandoned precaution.

Chellapah's testimony reflected a strong undercurrent of violence and fear in the DDT experiments. He observed large numbers of birds dying in Charbatia after feeding on insects poisoned by the insecticide. On returning to Ceylon, he was placed in a concrete room already sprayed with DDT and tasked with collecting fallen mosquitoes. Fumes from the pesticide affected his health, causing tremors that lasted for five years, until 1949. In a frightening episode, Chellapah witnessed two Sinhalese workmen who were brought into the office by a naval officer. The officer soaked cotton wool in DDT solution, slit the first workman's arm with a razor blade, and bandaged it. For the second worker, who served as a control, kerosene-soaked cotton wool was applied to the wound. Both men collapsed and suffered tremors.[74] From military bases, DDT gradually reached civilian populations by 1945.[75]

On September 19, 1945—a week after Britain reoccupied Singapore—the Royal Air Force sprayed 640 acres of rubber estates, gardens, marshes, and Changi Gaol Camp with DDT from a Dakota aircraft. The operation lasted four minutes.[76] Health authorities hoped the aerial spray of DDT would reduce the incidence of malaria and dysentery. But an article by W.E. Hutchinson on August 5, 1946, entitled "The War against Mosquitoes in Singapore" was skeptical toward the efficacy of DDT in eliminating malaria. He argued:

> Unfortunately DDT does not appear to confine its deadly effects to the insect 'enemies' of man but it may also kill off his 'friends' and there are sound warnings of its possible interference with nature's pollenisation. What may be justifiable measures under war conditions are not necessarily so in times of peace. The duration of its effects are limited: repeated applications are necessary; and until the whole question is more fully investigated, the costs would seem to be out of all proportion to the benefits derived at least where the local control of malaria is concerned.[77]

Postwar fiscal stringency and staffing shortages restricted the Singapore health department from conducting mass DDT spraying.

Despite local reservations and resource constraints in Singapore, DDT's worldwide reception ushered in an epistemic shift in international health—from experimental public health strategies of the interwar years to postwar technological determinism. Wartime innovations—such as the insecticide DDT and the wonder drug streptomycin against TB—epitomized an era in which medical advances were hailed as the proverbial magic bullet against disease. This transformation reflected a gravitation toward administrative rationality and a preference for narrow technical interventions.[78]

From Relief to Rehabilitation: The Work of the United Nations Relief and Rehabilitation Administration (UNRRA), 1943–1947

Multilateral relief for the postwar era was initiated during wartime. In 1941, Britain proposed an Inter-Allied Committee on Postwar Requirements as a UK agency, but the Soviets refused to participate, instead advocating an international body with formal representation for all states.[79] The UNRRA—active between 1943 and 1947—was a US-led initiative reflecting the American view that the administration's staff should be international civil servants accountable to all member states. But the Soviets insisted on securing member-state consent for aid administration. Given political differences between the US and the USSR, UNRRA sought to portray itself as an apolitical body and urged its staff to respect different working methods and ways of life. Jessica Reinisch argues that although the organization was expected to deliver more than soup-kitchen charity, reconstruction lay beyond its remit. Rather, the UNRRA was to provide relief and immediate rehabilitation. Even in 1943, the broad terms—relief, rehabilitation and reconstruction—left substantial room for disagreement.[80] UNRRA navigated the interlude between the end of World War II and the onset of the Cold War, operating within a contested relief mandate shaped by divergent member-state expectations.

Many national health departments were devastated by World War II. There were unprecedented shortages of materials, apparatus, transport, buildings, and essential medicines. This was compounded by the loss of trained medical personnel and isolation from the latest medical developments. The LNHO and the Office International d' Hygiène Publique (OIHP), to which most national governments would have turned for medical assistance became moribund. To tackle wartime health challenges, the UNRRA Health Division was created in December 1943. The functions of the division included:

(a) prevention of war-engendered epidemics;
(b) restoration of national health departments;
(c) determination of medical and sanitary requirements to replace losses due to destruction and looting;
(d) revision of International Sanitary Regulations;
(e) provision of technical supervision and care for displaced persons under UNRRA's jurisdiction;

(f) training of medical personnel overseas.[81]

UNRRA's lifespan was ephemeral, shaped by its mandate to correct the deleterious effects of World War II. The San Francisco Conference, convened by the Allied nations in 1945, introduced the United Nations (UN) Charter. Furthermore, conference delegates proposed the establishment of an international health organization.[82] The Conference redefined the niche of the UNRRA in international health and its evolving relationship with the would-be World Health Organization (WHO). UNRRA's principal functions included direct assistance to the health services of liberated countries—not only in the field of maternal and child health, but also in managing outbreaks of typhus fever, malaria, and TB. The organization also controlled epidemics of enemy or ex-enemy states to prevent contagion among UN members. As an intergovernmental agency, UNRRA channeled aid through recipient governments.

The 1943 UNRRA agreement established two regional policy-making bodies: a Committee of the Council for Europe and a Committee of the Council for the Far East.[83] Operationally, this translated into relief and rehabilitation, each calibrated to the exigencies of occupied and liberated countries. Operations in devastated territories essentially involved: (1) determining the needs of occupied territories and the policies of occupying forces toward the civilian population; (2) procuring essential supplies to fulfil those needs; (3) restoring health and welfare services disbanded due to enemy occupation; (4) rehabilitating agricultural and industrial equipment to support postwar recovery.

To illustrate the need for regionalization of the UNRRA, L. Larry Leonard pointed out that China's wartime devastation necessitated a distinct relief strategy from Yugoslavia's. Other considerations that supported the regional approach to UNRRA's functioning included the Soviet Union's neutrality in the Far Eastern conflict and the expectation that China's liberation would follow Europe's.[84]

In 1944, although the preoccupation of China's Nationalist government was winning the war against Japan, the government established the Chinese Rehabilitation Planning Commission to survey wartime dislocation, estimate import requirements, and draft a practical postwar relief and rehabilitation strategy. UNRRA dispatched agricultural, economic, and medical experts to China to collaborate with the Commission. China's original request to the UNRRA for relief and rehabilitation in 1944 totaled approximately US$ 945 million, with one-sixth earmarked for food.[85] UNRRA's deliveries fell short of requisition. Nonetheless, food supplies from the agency stimulated the country's economic rehabilitation.

UNRRA flour, used as miners' wages, doubled coal output in Tongshan.[86] A key component of China's agricultural rehabilitation was the Yellow River Flood Control Project. Breakage of dikes along the Yellow River during the Second Sino-Japanese War in 1938 resulted in the inundation of two million acres of fertile farmland.[87] While the Chinese government funded flood control, UNRRA dispatched river conservancy engineers and seed stock.

The health and medical section of UNRRA's China program consisted of rehabilitating 500 health centers throughout formerly Japanese-occupied territories. Additionally, the section planned to establish 650 hospitals and 5 sanatoria; 10 epidemic control units; maternity hospitals with a total of 10,000 beds; 400 maternal and child health centers with 1000 field midwifery units; 5 pharmaceutical plants; 4 biological institutes; and 5 centers for training workers in sanitary engineering, nursing, and midwifery.[88] The health and medical section aimed to redress the acute shortage of physicians in the aftermath of the Pacific War.

During the summer of 1945, China suffered a cholera epidemic. UNRRA was called upon for emergency measures in Chungking. A UNRRA team—seven physicians and two sanitary engineers—with six tons of medical supplies was flown from British India to China over The Hump, the name given by Allied pilots to the Eastern Himalaya section in Burma.[89] Unfortunately, one batch of supplies was lost over the Himalayas. During the 1946 mid-summer cholera epidemic, the UNRRA medical staff assisted Chinese authorities in mass immunizations. Neglect of public health during the war aggravated the prevalence of Kala Azar or visceral leishmaniasis, transmitted by a blood-sucking fly *phlebotomus*. Nearly 300,000 persons in Honan, Kiangsu, and adjacent provinces were in urgent need of treatment but were cut off from drug supplies due to the war. UNRRA initially assisted Chinese health authorities with procuring supplies of antimony drugs used in treating Kala Azar cases but soon switched to DDT in a concerted attack against *phlebotomus*.

In UNRRA's health and welfare programs, western specialists and western-educated Chinese often devised programs misaligned with China's needs. Profound linguistic and operational differences were insurmountable. Without a rationing system, equitable distribution of essentials remained unworkable.[90] So what was the significance of the UNRRA's

China chapter? First, the division of responsibilities between the Chinese government and UNRRA. At China's request, UNRRA deployed personnel from 25 nationalities to liaise with the Departments of Health, Communications, Agriculture, Forestry, and Interior. Second, UNRRA personnel accelerated program implementation and shared technical expertise with local counterparts. Third, the UNRRA's China program concentrated on localized relief efforts, including the development of a low-cost demonstration plant for the treatment of night soil and garbage at Shaoyang, Hunan.[91]

Beyond China, UNRRA's Committee of the Council for the Far East received requisitions between 1944 and 1945 from the governments of the Netherlands Indies, French Indochina, and British India. Authorities in the Netherlands Indies sought assistance to contain widespread epidemics, while French Indochina and British India requested support for repatriating displaced persons.[92]

UNRRA's health activities were transitional in scope. International health problems that exceeded its mandate were transferred to the Economic and Social Council of the UN. These included: (a) strategies for international cooperation against disease, including the formation of expert committees; (b) the revision of quarantine regulations; and (c) international biological standardization of drugs.[93]

Contemporary political commentators such as Philipp Weintraub view UNRRA as a failure due to its dependence on the licet of national governments.[94] The subordination of UNRRA's activities to state sovereignty implied recognition of national authority over supranational unification. The transfer of relief and rehabilitation duties to individual states eroded the moral and collective foundation of international welfare. In contrast, historians offer a more nuanced account of UNRRA's shortcomings. Samantha Knapton and Katherine Rossy argue that the agency's creation marked the first step in state-led international humanitarianism. Its principle to "help the people help themselves" influenced subsequent aid agencies. United Nations Children's Fund (UNICEF) Executive Director Maurice Pate, for example, applied the UNRRA dictum to maternal and child health.[95] Yet UNRRA aid was politically constrained, serving only nationals of UN member states displaced by war, while excluding enemy or ex-enemy nationals from Germany, Austria, Bulgaria, Hungary, Romania, Japan, and Siam (Thailand).

Planning for Health of the Future Nation: India

By late 1944, as World War II drew to a close, several countries were charting plans for postwar reconstruction. In Britain, the Beveridge Report proposed universal protection as a right—from cradle to grave—abolishing the household means test that had defined public relief during the Slump years (1930s).[96] While South Africa had its Medical Association and Planning Committee since 1941, British India appointed a Health Survey and Development Committee (widely known as the Bhore Committee) in 1943.

Planning for national health in British India arose due to wartime exigencies. The resignation of provincial Congress ministries in 1939, in protest of Viceroy Lord Linlithgow's declaration of war without the consent of Indians, left the British desperately searching for allies. While suppressing the Quit India Movement (1942), the British turned to postwar reconstruction to display their concern for national welfare.

In October 1943, the Government of India appointed the Bhore Committee, chaired by Indian Civil Service (ICS) officer Sir Joseph Bhore, to assess national health conditions and draft a blueprint for service development. Influential Indian members included Diwan Bahadur Arcot Lakshmanaswami Mudaliar, prominent during the WHO's formative period (1946–1948), and K.C.K.E. Raja, a medical statistician at the All India Institute of Public Health (AIIHPH). British members included John Ryle, a founder of social medicine as an academic discipline at Oxford, and Janet Vaughan, who organized Britain's blood bank during the Blitz.[97] Prominent foreign experts such as Henry Sigerist (Johns Hopkins) and John Grant (Rockefeller Foundation) also contributed (Image 3.4).

The Bhore Committee's incorporation of social medicine was not incidental—it reflected a recalibration of international health to Indian conditions. Social medicine emphasized the role of socioeconomic factors on health outcomes. It advocated structural interventions: improved nutrition, housing, education, and reduced industrial fatigue. It aimed to prevent noninfectious diseases in the community, particularly rickets, chlorosis, and nutritional anemias—conditions impairing physical and mental well-being.[98] By prioritizing preventive over curative care, social medicine provided the theoretical bedrock for integrating both within a national health service.

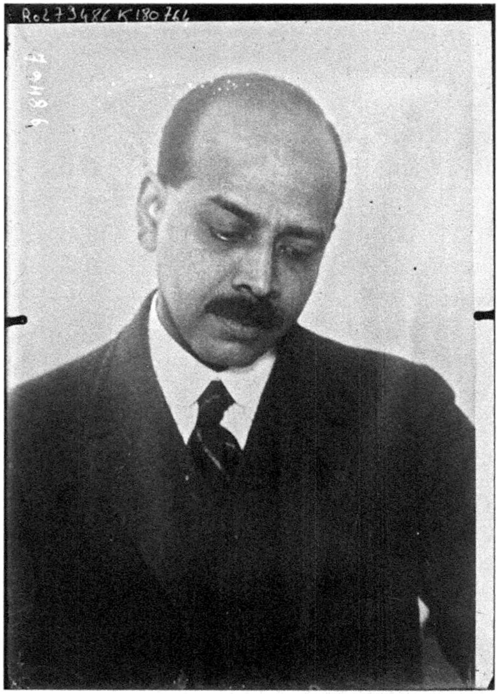

Image 3.4 Sir William Joseph Bhore (1878–60), Chair of the Landmark 1946 Health Survey and Development Committee. Source: Bibliothèque nationale de France, Département Estampes et Photographie, EI-13 (955); Rol, 79486. Identifier: ark:/12148/btv1b530960667. Public domain

The Bhore Committee's recommendations did not emerge in isolation but appropriated international health models—particularly Soviet socialized medicine, described by Sigerist. He advocated universal, free access to protective and restorative care. A defining feature of Soviet socialized medicine, which Sigerist outlined in *Medicine and Health in the Soviet Union*, was the erasure of the traditional divide between preventive and curative health services.[99] The Bhore report integrated this principle—collapsing the preventive-curative dichotomy—in an indelible imprint of Sigerist (Image 3.5).[100]

Sigerist was closer to socialist ideology than Grant, but in practice they were broadly aligned in their approach to social medicine.[101] Grant's work in China established the Beijing First Health Station, which addressed health problems by integrating curative and preventive care in a community setting.[102] Grant's familiarity with malaria and hookworm stations in the US South, in conjunction with regular correspondence with Rockefeller

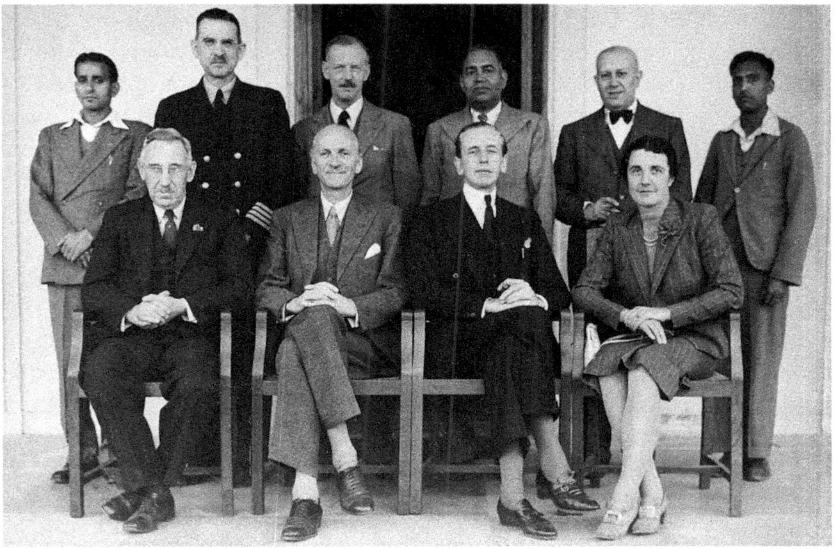

Image 3.5 M0016030: The Medical Mission of Experts on their visit to India. Wellcome Collection. The Medical Mission for Experts, visiting Sh. Janki Devi Jamiat Singh Free Maternity Hospital in Lahore (c. 1944), to advise the Health Survey and Development Committee of the Government of India. Those present include Henry E. Sigerist (back row, second from right), and John Ryle (front row seated, second from left). Reference no WT/D/1/20/1/145/73. The image is under a CC-BY-4 license. URL: https://wellcomecollection.org/works/ydau4cnt/images?id=c3fr6ewp

Foundation officials, shaped the Beijing station's design—combining medical services, disease prevention, and the collection of vital statistics.[103]

In 1939, drawing on Grant's experience in China, the Rockefeller Foundation deputed him to reorganize the AIIHPH, Calcutta. At the AIIHPH's Singur unit, Grant operationalized community-centered health principles. As a Bhore Committee member (1943–1946), he acquainted Indian colleagues with emerging international health paradigms. The Committee's rural health recommendation—*panchayat*-led community mobilization around targeted priorities—was partly inspired by Grant's Singur model.[104]

The Bhore Committee articulated a framework for postcolonial health policy. In the words of the Committee, "The term health implies much more than an absence of sickness in the individual and indicates a state of harmonious functioning of the body and mind in relation to his physical and social environment, so as to enable him to enjoy life to the fullest possible extent and to reach his maximum productive capacity."[105] The Committee defined health in holistic terms, later echoed in the WHO Preamble.

Despite endorsing comprehensive health systems, the Bhore Committee confined its remit to disease control—recognizing structural determinants, yet excluding them from its actionable scope.[106] In the case of tuberculosis, the Committee recommended: (1) raising socioeconomic standards through improvements in housing, sanitation, and nutrition; and (2) curbing transmission from infected individuals.[107] This perspective was shaped by resource scarcity toward the twilight of colonial rule and the urgency of infectious disease containment.

To counteract entrenched rural healthcare neglect, the Bhore Committee envisioned a district-level framework, serving administrative units of three million.[108] The primary health unit would serve a population of 20,000. A cluster of 15–25 primary units constituted a secondary health node within a stratified service delivery system. Each district was anchored by three to five secondary nodes. Provincial health ministries ensured that district-level activities aligned with national directives, permitting only limited local adaptations. The Committee delineated a three-tier decentralized structure with a well-articulated referral system. Post-independence fiscal constraints derailed the Committee's vision, reinforcing a bias toward curative care.[109]

Equitable care, the Committee contended, demanded engagement with the broader structural determinants of health. They were unanimous that under prevailing conditions in India—active disease, diets deficient in calories, vitamins, and proteins, inadequate housing and sanitation—medical care should be free to all and provided by a salaried service.[110] The Committee argued for a national health service led by salaried doctors, asserting that private practice was antithetical to the ideal of socialized medicine.[111]

Committee members diverged on expanding health insurance to the entire population.[112] Following extensive debates on adapting foreign insurance models to Indian conditions, the Bhore Committee resolved:

> In India it is recognised that there are difficulties in the way of introducing at present a scheme of health insurance either by itself or as a part of a universal social insurance scheme. We feel that a very large section of the people are living below the normal subsistence level and cannot afford as yet even the small contribution that an insurance scheme will require. We therefore consider that medical benefits will have, in any case, to be supplied free to this section of the population until at least its economic condition is materially improved.[113]

The Bhore Committee's vision for universal healthcare aimed to correct existing health disparities but also grappled with broader structural concerns, including India's growing population and its strain on food supplies. The Committee adopted a cautious stance toward population policy.

Sir John Megaw, a British member of the Bhore Committee, introduced a distinctly Malthusian perspective to its deliberations. He argued that India's rising population was the root cause of the country's health problems. As there was a gap between the amount of food available and the number of mouths to be fed, malnutrition was inevitable.[114] Megaw's perspective informed the Bhore Committee's approach to birth control—not as an immediate solution but as a long-term strategy constrained by India's socioeconomic realities.[115] Underlying Megaw's reasoning were late colonial anxieties about India's demographic pressure—framing limitation of family size as a mechanism for managing scarcity and alleviating administrative burden.

The Bhore Committee report contained several contradictions. For example, the tension between demographic concerns and resource limitations was reflected in the Committee's discussion on public health expenditure. This duality—between aspirational investment and systemic constraints—revealed the fragilities underlying technocratic optimism embedded within India's postwar planning framework. While the Committee contended that expenditure on improving the nation's health was a "gilt-edged investment," yielding substantial increases in productivity, it also acknowledged bottlenecks in implementation due to entrenched socioeconomic asymmetries and budgetary constraints.[116]

The dilemma of reconciling the lofty aspirations of the Bhore Committee with economic realities persisted in the post-independence period. Between 1946 and 1957, there was a conspicuous shift in public health priorities of the postcolonial state in India from rural sanitation and nutrition to disease control. Public health—deemed relatively unimportant by the central government compared to either defense spending or industrialization—was delegated to the cash-strapped provinces. Provinces such as Assam witnessed a steady influx of refugees from East Pakistan in the aftermath of Partition. Rather than providing relief to displaced persons, the Assam government was engaged in a game of one-upmanship with the center. The central and state governments' lackadaisical approach to refugee rehabilitation compounded epidemic vulnerability, resulting in belated responses to malaria, smallpox and cholera outbreaks.[117] India had to adapt its health strategy to meet the Partition-induced humanitarian emergency. Under such circumstances, spraying DDT or mass vaccinations were significantly cheaper than investing in primary health infrastructure, reflecting economic constraints first acknowledged by the Bhore Committee.

New Delhi, 1947

In 1946, Jawaharlal Nehru led an interim government to assist in the transition of British India to independence. The Indonesian Republican Government was at the time embroiled in military confrontation with the Dutch after the latter reimposed military control on the archipelago in October 1945, following the Japanese surrender. The Republican Government was eager to secure *de jure* recognition from India, as soon as a future government would be constituted in New Delhi. To expedite diplomatic recognition for the fledgling republic, Premier Sjahrir from Partai Sosialis Indonesia (Indonesian Socialist Party) pledged to send half a million tons of rice to India to alleviate food scarcity resulting from the Bengal Famine.[118] In exchange, Sjahrir asked for textiles and medicines from India. Indonesia-India rice diplomacy—described by Indonesian Vice President Mohammed Hatta as motivated by humanitarian ideals—enabled the Indonesians to defy the Dutch military blockade.

Indonesia's humanitarian gesture toward India exemplified Sjahrir's and Nehru's shared vision of cementing regional solidarity, a principle that would subsequently shape the agenda of the First Asian Relations Conference (1947). India hosted the First Asian Relations Conference with the aim of reviving the Asian region as a connected space after centuries of fragmentation under colonial rule.[119] The months leading to the Asian Relations Conference (March 23 to April 2, 1947) witnessed communal riots in the provinces of Punjab, adjacent areas of Delhi, Bengal, and Assam. Gopa Sabharwal notes that, at the time of hosting the forum, no one had a clue that Indian independence would be fast-tracked from June 1948 to August 1947 and that the country would be partitioned at birth.[120] Despite the volatile political environment, Nehru went ahead and hosted the conference. The All-India Muslim League declined the invitation. The Working Committee of the Asian Relations Conference issued a rebuttal clarifying the forum's nonpolitical orientation.

Among the topics discussed at the conference included agricultural and industrial development, labor problems, social services, inter-Asian migration, the status of women, and cultural problems, particularly in education and scientific research. In all these matters, there were several similarities between Asian countries. Nehru suggested that a review of ideas to deal with common problems afflicting Asian countries would yield incomparable results for quickening the pace of economic and social emancipation of the people of Asia, who constituted half the world's population.[121]

Nehru's opening address at the conference was riddled with contradictions. He stated that at the Asian Relations Conference there were no leaders and followers. Yet, he carved out a niche for would-be independent India in the new phase of Asian decolonization.[122] Nehru's opening address presented India as central to Asia's future.[123] Vineet Thakur notes that while Nehru's calls for an Asian federation were endorsed by Ceylon's Solomon Bandaranaike, Southeast Asian leaders—particularly from Indonesia, Malaysia, and Vietnam—expressed reservations about an uncritical and rhetorical romanticism about Asia that Nehru espoused. Instead, they appealed for measures to advance decolonization and keep Asia away from bloc-politics.[124]

Within Southeast Asia, there were growing apprehensions that European colonialism would be replaced by Indian or Chinese imperialism in the aftermath of the Pacific War. On the question of inter-Asian Migration—one of the themes broached by the Asian Relations Conference—it was noted that of Burma's decennial population increase of two million, nearly half were of Indian or Chinese descent.[125] There were concerns within Burma that the country was being demographically overwhelmed by Indian or Chinese migrants—an apprehension amplified by fears of economic domination and cultural dilution.

During the First Asian Relations Conference, public health was discussed in the joint session related to Social Services and Status of Women and Women's Movements respectively. Raja delineated that the purpose of the conference was to stimulate collaboration between Asian countries—social, cultural, and intellectual—in which mutual interests could be advanced through a harmonization of national aspirations. Simultaneously, Raja argued that while epidemics did not respect international frontiers and necessitated interstate collaboration, the scope of a modern health program transcended disease control. At the heart of such a program was the achievement of a growing measure of positive health for individuals, whereby their productive capacity and ability to enjoy life progressively increased.[126]

Raja recognized India's strategic geographical position in coordinating quarantine measures, especially with the growth of air travel. He delineated shared health challenges—particularly a high incidence and prevalence of infectious diseases, inadequacy of preventive and curative services, unhygienic living conditions, endemic malnutrition, and illiteracy—as commonalities affecting Asian states.[127]

Building on Raja's observation, Maung Sein, the Burmese delegate, outlined a Common Organization, pooling regional expertise for infectious disease coordination.[128] Likewise, Abdul Majid, president of the University of Kabul, noted that cholera was endemic to certain parts of Afghanistan. He implored Afghan authorities to prevent outbreaks through mass immunizations and pursue collaborative epidemiological surveillance with India.[129]

Recognizing the magnitude of public health challenges, delegates to the Asian Relations Conference emphasized that these issues needed state intervention rather than reliance on private enterprise. N.M. Joshi, a prominent trade union leader from Bombay and chairperson of the joint session, underlined the broad consensus amidst delegates that public health was a state responsibility. He observed:

> First, except a few regions in Asia the rest of the continent was in need of transformation—if not a revolution—in the matter of health, hygiene, housing and education. Secondly, we cannot rely very much on private enterprise for the betterment of social services. Conditions can be changed only by throwing the obligation to governments.[130]

So, what was the significance of the Asian Relations Conference? The conference —held on the eve of Indian independence—aimed to forge solidarities among Asian states amid political upheaval. While the conference lacked an overarching agenda, delegates emphasized shared health challenges concerning tropical diseases and actionable solutions on lines distinct from the West. Nonetheless, they remained ambiguous about delineating non-Western alternatives.

The conference also highlighted the limits of Pan-Asian unity, offering political support rather than material assistance for the region's decolonization. Nehru's vision for a regional association consisting of India, Southeast Asia, Afghanistan, Iran, and the Arab world reflected India's broader ambitions for a larger Asian federation. However, Southeast Asian leaders were unnerved about potential Indian domination. In response to these concerns, Indonesian leader Abu Hanifah noted that the notion of a Southeast Asian grouping emerged at the conference.[131]

Coda

The Japanese occupation of Southeast Asia resulted in severe dislocation and deprivation which intensified political unrest after the war. All postwar governments of the area were forced to introduce relief measures. According to Virginia Thompson and Richard Adloff, these measures were accelerated by the breakdown of the traditional family, communal, and religious systems, which posed fresh problems and released synergies for their solutions.[132] Because of its enormous population, Java arguably suffered more than any other area during the Pacific War, particularly from Japanese depredations on its human resources. A number of young Javanese were conscripted into forced labor in Japanese factories; not more than 10percent of the workers were repatriated toward the end of the war.[133]

The advent of socialist-minded governments after the war—particularly in Indonesia (1945), India (1947), Burm (1948), and Ceylon (1948)—was animated with a sense of responsibility to ameliorate living conditions. The political will to better people's living conditions was stronger in postwar Asia than before the war, but material means were never weaker. As Indonesian physician Sulianti Sukanto (Saroso), who headed the Division of Maternal and Child Health during the 1950s, noted:

> Indonesia was a Dutch colony for 350 years. On the 17th of August 1945 we declared our independence and established the Republic of Indonesia. But we know that a declaration does not mean anything unless the whole population is conscious of its responsibility. Independence is meaningless if a people are still submerged in ignorance and does not get the opportunity of learning to read, of knowing the world outside or if the living conditions do

> not improve. Therefore our constitution has accorded the same rights to every subject of the Indonesian Republic and provided that every subject was entitled to employment and human living conditions.[134]

Following independence, the nascent Indonesian Ministry of Health announced an urgent campaign against communicable diseases, but program implementation was constrained by entrenched shortages of physicians and paramedical personnel.

In 1947, when the Dutch launched their first military aggression to suppress the ambitions of the Indonesian Republic, the Rockefeller Foundation-sponsored Demonstration Unit in Poerwokerto was occupied. Hygiene mantris, under the leadership of Rockefeller-trained physician Raden Mochtar, resurrected a health education program in a new hygiene mantri school in Magelang, central Java. Casting aside the colonial-era appellation of *mantri*, the new rural hygiene workers called themselves health educators (Bahasa Indonesia: *pendidik hygiene*).[135] During the revolutionary war, the Magelang school aided the Republican Government in combating a plague outbreak in Central Java.[136]

The end of the Pacific War triggered mass internal displacement, particularly in Indonesia and Vietnam, partly due to political factors. More than three million Annamese fled French-controlled territory to sparsely populated Việt Minh-administered highlands in Tonkin, a malarious region, during the First Indochina War.[137] Due to the sudden influx of displaced persons, Việt Minh authorities were unable to clear dense highland vegetation, and a number of migrants succumbed to malaria. In Indonesia, revolutionary troops demobilized by the Renville agreement made unreasonable demands on the public distribution system.[138] The Dutch-held town of Surabaya lost several residents during the Battle of Surabaya (1945), but evacuees soon returned to their homes. The ebb and flow of displaced people took placein Hanoi, Saigon, Singapore, Batavia, and Rangoon.[139] All these cities experienced at least a temporary doubling of population.

During the interwar period, colonial governments generally kept epidemics under control. This was particularly true of the Netherlands Indies, which succeeded in eliminating smallpox by 1940 due to systematic vaccination efforts.[140] But during the Japanese occupation, routine vaccinations were disrupted. By 1947, smallpox was reintroduced into the Indonesian archipelago from neighboring Malaya, then smallpox endemic. Apart from the recrudescence of communicable diseases, particularly smallpox, overall immunity of Southeast Asians deteriorated during the Pacific War. Toward the close of the Pacific War, malaria became rampant in the region; localized epidemics of smallpox and plague were also reported. Given limited financial resources at the disposal of health authorities, each country emphasized the campaign against endemic diseases: for e.g., malaria in India; yaws in Indonesia; and TB in the Philippines. Such diseases could not be handled effectively without long-term investments in improving living conditions. Yet, in the struggle between strengthening the nation's public health and the need for economy, the availability of new medical discoveries enabled postwar planners to paper over underlying socioeconomic causes.

Notes

1. For understanding transitions in public health in Southeast Asia during the Pacific War, see Sunil Amrith, *Decolonizing International Health: India and Southeast Asia, 1930-65* (Basingstoke: Palgrave Macmillan, 2006), 47–71. For understanding continuities, see Eric Stein, "Hygiene and Decolonization: The Rockefeller Foundation and Indonesian Nationalism," 1933–58 in *Science, Public Health and the State in Modern Asia*, Liping Bu, Darwin Stapleton and Ka-che Yip edited (Abingdon, Oxon: Routledge, 2012), 51–70.
2. See Stein, "Hygiene and Decolonization," 57.
3. Peter Duus, "Diplomacy and Statecraft: The Vision of a Greater East Asia Co-Prosperity Sphere," *Diplomacy and Statecraft* 7, no. 1 (2007): 54–72.
4. Duus, "Diplomacy and Statecraft," 63.
5. Shigeru Sato, "Oppression and Romanticism: The Food Supply in Japan during the Japanese Occupation," in *Food Supplies and Japanese Occupation in Southeast Asia*, Paul Kratoska edited (Basingstoke: Macmillan, 1998), 167–86.
6. G.M. Kahin, *Nationalism and Revolution in Indonesia* (Ithaca: Cornell University Press, 2003), 102.
7. Ibid., 102.
8. Kahin, *Nationalism and Revolution*, 103.
9. Hans Pols, *Nurturing Indonesia: Medicine and Decolonisation in the Dutch East Indies* (Cambridge: Cambridge University Press, 2018), 164.
10. Pols, *Nurturing Indonesia*, 165.
11. Pols, *Nurturing Indonesia*, 166.
12. "Oepatjara Pemberian Idjazah Sekolah Kedokteran Tinggi," *Berita Ketabiban* nos.7–8 (2603 [1943]), Leiden University Library KITLV

Collection (hereafter KITLV); See also T. Sato, "Persatoean Kebaktian Dokter Dokter," *Berita Ketabiban* nos. 1–2–3 (2604 [1944]), KITLV.

13. "Pidato Toean Ir. Soekarno," August 30, 1943, *Berita Ketabiban*, nos. 1–2–3 (2604 [1944]), KITLV.
14. Ibid.
15. Pols, *Nurturing Indonesia*, 168.
16. Ibid., 168.
17. Boentaran Martoatmodjo, cited in "Persidangan Oemoem Izi Hookoo Kai," *Berita Ketabiban*, nos. 1–2–3 (2604 [1944]), KITLV.
18. Ibid.
19. Hendarmin "Mempertegoeh Djasmani," *Berita Ketabiban*, nos. 1–2–3 (2604 [1944]), KITLV; See also "Menjehatkan Bangsa," *Berita Ketabiban*, nos. 1–2–3 (2604 [1944]), KITLV.
20. Ethan Mark, Japan's *Occupation of Indonesia during the Second World War: A Transnational History* (London: Bloomsbury, 2018), 145–46.
21. See, for example, "Penjakit Lapar Warisan Pemerintah Belanda: Sekarang Diberantas Dengan Giat," *Asia Raya*, March 17, 1943 [2603], 1, Digital Collections Leiden University (hereafter Leiden University).
22. Ibid., 1.
23. R. Kodijat, "Menoedjoe Djawa Sehat dan Koeat," *Asia Raya*, April 15, 1944 [2604], 2, Leiden University.
24. Ibid., 2.
25. Ibid., 2.
26. Pols, *Nurturing Indonesia*, 174.
27. Sato, "Oppression and Romanticism," 176.
28. Ibid., 176.
29. Sato, "Oppression and Romanticism," 177.
30. Benedict Anderson, *Java in a Time of Revolution: Occupation and Resistance, 1944–46* (Ithaca: Cornell University Press, 1972), 10–11.
31. Gregg Huff, "The Second World War Vietnam and Java Famines," *Modern Asian Studies* 53, no. 6 (2019): 1–36, 17.
32. Huff, "The Second World War," 2–21. See also Amartya Sen, "Famines as Failures of Exchange Entitlements," *Economic and Political Weekly* 11, no.31/33 (1976): 1273–80.
33. Huff, "The Second World War," 24.
34. Gregg Huff, *World War II and Southeast Asia: Economy and Society Under Japanese Occupation* (Cambridge: Cambridge University Press, 2020), 248.
35. Huff, *World War II and Southeast Asia*, 249.
36. Huff, *World War II and Southeast Asia*, 255.
37. Huff, *World War II and Southeast Asia*, 256.
38. Ibid., 256.

39. Ibid., 256.
40. Ricardo Trota Jose, "Food Production and Food Distribution Programmes in the Philippines during the Japanese Occupation," in *Food Supplies and the Japanese Occupation in South-East Asia,* Paul Kratoska edited (Basingstoke, Oxon: Macmillan, 1998), 67–100, 77.
41. Ibid., 77.
42. Jose, "Food Production," 78.
43. Jose, "Food Production," 89.
44. Ibid., 89.
45. Jose, "Food Production," 89–90.
46. Huff, *World War II and Southeast Asia*, 275.
47. Huff, *World War II and Southeast Asia*, 276.
48. Huff, *World War II and Southeast Asia*, 279.
49. M. Gullick, "Recollections of My Time in Malaya (1945–1956) Part 2," *Journal of the Malaysian Branch of the Royal Asiatic Society* 87, no. 1 (2014): 53–81, 66.
50. Huff, *World War II and Southeast Asia,* 280.
51. J.M. Gullick, "Recollections," 68.
52. Gullick, "Recollections," 66.
53. Huff, *World War II and Southeast Asia*, 294.
54. Ibid., 294.
55. For details see Arjun Subrahmanyan and Michael Sturma, "Asian Labourers, the Thai Government and the Thai-Burma Railway," *Journal of Contemporary History* 56, no. 2 (2020): 364–85.
56. Huff, *World War II and Southeast Asia*, 295.
57. Ibid., 295. In Lower Burma, especially the Irrawaddy delta, was a major rice surplus region and imported clothing and other foodstuffs from the Upper Burma Dry Zone.
58. Huff, *World War II and Southeast Asia*, 303.
59. Paul Greenough, "Indian Famines and Peasant Victims: The Case of Bengal in 1943–1944," Modern *Asian* Studies 14, no. 2 (1980): 205–35, 209.
60. Greenough, "Indian Famines and Peasant Victims," 210–11.
61. Greenough, " Indian Famines and Peasant Victims," 211.
62. Greenough, " Indian Famines and Peasant Victims," 212.
63. Ibid., 212.
64. Ibid., 212.
65. Greenough, " Indian Farmers and Peasant Victims," 213.
66. Ibid., 213.
67. Randall Packard, *The Making of a Tropical Disease: A Short History of Malaria* (Baltimore, MD: Johns Hopkins University Press, 2007).

68. "Big Moves Expected: Sequel to Establishment of South-East Asia Command," *Warwick Daily News*, August 27, 1943, 2. National Library of Australia. Accessed July 7, 2024. https://trove.nla.gov.au/newspaper/article/191821640?searchTerm=SOutheast%20asia%20command.
69. Wilfred Chellapah, Interviewed by Daniel Chew (1983), Communities of Singapore (Part II), Accession No. 0000353, Reel 9, National Archives of Singapore Oral History Collections. Accessed July 7, 2024. https://www.nas.gov.sg/archivesonline/flipviewer/publish/e/e7c21add-115d-11e3-83d5-0050568939ad-OHC000353_009/web/html5/index.html?launchlogo=tablet/OralHistoryInterviews_brandingLogo_.png&pn=1.
70. Ibid.
71. Ibid.
72. Ibid.
73. Ibid.
74. Ibid.
75. Amrith, *Decolonizing International Health*, 52.
76. Straits Times Reporter, "Bombing Malarial Mosquitoes," *The Straits Times*, September 20, 1945, 2, National Library Board, Singapore (hereafter NLB).
77. W.E. Hutchinson, "War against Malaria in Singapore," *The Straits Times*, August 5, 1946, 4, NLB.
78. Darwin H. Stapleton, "A Lost Chapter in the Early History of DDT: The Development of Anti-Typhus Technologies by the Rockefeller Foundation's Louse Laboratory, 1942–44," *Technology and Culture* 46, no. 3 (2005): 513–40, 514.
79. Andrew Harder, "The Politics of Impartiality: The United Nations Relief and Rehabilitation in the Soviet Union, 1946–47," *Journal of Contemporary History* 47, no. 2 (2012): 347–67.
80. Jessica Reinisch, "Auntie UNRRA at the Crossroads," *Past and Present* 218, supplement 8 (2013): 70–97.
81. Wilbur A. Sawyer, "Achievements of UNRRA as an International Organization," *American Journal of Public Health* 37 (1947): 4158.
82. See A.E. Feller, "Memorandum on the International Health Activities of the UNRRA," UNRRA and San Francisco Conference, Folder S-1271-0000-0066-00001 [Undated], United Nations Archives, New York (UNA).
83. L. Larry Leonard, "UNRRA and the Concept of Regional International Organization," *Iowa Law Review* 30 no. 4 (1945): 489–514, 490.
84. Leonard, "UNRRA," 500.
85. Ruth E. Pardee, "First Aid for China," *Pacific Affairs* 19, no. 1 (1946): 75–89.

86. Ibid., 80.
87. Pardee, "First Aid," 81.
88. Pardee, "First Aid," 83.
89. Sawyer, "Achievements," 30.
90. Katrine R.C. Greene, "UNRRA's Record in China," *Far Eastern Survey* 20, no. 10 (1951): 100–105.
91. Greene, "UNRRA's Record," 102.
92. "Undated Report to the Committee of Council for the Far East," Feb 20 to Aug 1, 1945, Committee for the Far East: General, Doc. S-1241-0000-0047-00001, UNA.
93. "Undated Memorandum on the International Health Problems," UNRRA and San Francisco Conference, Doc. S-1271-0000-0066-00001, UNA.
94. Philipp Weintraub, "UNRRA: An Experiment in International Welfare Planning," *The Journal of Politics* 7, no. 1 (1945): 1–24.
95. Samantha Knapton and Katherine Rossy, "Introduction," in *Relief and Rehabilitation in a Post-War World*, Samantha Knapton and Katherine Rossy edited (London: Bloomsbury, 2024), 1–16, 4.
96. Noel Whiteside, "The Beveridge Report and its Implementation: A Revolutionary Project?" *Dans Histoire et Politique* 3 (2014): 24–37.
97. Amrith, *Decolonizing International Health*, 58.
98. John A. Ryle, "Social Medicine: Its Meaning and Its Scope," *The Milbank Memorial Fund Quarterly* 22, no. 1 (1944): 58–71.
99. Henry Sigerist, *Medicine and Health in the Soviet Union* (New York: Citadel Press, 1937).
100. *Report of the Health Survey and Development Committee*, volume I (Delhi: Government of India, 1946), 32.
101. Rama V. Baru, " The Bhore Committee and Recent Debates," *Seminar* 714 (2019). Accessed July 14, 2024. https://www.india-seminar.com/2019/714/714_rama_v_baru.htm.
102. Liping Bu, " Beijing First Health Station: Innovative Public Health Education and Influence on China's Health Profession," in *Science, Public Health and the State in Modern Asia*, in Liping Bu, Darwin Stapleton and Ka-Che Yip edited (Abingdon, Oxon: Routledge, 2012), 129–43.
103. Bu, "Beijing First Health Station," 133.
104. *Report of the Health Survey and Development Committee: Recommendations*, volume II (New Delhi: Government of India Press, 1946), 45. *Panchayat* in South Asia loosely translates as village council.
105. *Report of the Health Survey and Development Committee*, volume II, 7.
106. *Report of the Health Survey and Development Committee*, volume II, 158; See also Niels Brimnes, "Rallying around the Magic Wand: Visions of Social Medicine, Public Health and Disease Control in India," in *Yearbook*

for the History of Global Development: Health and Development, Iris Borowy and Bernard Harris edited (Oldenburg: de Gruyter, 2023), 175–91, 183.

107. *Report of the Health Survey and Development Committee*, volume II, 158.
108. "Health Plan for India," *Amrita Bazar Patrika*, March 4, 1946, JSTOR South Asia Open Archives, https://www.jstor.org/stable/saoa.crl.34615662.
109. Rama V. Baru, "Changing Avatars of Social Medicine in the Indian Subcontinent," in *Medicine on a Larger Scale: Global Histories of Social Medicine*, Anne Kveim Lie, Jeremy Greene, and Warwick Anderson edited (Cambridge: Cambridge University Press, 2025), 278–96, 280.
110. "Health of India," *British Medical Journal* no. 4444 (March 16, 1946): 395–96.
111. Baru, "The Bhore Committee."
112. See, for example, John B. Grant, "All India Policy and Initial Steps for Medical Research Relating to Industry," January 28, 1944, Reports and Memoranda Circulation: Health Survey and Development Committee (1943), File No. 24-2/43 G, Identifier PR_000005014082, NAI. Accessed July 15, 2024. https://www.abhilekh-patal.in/jspui/handle/123456789/2753875?searchWord=sokhey&backquery=[query=sokhey&originalquery=&sort_by=dc.date.accessioned_dt&order=desc&rpp=20&etal=0&start=0]; See also Henry E. Sigerist, "Undated Report on India: On the Sociology of Medicine," 1960, Box 35, Folder 74, Henry Ernst Sigerist Papers, MS 788, Yale University Archives.
113. *Report of the Health Survey and Development Committee*, volume II, 14.
114. "Health of India."
115. *Report of the Health Survey and Development Committee*, volume II, 488.
116. G. Borkar, *Health in Independent India: A Decade of Progress* (New Delhi: Ministry of Health, 1958).
117. For details, see Binayak Dutta, "Challenging Times, Challenged Body: Decolonization, Displacement and Disease among East Pakistani Refugees in South Assam, 1947–54," in *Playing with Nature: History and Politics in North-East India*, Sajal Nag edited (Abingdon, Oxon: Routledge, 2018), 255–72.
118. "Publication of Radio Broadcast by Mohammad Hatta, Vice President of Indonesia," June 22, 1946, PRS Mani Collection, UTS Library Special Collections. Accessed July 15, 2024. https://opus.lib.uts.edu.au/handle/10453/28096.
119. Sharinee Jagtiani, "'Foreign Armies are Functioning on Indian Soil': India, Indonesian Decolonization and Onset of the Cold War (1945–49)," *Cold War History* 22, no. 3 (2022): 305–24.
120. Gopa Sabharwal, "In Search of an Asian Vision: The Asian Relations Conference of 1947," in *Imagining Asia(s): Networks, Actors, Sites,*

Andrea Acri, Kashshaf Ghani, Murari Jha and Sraman Mukherjee edited (Singapore: ISEAS, 2019), 60–90.

121. "Asian Conference," *The Hindustan Times*, March 14, 1947, Inter Asian Relations Conference held at New Delhi in March and April 1947, Identifier: PR_000001593212, File No. Progs.. Nos.62 (6)-OS III, 1947, NAI. Accessed July 25, 2024. https://indianculture.gov.in/archives/inter-asian-relations-conference-held-new-delhi-march-april-1947.
122. *Asian Relations: Being the Proceedings and Documentation of the First Asian Relations Conference, New Delhi, March-April 1947* (New Delhi: Asian Relations Organization, 1948), 23.
123. Ibid., 23.
124. Vineet Thakur, "An Asian Drama: The Asian Relations Conference, 1947," *International History Review* 41, no. 3 (2019):673–95.
125. *Asian Relations*, 96.
126. K.C.K.E. Raja, *Health Problems of India* (New Delhi: Indian Council of World Affairs, 1947).
127. Ibid.
128. Maung Sein, *Health Problems of Burma* (New Delhi: Indian Council of World Affairs, 1947).
129. Abdul Majid, *Public Health Activities in Afghanistan* (New Delhi: Asian Relations Conference, 1947).
130. *Asian Relations*, 183.
131. Amitav Acharya, "Asia is Not One," *The Journal of Asian Studies* 69, no. 4 (2010): 1001–13, 1008.
132. Virginia Thompson and Richard Adloff, "Social Welfare in Southeast Asia," *Far Eastern Survey* 18, no. 2 (1949): 136–40.
133. Thompson and Adloff, "Social Welfare."
134. Julie Sukanto, "Education and Welfare in Indonesia," *Pakistan Horizon* 1, no. 2 (1948): 131–36.
135. Stein, "Hygiene and Decolonization," 58.
136. Ibid., 58.
137. Thompson and Adloff, "Social Welfare."
138. The Renville Agreement (1948) was a political accord brokered by the United Nations Security Council between the Netherlands, which was seeking to reestablish its colonies in the Indonesian archipelago, and the Indonesian Republicans who were determined to secure Indonesian independence from colonial rule.
139. Thompson and Adloff, "Social Welfare."
140. Vivek Neelakantan, "Eradicating Smallpox in Indonesia: The Archipelagic Challenge," *Health and History* 12, no. 1 (2010): 61–87.

CHAPTER 4

Coming to Terms with the Cold War: The WHO in Southeast Asia

Introduction

Since it was established as a specialized UN agency in 1948, the World Health Organization (WHO) faced two major challenges. The first was the Cold War—a period of geopolitical tensions between the USSR, the US and their allies. During this time, the USSR and its East European allies withdrew from the agency (1949 and 1956), citing irreconcilable differences with the US regarding socialized medicine.[1] The second challenge emerged in response to the collapse of colonial empires, including the Dutch, French, British, and Portuguese, who were eager to maintain their foothold in Southeast Asia. Meanwhile, the WHO had to accommodate the aspirations of nationalist leaders of newly independent nations in Southeast Asia who pushed for public health to be linked to wider concerns of postwar state-building. To balance the interests of colonial empires in Southeast Asia with the requirements of recently independent states, the WHO began a decentralization policy.

At the 1946 International Health Conference in New York, delegates affirmed the need for a decentralized organization to address worldwide health disparities. Rather than delegating authority to branch offices, the WHO endorsed regionalization—shaped by Latin American insistence on preserving the autonomy of the Pan American Sanitary Bureau (PASB).[2] The WHO Constitution empowered the World Health Assembly (WHA)

V. Neelakantan, *The Emergence of International Health Policy in Southeast Asia, India, and Sri Lanka, 1937–1978*,
https://doi.org/10.1007/978-3-032-21233-7_4

to designate geographical areas for the establishment of regional organizations.[3]

Between 1948 and 1951, the WHO Regional Office for South-East Asia (SEARO) and the WHO Regional Office for Western Pacific (WPRO) assumed responsibility for the organization's Asian operations. During this period, the agency also moved away from the broader social medicine mandate, instead prioritizing targeted campaigns against malaria, tuberculosis, and yaws. This shift exemplified the WHO's allegiance to the proverbial magic bullet approach—a quick technical fix that papered over the structural determinants of health.

Since 2006, the regional histories of the WHO have received limited attention.[4] In his monograph *Decolonizing International Health: India and Southeast Asia, 1930–65*, Sunil Amrith contends that India played a disproportionately influential role in shaping approaches to Asia's health challenges. Burma and Indonesia, by contrast, were contending with fragile state authority and ethnic insurgencies. International health biopolitics mediated Indian aspirations for regional leadership while navigating Southeast Asian anxieties over Indian imperialism and American influence.[5] Yet, this perspective overlooks the Philippine initiative in establishing WPRO and the broader imbrications of Cold War diplomacy on health governance in Southeast Asia. In crafting a regional health plan, both SEARO and WPRO balanced member states' compliance with aid agency directives against the imperative to secure increased WHO budgetary appropriations for Southeast Asia.[6]

From Interim Commission to Regional Office: The WHO's Journey in Southeast Asia

The WHO's planning phase unfolded amidst postwar optimism for a world free of disease. Between March and April 1946, the Technical Preparatory Committee—which included representatives from the League of Nations Health Organization (LNHO), PASB, and United Nations Relief and Rehabilitation Administration (UNRRA)—convened in Paris. Its primary responsibility was drafting the WHO Constitution and decentralizing international health governance through regional offices.

The Technical Preparatory Committee established the Interim WHO Commission (1946–1948) to prepare for the First World Health Assembly, oversee the amalgamation of health functions from pre-existing organizations—including the LNHO, Office International d' Hygiène Publique (OIHP), and UNRRA—and revise international sanitary conventions.[7] Its other mandate included negotiating the WHO's accession to the UN framework.

The San Francisco Conference (1945) set the stage for WHO's formation, although the US and UK had reached a tacit agreement to strategically sideline health from its formal agenda.[8] Hugh Cumming—then director of the PASB—assumed that health would be folded into broader social policy discussions.[9] However, Chinese diplomat Szeming Sze, Brazilian professor Geraldo de Paula Souza, and Norwegian physician Karl Evang lobbied independently for an autonomous health organization. They inserted the concept of a health agency into the UN constitution.[10] Their efforts secured the WHO's placement within the jurisdiction of the UN Economic and Social Council.

Marcos Cueto, Theodore Brown, and Elizabeth Fee argue that the British and Americans had considered setting up an international health organization even before the San Francisco Conference.[11] The US Department of State ensured that the UN Charter was amended to facilitate handover of the UNRRA's assets to the UN Economic and Social Council as a preparatory step toward the constitution of the new health agency.[12]

While the Technical Preparatory Committee was drafting the WHO Constitution in Paris, it initially referred to the prospective health agency as the United Nations International Health Organization, leaving the final name unresolved.[13] According to one view, Sze recommended replacing United Nations from the title in favor of World Health Organization, as he was of the conviction that health was a global concern and should not exclude any nation.[14]

According to the established historical view, Croatian physician Andrija Štampar—founder of the School of Public Health in Zagreb (1927) and President of the First WHA— helped draft the Constitution of the WHO, most notably the preamble.[15] The Preamble of the

WHO states, "Health is a state of complete physical, mental and social well-being and not merely the absence of disease or infirmity." The full preamble contained nine principles, including the enjoyment of the highest attainable standard of health as a fundamental right of every human being without distinction of race, religion, political belief, or social condition.[16] In his 1943 unpublished document, Raymond Gautier—director of the Eastern Bureau of the LNHO, Singapore (1926–1931)—defined health as a positive condition comprising physical, mental, and moral fitness. This formulation subsequently influenced the WHO Preamble (Image 4.1).[17]

Štampar recognized the need for a comprehensive reappraisal of the architecture of pre-existing international health organizations to shape the WHO's operational framework— preserving their institutional strengths while remedying their structural limitations.[18] He noted that before World War I, international health was a patchwork of activities dominated by organizations, particularly the Maritime Sanitary and Quarantine Board of Egypt (established in 1831), the Constantinople Health Board

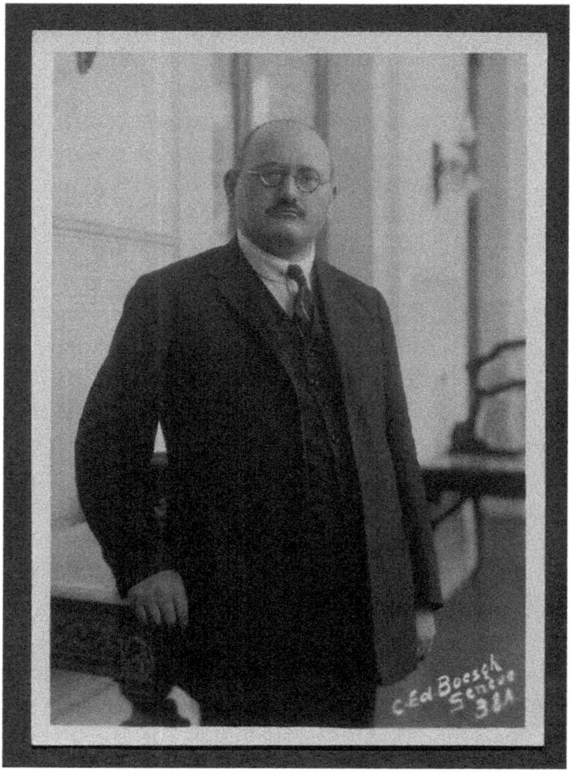

Image 4.1 Andrija Štampar. Reference Code: P070_01_053. League of Nations Visual Materials Collection. UN Library and Archives Geneva. With Permission

(1838–1914), the OIHP, and the PASB. However, the scope of these organizations was restricted to the collection and dissemination of epidemiological intelligence. Between 1921 and 1939, the LNHO expanded its scope beyond epidemic containment, embracing holistic health initiatives such as nutrition, sanitation, and housing. However, overlaps between the jurisdiction of the LNHO Epidemiological Intelligence Section and the OIHP frustrated coordinated efforts in international health governance. The LNHO's strengths lay in leveraging expert committees and liaising with government authorities, particularly in housing, nutrition, and health insurance. Štampar faced the dilemma of how the new international organization might reconcile the competing agendas of the US and the USSR—while also engaging local governments in regional operations. As a way out, he proposed a single central organization coordinating the work of strong, flexible regional branches.[19]

Štampar's advocacy for a decentralized model in international health aligned with the Mani-Sze proposal. The proposal incorporated regional arrangements into the constitution of the future WHO, ensuring that the organization reflected local needs. Chandra Mani played the defining role as the chief architect of regionalization. Mani joined the Indian Medical Service in 1927 as a medical officer and commanded military hospitals during the Pacific War.[20] After his brief stint in leading the provincial health services of Orissa in 1945, Mani officiated as public health commissioner for the Government of India (1945–1947) and was subsequently promoted to the position of deputy director of public health (1947–1948). He was a member of the Technical Preparatory Committee (1946) and the Interim Commission (1946–1948). He was the founder-director of SEARO, a position he held for two decades.

The Mani-Sze proposal envisaged the creation of Regional Committees to articulate country-specific health needs, supervise region-specific activities, liaise with UN regional commissions, and recommend budgetary supplements if the central organization's allocations were inadequate.[21] The Director-General of the proposed international health organization could delegate specific tasks—such as rural sanitation—to regional offices. Transitional regional arrangements were outlined in cases where regional health agencies—such as the PASB—predated the WHO's formation. This allowed pre-existing regional agencies to retain autonomy while their integration into the post-World War II international health architecture was finalized.

The proposals for regional arrangements generated heated discussion in Paris. The Mani-Sze proposal represented a compromise between the PASB's preference to maintain regional autonomy and the centralized approach espoused by some European nations.[22] At the International Health Conference in New York (June 19 to July 22, 1946), delegates determined the fate of pre-existing international organizations— namely, the OIHP, LNHO, and UNRRA. The conference resolved to dissolve these organizations and entrust their functions—particularly maintaining epidemiological surveillance and implementing provisions of the International Sanitary Conventions—to the Interim Commission of the prospective WHO.[23]

One of the Interim Commission's key priorities—alongside disease control, infant mortality reduction, and biological standardization—was integrating the PASB and other intergovernmental organizations, such as the Eastern Bureau, into the WHO framework.[24] Incorporating regional bodies into the WHO's decentralized structure ignited membership debates, exposing geopolitical fault lines dictating the inclusion—or exclusion—of colonial powers and newly independent states.

The Americans proposed that the WHA admit nations on a simple majority vote. In contrast, the Soviets argued that non-UN members should require a two-thirds vote for admission. The notion of Associate Membership—participation of non-self-governing territories not eligible for full WHO membership—shaped the accession of dependencies, trust territories, and protectorates. At the insistence of the Chinese delegation, the International Health Conference's Legal Committee proposed admitting associate members "with all rights and privileges except voting and holding office." These included territories ineligible for separate UN membership but large in area and population, affected by international health concerns, and staffed by Indigenous administrations.[25] Delegates affirmed the WHA's authority to appoint such territories as associate members that were not responsible for the conduct of their international relations by simple majority vote. Applications for Associate Membership would be submitted via WHO members or other entities responsible for their external affairs.[26]

Perhaps, the most contentious issue before the International Health Conference was regionalism—complicated by the existence of the PASB and the American states' vigorous support for preserving its institutional autonomy. Soviet delegates urged "immediate and complete adsorption" of the PASB into the WHO.[27] However, no such drastic solution was acceptable to the US and Latin American states. To arrive at a satisfactory solution, Thomas Parran—who served as president of the International Health Conference—introduced a draft resolution. The resolution recommended that pre-existing bodies be transformed into WHO regional offices or that their facilities be integrated into the WHO, subject to a phased institutional merger.[28]

In its first session, the Interim Commission constituted a sub-committee for negotiation with the PASB. Under the draft agreement, the PASB would become the WHO Regional Office for the Americas.[29] On April 1, 1947, the Interim Commission assumed responsibility of the Eastern Bureau.[30]

On August 15, 1945—following the end of the Japanese occupation of Singapore—the UN made several attempts to resuscitate the LNHO's Eastern Bureau, which ceased operations during the Pacific War. However, attempts to reestablish the Eastern Bureau had to contend with the geopolitical realities of the time, particularly decolonization. The Indians and Chinese balked at locating the Eastern Bureau outside their respective countries.[31] The Americans did not prefer a League vestige but an entirely new regional health organization. By early 1946, the League of Nations was liquidated.

In January 1947, Allied Nations requested the UNRRA to reestablish the Eastern Bureau, given the recrudescence of cholera in China, Laos, Cambodia, and Indonesia.[32] However, UNRRA's institutional ephemerality limited its response. Faced with a difficult situation, the Supreme Allied Commander in Southeast Asia, Lord Louis Mountbatten, established a port health section in Singapore and instructed high commanders stationed in various parts of Southeast Asia to collect epidemiological intelligence. In April 1947, shortly after the Interim Commission's assumption of authority, the Eastern Bureau was renamed the Singapore Epidemiological Intelligence Station. The Station monitored infectious diseases in East Asia and implemented provisions of the International Sanitary Conventions.

By 1949, the Intelligence Station was unprepared to take on the responsibilities of a WHO regional office for Asia when the WHO announced plans to open the Western Pacific Regional Office. P.M. Kaul—Head of the Singapore Epidemiological Intelligence Station—expressed reservations. As the Station restricted itself to collecting and transmitting information related to infectious diseases, it was, therefore, ill-equipped to handle vast amounts of statistical data for a region as expansive as the

Western Pacific.[33] In 1956—following negotiations between the WHO headquarters and the WPRO regional office in Manila—the latter took over the functioning of the Epidemiological Intelligence Station in Singapore.[34] This administrative shift signaled the WHO's evolving regionalization approach.

By 1947, the Interim Commission divided the world into various health areas—considering the prevalence of endemic and epidemic diseases—providing a strong foundation for the WHO's regional architecture. Members of the Interim Commission imagined South-East Asia as a geopolitical construct:

> The Central and Southeastern parts of Asia together with Indonesia, i.e. the 'Monsoon Asia of Geographers,' should be considered as one epidemiological area. It would include the endemic foci of cholera and territories most readily infectible by that disease, also foci of plague endemic and epidemic. It is free from yellow fever but severely affected by malaria, by fleaborne and miteborne rickettsioses and by the ubiquitous smallpox. Most of the area suffers from the food deficiencies of rice eaters, from a high tuberculosis morbidity and mortality in its cities and an extension of that disease in the more backward districts of this area.[35]

Indian delegates impressed the Interim Commission on the need for early regionalization of international health. After vigorous discussions at the First WHA, three Working Parties were appointed to make recommendations concerning the three main regions: South-East Asia, the Far East, and the Middle East.[36] Each Working Party would consist of members from the interested countries of that region. At the time of the First WHA, regional boundaries were fluid; states exercised considerable autonomy in selecting geopolitical affiliations in international health.[37] The WHO confronted complex cartographic and geopolitical challenges in demarcating South-East Asia and the Western Pacific. Pakistan was originally assigned to the Working Party for South-East Asia. However, the country was subsequently transferred to the Working Party for the Middle East due to the escalating tensions with India over Kashmir—a move reflecting the diplomatic fallout triggered by the 1947 Partition. The reassignment signaled Pakistan's strategic distancing from India-led regional health governance and its alignment with the Eastern Mediterranean, reflecting its evolving postcolonial orientation toward the Middle East.

Between 1948 and 1959, the WHO's regionalization efforts were punctuated by protracted negotiations concerning member state affiliations, demarcation of health regions, and the institutional logic of regional offices. The First WHA codified WHO's regional architecture by delineating six geographical areas. While South-East Asia, the Eastern Mediterranean, and the Western Pacific were listed by enumerating individual member states, Europe and the Americas were delineated by reference to a continental mass. Africa was defined through its natural and political boundaries.[38]

The First WHA resolved that the region comprising India and the surrounding countries in South-East Asia formed a homogeneous area with common complex health problems.[39] This epidemiological framing justified establishing a regional office—with New Delhi positioned as its administrative anchor. Conference delegates from India, Ceylon, Siam, Burma, and Afghanistan unanimously nominated Mani as SEARO's first regional director.[40]

The inclusion of the Netherlands as an Associate Member representing its colonial interests in Indonesia within SEARO experienced geopolitical complications due to the Dutch Military Action against the Indonesian Republic (1947–1949). The Netherlands Indies Department of Health (Dutch: Departemen van Gezondheid) expressed concern that SEARO would be of little value to Indonesia, as Batavia (now known as Jakarta) was geographically closer to the would-be headquarters of WPRO at Manila than New Delhi.[41] But India supported the revolutionary government—then based at Yogyakarta—to accede to SEARO. At the Third WHA (1950), Indonesia declined accession to the Western Pacific region, opting instead for the South-East Asia area to deepen solidarity with India, whose antipathy toward imperialism echoed Indonesia's anti-colonial struggle.[42] Indonesia's SEARO accession—despite Dutch objection—marked a symbolic defiance of metropolitan oversight.

The Indian community in Malaya was no less influential in steering Malaya toward the South-East Asian grouping at the First WHA.[43] SEARO provisionally included Malaya and Singapore as Associate Members, as both were non-governing territories.[44] However, given the undercurrent of Indian domination of British Malaya—highlighted at the Asian Relations Conference in New Delhi (1947)—Malaya and Singapore acceded to the newly founded WPRO in 1951.[45] As WPRO was not yet established in 1950, the State of Vietnam and the Kingdoms of Cambodia and Laos were provisionally assigned to the South-East Asia area.[46]

WPRO's launch was delayed due to political upheavals in East Asia—namely, the Chinese Civil War (1945–1949) and the Korean War (1950–1953). By 1949, the Chinese Communists had expelled the Nationalists to Taiwan, which—despite its smaller population—held China's WHA seat until 1972. After the Korean War, South Korea retained sole WHO representation until North Korea joined WHO in 1973.

At the First WHA (1948), Chinese and Filipino delegates proposed the establishment of a regional office for the Western Pacific. Yet, the assembly did not affect the proposal of the Chinese and Filipino delegates, as most states in that area had not yet expressed their support for such a regional health arrangement. At the Second WHA in Rome (1949), Filipino Health Secretary Antonio Villarama put forward a compelling rationale for a WHO regional office for the Western Pacific area:

> I believe that the Philippine position is unique: it cannot be considered properly as one with India, because of its great distance from that vast country; it is, geographically and commercially, the hub of the wheel in the Far East, Australia and New Zealand being far down south in the Western Pacific Area, and thus being not quite disposed to join hands with us in the consideration of the establishment of a regional organization in that area, with headquarters in the Philippines.[47]

Villarama made a strong case for setting up the regional office for the Western Pacific in the Philippines. Yet, the WHO deferred the Filipino proposal to the Third WHA, pending approval of three constituent states of the area.[48]

In 1950, during the Third WHA, France objected to the setting up of a regional office for the Western Pacific, arguing that the Singapore Epidemiological Intelligence Station was sufficiently protecting the Western Pacific's regional interests.[49] Australia and New Zealand sided with France.[50] Delegates from both countries observed that the proposed WHO Regional Office for the Western Pacific was heterogeneous. They recommended assigning the northern arc—Japan, Korea, China, Vietnam, Laos, Cambodia, and the Philippines—to the South-East Area, while Australia, New Zealand, New Guinea, and the South Sea Islands could constitute the Western Pacific.[51]

W. de Leon—Director of Laboratories from the Philippine Department of Health and a delegate to the Third WHA—drew on the trope of contagion to emphasize the urgency of a regional health organization for the

Western Pacific. He observed that countries that suffered most during the War, including the Philippines, were located in the central portion of the Western Pacific. He complained, "Feeling the need of more immediate material help, our neighbours in the Western Pacific Region have already been leaving or are intending to leave our regional area and to realign themselves with another already established regional group [South-East Asia] in the hope thus to expedite relief."[52] In expediting the establishment of the regional organization for the Western Pacific, de Leon contended that the WHO would prevent "more prosperous, undamaged and well-developed countries from the danger of epidemics which would result if the under-developed countries were left alone, unaided to become the foci of diseases."[53]

Soon after the Third WHA, the WHO instituted a provisional office for the Western Pacific in Hong Kong—under I-Chi Fang's leadership, between 1950 and 1951—before the regional headquarters were established in Manila.[54] Countries that expressed their interest to join the Western Pacific included Australia, China, New Zealand, British Territories, Japan, the Philippines, Vietnam, Cambodia, Laos, and South Korea.[55]

Fang served as the WPRO regional director between 1951 and 1965. After graduating from Peking Union Medical College (PUMC) in 1922, he earned a master's degree in public health from Harvard in 1931. During the 1930s, Fang served as medical officer of the Peking Health Demonstration Center and taught public health between 1934 and 1935 at PUMC. In 1937, he was appointed provincial health commissioner of Kiangsi, a position he held until 1945. After World War II, Fang worked for the Nationalist Health Administration as deputy director (1946–1947) and briefly held the position of Chief Medical Officer of Nationalist China before being appointed as WPRO regional director in 1951.[56]

His appointment came at a time when the WHO was expanding its mandate across Asia. By 1950, the agency had instituted the BCG vaccination against TB in Singapore, Malaya, the Philippines, Hong Kong, and Taiwan. Additionally, the agency collaborated with UNICEF to organize maternal and child health services in the British territories of Sarawak, Brunei, and North Borneo.[57] The activities of the temporary WPRO office in Hong Kong coincided with the progress of the First Indochina War (1946–1954). Twenty-five percent of the sanctioned US$ 230 million to WPRO's Hong Kong office was diverted toward Indochina's medical and health rehabilitation.[58] WPRO developed a partnership with the United States Public Health Service (USPHS) to undertake mass campaigns against endemic diseases, notably malaria, trachoma, venereal diseases, and TB.[59] Given the context of war, USPHS authorities and Fang devised a slogan, "Immediate implementation, money no concern, and quick results."[60] Fang aimed to position the regional image of the WHO as responsive to local needs.

Fang's regional dynamism stood in stark contrast to the geopolitical realities that confronted the WHO during its formative years. Between 1948 and 1958, the organization was a prisoner of US strategic interests. The US government—preoccupied with addressing the perceived geopolitical threat posed by the USSR—dampened the enthusiasm for a strong central organization with a wide-ranging mandate.[61] Cold War tensions between the US and the USSR exposed the schism between those who envisioned an organization that embraced the values of social medicine and those who sought to circumscribe the WHO mandate to disease surveillance. The first decade of the agency witnessed a complex entanglement of international health initiatives with Cold War maneuvering, oscillating between aspirational social medicine ideals and efforts to restrict its scope to disease eradication.

At the First WHA, the USSR Deputy Health Minister N. Vinogradov leveled criticisms against the work of the Interim Commission. The commission allocated over US$ 500,000 solely in 1947 on technical assistance missions.[62] Vinogradov contended that the Interim Commission's technical missions could not ameliorate national health services since they were unfamiliar with local quirks. He pointed out that the arbitrary exploitation of populations deprived of their rights and the inadequate organization of health services in colonies and dependent territories were responsible for epidemic outbreaks. Vinogradov posited that the WHO needed to attack the root cause of illness, notably poverty, rather than imposing quarantines.[63] Soviet delegates suggested that combining social reform and building stronger national health services might address global health challenges.

The Soviet Union and the Ukrainian and Byelorussian Soviet Socialist Republics withdrew from the WHO in 1949 due to the Cold War, citing irreconcilable differences with capitalist ideologies. At the same time, the Soviet's Eastern European allies, namely, Albania, Bulgaria, Czechoslovakia, Hungary, Poland, and Romania, boycotted the organization. The Soviets and their allies alleged that although they had paid a high price during World War II, they received little help from either the Marshall Plan for the reconstruction of Europe or the WHO (Image 4.2).[64]

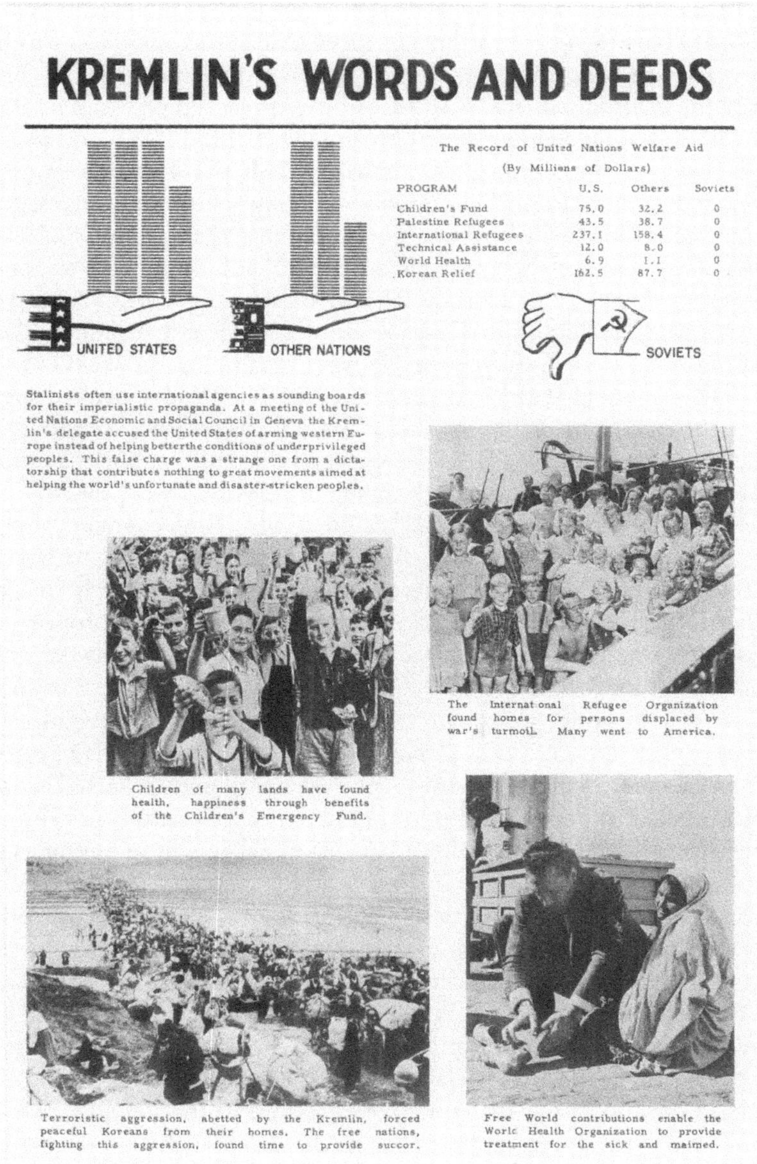

Image 4.2 Kremlin's Words and Deeds. NAID: 5729981. Local ID: 306-PPA-80. Produced: January 9, 1952. Records of the US Information Agency. Series: Propaganda Posters Distributed in Asia (1950–55). NARA. URL: https://catalog.archives.gov/id/5729981. Access: Unrestricted (Public Domain)

The decision of the USSR and its Eastern European allies to boycott the WHO hurt the organization's finances. The absent members withheld their assessed contributions.[65] The WHO Director-General Brock Chisholm asserted that the WHO Constitution lacked provisions for formal withdrawal by member states. He argued that the USSR and its allies were "inactive" rather than withdrawn.[66] With the withdrawals of the USSR and its allies from the international body, Chisholm expressed disappointment that "somehow the World Health Organization would have to get along without the emphasis on 'World' and do its best to control epidemics on *this* [East European] side of the iron curtain."[67] Several WHO leaders, including the Indian Minister of Health Rajkumari Amrit Kaur reassured the USSR that the US was not running the WHO.[68]

USSR—upon its readmission into the WHO in 1956—invoked Article 47 of the WHO to secure Associate Membership within SEARO. The Soviet delegate to the Twelfth WHA argued that the five Soviet republics (Uzbek, Tadzhik, Turkmenian, Kazakh, and Kyrgyz) were directly contiguous to Afghanistan, then a SEARO member. The geographical proximity of the Soviet republics to Afghanistan led the USSR to have an interest in joint solutions to Asia's health problems, particularly smallpox eradication. But the Twelfth WHA deferred the USSR proposal for SEARO Associate Membership because the five Soviet republics were contiguous with the USSR and not constitutionally self-governing countries situated within South-East Asia.[69] The USSR subsequently withdrew its proposal. The criteria for assigning member states to WHO regional offices remained ambiguous until 1959.[70] This ambiguity reflected broader tensions between geopolitical positioning and public health priorities—a theme that shaped the organization's institutional evolution during its formative years (1946–1953).

Despite the charged political and ideological environment, WHO founders, particularly Štampar and Chisholm, were unwavering in their optimism about integrating social medicine into the agency's core priorities. Štampar advocated for WHO policies that focused on social and economic security, education, nutrition, and housing—key elements of holistic public health.[71] A social medicine perspective, if taken seriously, would imply addressing structural issues related to the unequal distribution of land in rural areas and a multitude of inequities that produced poor housing and ill health. To skirt these sensitive issues and to avoid antagonizing the US, the WHO introduced a technical assistance program that emerged from US governmental discourses at the end of World War II.[72]

Historian Sunil Amrith highlights this transition by observing that "The new emphasis on technical assistance, and the subordination of social goals to that of economic growth, found a sympathetic echo within the new post-colonial states of Asia."[73] Technical assistance was rooted in the premise that development hinged on transferring science and technology, sidestepping structural determinants of underdevelopment.

"The Health Problem in South-East Asia"

At the First WHA, US delegate and WHO Assistant Director General Martha May Eliot recommended that the organization concentrate on a limited number of health problems of international significance. These problems included malaria, tuberculosis, maternal and child health, and venereal diseases, where scientific knowledge and practical experience justified the hope of early positive results at minimum cost.[74] Furthermore, she proposed that the WHO address the problem of environmental hygiene. Between 1948 and 1951, SEARO's priorities were identical to those emphasized at the WHA. The regional organization emphasized the "big six." These included malaria, tuberculosis, venereal diseases, maternal and child health, nutrition, and environmental sanitation.[75] However, by 1951, the organization switched its focus to long-term technical assistance and training health personnel. By the late 1950s, SEARO programs revealed two distinct public health approaches: (1) the broader social medicine approach that correlated ill health with social deprivation, and (2) the proverbial magic bullet approach that emphasized disease eradication.

Since its inception, SEARO has compiled and addressed technical assistance requests from member states, while calibrating WHO Expert Committee recommendations to local conditions. During the first year of the regional organization, India and Ceylon requested technical assistance from SEARO relating to challenges such as malaria, tuberculosis, and maternal and child health.[76]

In 1949, three epidemic outbreaks in South-East Asia attracted the assistance of the regional office.[77] The first emergency was a typhus outbreak in Afghanistan in August of that year. SEARO recommended widespread application of dichloro diphenyl trichloroethane (DDT) to arrest the spread of infection. The regional office liaised with the Government of India to procure vaccine supplies for Afghanistan. The second was an outbreak of acute anterior poliomyelitis in Bombay State, western India.

SEARO liaised with the WHO headquarters in Geneva to arrange timely shipment of respirators for Bombay. The third epidemic was an outbreak of plague in Shimoga district, in Mysore State's hilly Malnad region. SEARO diverted its malaria control team from neighboring Mysore district for firefighting plague, demonstrating its ability to coordinate resources across concurrent disease outbreaks.

The experience of a WHO Nurse, assigned to Sagar village, Mysore in 1949 underscored that the effectiveness of DDT in malaria and plague control depended on the participation of rural communities. Her program schedule included spraying DDT and collecting blood specimens from sprayed and non-sprayed areas to determine parasite levels in villagers' blood. The nursing team enlisted the support of village headmen and devised creative slogans:

(a) "Mosquito is the carrier of malaria."
(b) "DDT sprayed on the wall will kill the mosquito."[78]

The institution of school health education and roadside clinics ensured consistent community support for malaria elimination.[79] In October 1949, the Mysore government mobilized the WHO nursing team to contain the spread of the plague. The words of the WHO nurse captured the exhaustion and resolve of fieldwork:

> We talked on the streets, playgrounds and sportsfields and were quite hoarse, when dead tired we returned to Sagar the following week. But our efforts were well paid.[80]

Beyond Mysore, SEARO instituted a malaria control project in the Terai district of the United Provinces (now Uttar Pradesh) in northern India, collaborating with the United Nations Children's Fund (UNICEF), the FAO (Food and Agricultural Organization of the UN), and the Government of India. The Terai region was designated a model malaria control and demonstration site. Malaria impeded economic productivity in this agriculturally rich zone, south of the Himalayan foothills. Beyond disease control, the project aimed to improve living standards. As part of the project, the Government of India encouraged resettlement of Hindu and Sikh families displaced during Partition in 1947.

The Terai malaria control project was undertaken in the western part of the district between May and July 1949, coinciding with the start of the transmission season.[81] But due to a delay in funding allotment from the United Provinces government, SEARO was unable to expand anti-malarial activities to the adjacent Bhabar (a region to the south of the Himalayan foothills).[82] By 1953, international aid agencies withdrew from the project and relinquished operational control to the Indian government. Although the project succeeded in halting malaria transmission, the Indian government fell short of training auxiliary health personnel in complementary public health areas such as maternal and child health.[83] This gap revealed the limitations of vertical disease control programs when not supported by health systems strengthening.

Cultural Anthropologist Cora Du Bois—head of the US State Department's Southeast Asia Branch and assigned to the WHO between 1950 and 1951—was critical of the limited scope of the malaria control project in Terai. In her letter to C. Mani, Du Bois noted that despite SEARO's exclusive focus on malaria control, its staff—particularly public health nurses and malaria inspectors—actively cultivated relationships with rural communities to facilitate disease surveillance. However, the organization was unable to follow up on anti-malaria propaganda due to challenges resulting from the region's ethnic diversity.[84] Tharu and Buxa, indigenous people from the Terai, did not cooperate with the spray squads, fearing dispossession from their lands.[85] In her letters to Mani and S.F. Chellapah, then SEARO deputy director, Du Bois repeatedly emphasized that the Terai project should be considered an entering wedge in expanding the range of health services. That is, instead of trying to embed maternal and child health goals into malaria control projects with limited results, she posited that SEARO should prioritize the training of local health personnel for better results.[86]

Although Mani and Chellapah did not reply to Du Bois' criticisms of SEARO projects, by 1951, the regional organization reached a general agreement that the short-term demonstration projects focusing on individual diseases were unsustainable. Instead, the Regional Committee emphasized long-term assistance to member states, which included training health personnel.

The shift in SEARO's emphasis—from targeting endemic diseases to training health personnel—was particularly relevant for Thailand, which, alongside India, became a key beneficiary of international technical assistance from 1950 onward. Before 1945, malaria was the primary cause of morbidity and mortality in Thailand. Between 1945 and 1949, the disease afflicted nearly 18 million Thais, while 40,000 died.[87]

The collaborative SEARO-UNICEF malaria control and demonstration project at Saraphi, Chiang Mai province, emphasized the efficacy of spraying insecticide DDT in achieving control. Because Saraphi was situated in the rice bowl of northern Thailand, where malaria was hyperendemic, SEARO and UNICEF selected the district for a pilot intervention, showcasing vector control.

Despite initial challenges, the project showed promising results. SEARO undertook spraying activities between April and May 1950, prior to the monsoon. Spleen surveys revealed that parasite rates of infants born after spraying dropped to 0.47 percent.[88] The early successes with DDT fueled public demand for the insecticide in neighboring districts. Nevertheless, technical bottlenecks posed obstacles to the project. Village houses made of bamboo had smooth surfaces that lost DDT residue more rapidly. Additionally, the scale of insecticide application exceeded the Thai government's fiscal capacity. The dearth of curative health services in Saraphi impeded treatment of active cases.[89]

DDT was used in the elimination of not only flies but also bedbugs. As insects developed resistance after repeated sprayings, villagers became reluctant to cooperate with spraying teams. The weakest link in the malaria control operations chain of command lay in SEARO and UNICEF's inability to assess the health literacy of local personnel—sprayers, medical workers, and village headmen alike.

In Thailand, a cultural aversion to strong odors shaped villagers' preferences for odorless DDT. This sensory aversion contributed to localized pushback against spraying operations.[90]

These operational setbacks—rooted in both insecticidal resistance and cultural differences—exposed fault lines in malaria control, prompting the US to recalibrate its strategy in alignment with Cold War objectives.

Between 1955 and 1961, the country launched a national malaria control program. After USPHS officials convinced their Thai counterparts of DDT's efficacy, Thailand enlisted technical assistance from the International Cooperation Administration (ICA)—a US aid agency—active during the Eisenhower years (1955–1961). The ICA and the Thai government implemented the eradication program across all provinces except Bangkok, where malaria posed minimal public health risk.

ICA authorities addressed religious sensitivities, particularly the Buddhist proscription against killing living beings such as mosquitoes. Through sustained dialog, they convinced Buddhist monks that extirpating mosquitoes was essential for the sustenance of humans. When the

Thais saw their temples sprayed with DDT and their monks taking prescribed anti-malarial drugs, they emulated their religious leaders in taking medication and having their houses sprayed.[91] The ICA provided anti-malarial drugs to the country's health centers, Buddhist temples, and schools.

American technical assistance to Thailand—particularly through the MSA (Mutual Security Agency) and ICA—was shaped by geopolitical calculations. Beyond malaria control, these programs sought to purchase Thai allegiance for the US and countervail communist influence. Yet across both Thailand and India, this strategic emphasis on vertical disease eradication—malaria and tuberculosis—came at the expense of environmental sanitation. In 1949, Mani—in his correspondence with the WHO headquarters—emphasized that attention to environmental sanitation would decisively affect the control of ancylostomiasis (hookworm), typhoid, cholera, and malaria. He observed that prerequisites for cholera control—particularly a wholesome water supply and effective disposal of wastes—remained inadequate across South-East Asia.[92]

Beginning in 1950, Mani served as a liaison between SEARO member states, WHO headquarters, and the USPHS for technical health assistance. Representatives from the USPHS called on the Regional Director to discuss modalities of delivering health assistance to South-East Asia under President Harry S. Truman's Point Four Program. The program—framed as a Cold War initiative—sought to develop an economic basis for self-government and contain communist ascendancy across the region.[93]

In addition to the Point Four Program, Mani approached the Colombo Plan for Southeast Asia, founded in 1950, to administer technical assistance.[94] British officials feared that rising nationalism across Southeast Asia would provide an impetus to communist insurgency, prompting calls to buttress the region against ideological subversion.[95] The Colombo Plan was a system of mutual aid whereby member states helped each other and lobbied international bodies for increased funding. One of the main objectives of the Colombo Plan was to augment social capital in public health and education. SEARO-administered fellowships under the Plan enabled regional medical training.

Regional health architecture demanded embedded technical presence in member states. During the early 1950s, international health programs across South-East Asia were ad hoc and donor-driven. Mani appointed, in each SEARO member state, a public health expert to serve as the WHO Area Representative. These representatives—supervised by the SEARO

Regional Director—advised governments on effective health planning strategies.[96]

In a *Straits Times* article dated March 4, 1952, Mani delineated SEARO's challenges:

> The South-East Asia region of the WHO comprises Afghanistan, Burma, Ceylon, India, Indonesia and Siam [Thailand]. It contains more than 50 million people—more than three times the population of the United States in three-fourths of that area. More than 80 per cent of people live in villages; 80 per cent are illiterate and the average annual income is in the range of 150 Malayan dollars a year. All public health planning must start with these facts.[97]

He reframed the SEARO mandate not as an appendage of Geneva, but as an immediate response to poverty, epidemiological burden, and structural neglect.

This reframing of the SEARO mandate resonated with wider postcolonial sensibility, where national sovereignty, regional solidarity, and international aid were mediated not only through intergovernmental agencies but also articulated on diplomatic platforms such as Bandung. During the 1950s, foreign aid emerged as a sensitive political topic in Southeast Asia. Leaders of India, Ceylon, Burma, and Indonesia had to walk a tightrope between preserving their countries' sovereignty and increasing receptivity to international aid. The Asian-African Conference—known as the Bandung Conference, hosted by Indonesia at Bandung in April 1955—discussed problems of common concern to Asia and Africa. Although health was not explicitly on the Bandung agenda, the Communiqué urged UN-led cooperation to reduce nuclear weapons. Such reductions would facilitate peaceful uses of atomic energy and raise living standards, reflecting the aspirations of Asian and African leaders.[98]

The Eighth Regional SEARO Conference at Bandung coincided with the Asian-African Conference. In his opening address, Indonesian Minister of Health Johannes Leimena invoked shared priorities among regional leaders, as articulated in the Bandung Communiqué—including the imperative to improve living standards. Leimena's address espoused a holistic public health approach for South-East Asia, countering the magic bullet paradigm that undergirded postwar international health policy. He argued that communicable diseases emerged from three interrelated factors: (a) the host, with humans as the primary concern; (b) the disease agent; and (c) a constellation of biological, environmental, social, and economic determinants.[99] He maintained that addressing the host-agent-environment triad required concerted state action to integrate disease ecology into health policy.

Leimena acknowledged that rural health in Southeast Asia was deeply interwoven with living conditions. His host-agent-environment triad was congruent with SEARO's thrust on environmental sanitation. Yet such initiatives encountered systemic constraints: shortages of trained medical personnel and limited overseas aid.

Between 1948 and 1957, SEARO's sanitation programs originated within malaria control and rural health demonstration frameworks. Yet their progress rested on two fragile pillars: a limited pool of trained personnel and fluctuating US funding.[100] Administrative shifts—beginning with Truman's MSA in 1951—replaced by Eisenhower's Foreign Operations Administration (FOA)—tethered foreign aid to US geopolitical objectives.

Such geopolitical tethering of US assistance extended into ideological surveillance. Domestic right-wing elements led by J. Edgar Hoover undermined WHO's efforts to involve American public health experts in international health. When Du Bois joined the WHO, Hoover ordered the Federal Bureau of Investigation to scrutinize her activities.[101]

The failure of environmental sanitation and rural health did not impede the progress of malaria control across South-East Asia. If anything, American Cold War calculations bolstered support for malaria eradication. During the Eisenhower Era, the US reframed disease—especially malaria—as a generator of poverty, which, in turn, was seen as the breeding ground for communism. Thus, malaria eradication became an ideological weapon to stem the growth of communist ideology.[102]

The apparent speed with which DDT suppressed malaria further convinced US planners to pursue eradication.[103] Early elimination efforts seemed promising, particularly in Afghanistan and Indonesia.[104] But by the mid-1950s, in Indonesia and along Burma's Akyab coast, the malaria vector *Anopheles Sundaicus* developed resistance to DDT.[105] In response, SEARO member states adopted eradication as a formal national objective by 1955.[106] The ICA aided campaigns in Thailand and Indonesia with DDT supplies.

In 1959, President Soekarno inaugurated Indonesia's malaria eradication program. In his opening address, he substituted the word malaria with mal-mosquito to emphasize that malaria was not dictated by tropical climate but caused by mosquito bites that paralyzed the nation's economic potential. In Soekarno's vision, eradicating malaria would constitute a strong and healthy population (Bahasa Indonesia: *rakjat sehat*, *negara kuat*) (Image 4.3).

The Indonesian nationalist rhetoric on malaria eradication dovetailed with US technical assistance, which quantified the disease's economic

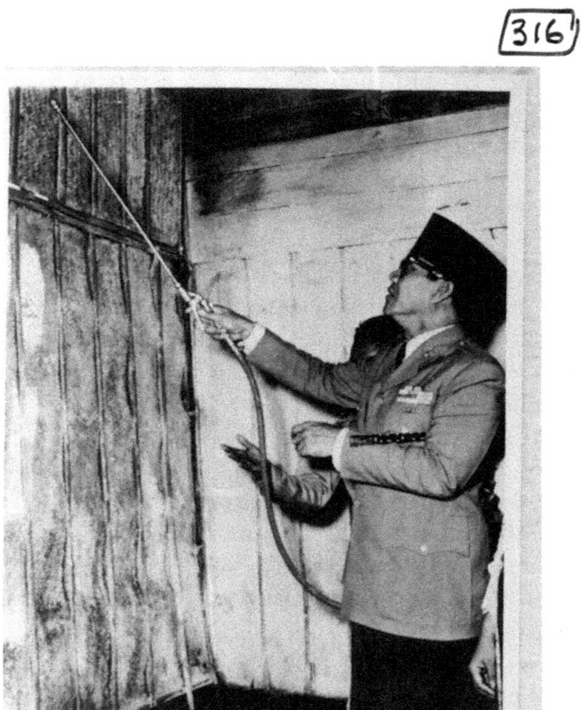

Image 4.3 Indonesia: DDT spraying inside a house (1959). President Soekarno wielding a hand sprayer to apply DDT to the walls of a house in central Java. Captured at a moment when US-Indonesian relations were at their nadir, the image symbolizes Indonesia wresting control over its malaria eradication program, distancing itself from US and WHO oversight. Courtesy of the National Library of Medicine. NLM Unique ID: A018331. Permanent Link: http://resource.nlm.nih.gov/101446953. Public Domain

impact on an international scale.[107] Nonetheless, the program suffered from several organizational bottlenecks. Compliance with bureaucratic procedures at the central, provincial, and local levels delayed access to DDT and other supplies. Consequently, the campaign stalled between 1959 and 1960. This forced the ICA to halve funding for the program—notwithstanding the then Minister of Health Satrio's struggle to expand coverage. As the SEARO Regional Director, Mani walked a diplomatic tightrope: ensuring the Indonesian Ministry of Health's compliance with the ICA's prescriptions, while preserving a degree of autonomy within the National Malaria Eradication Program.[108]

By 1957, as Indonesia's malaria control activities grappled with technical, administrative, and logistical bottlenecks, SEARO was simultaneously broadening its regional scope. This involved a shift from disease-specific interventions to an integrated approach. The new framework merged disease eradication programs, maternal and child health, nutrition, environmental sanitation, and health education—positioning these within the broader context of community development. SEARO convened the Rural Health Conference, New Delhi (1957), revisiting themes from the 1937 Bandoeng Conference. Key themes discussed included the organization of multipurpose health workers, the formation of village health committees to foster community participation, and the integration of health services into rural development.[109]

Two obstacles impeded the development of rural health services across South-East Asia. First, the lack of clear responsibility demarcation between SEARO and member states.[110] Second, constrained budgets led states to prioritize symbolic disease eradication campaigns. For instance, Indonesia focused on the campaign against the "Big Four Endemic Diseases," namely malaria, tuberculosis, yaws, and leprosy, which debilitated the population's productivity.

At the 1960 Thirteenth SEARO Meeting in Bandung, Mani acknowledged South-East Asia's remarkable progress in communicable disease control. However, he reaffirmed the regional body's longstanding concerns—malnutrition and poor environmental sanitation—which remained major morbidity drivers.[111] Mani asserted that while SEARO could assist member states in designing environmental sanitation projects, implementation hinged on governments' ability to secure funding (Image 4.4)[112]

SEARO's attention to environmental sanitation was just one dimension of the broader struggle to maintain momentum in regional health initiatives. Atsuko Naono notes that despite the official hype about rural health

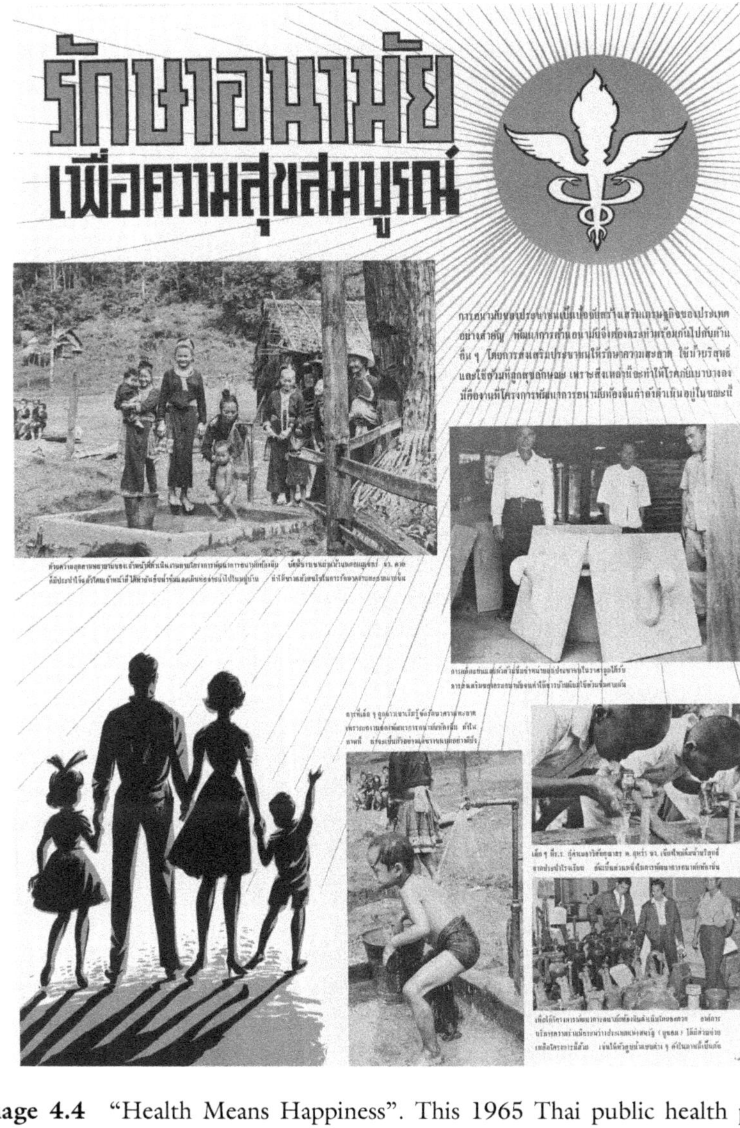

Image 4.4 "Health Means Happiness". This 1965 Thai public health poster stages hygiene as happiness, refracting the SEARO-UNICEF malaria control and demonstration project (1950s), where US technical assistance in health encountered rural idealism and infrastructural fragility. Record Group 306: Records of the U.S. Information Agency. Series: Propaganda Posters Distributed in Asia, Latin America and the Middle East. National Archives ID: 6949274. Local ID: 306-PPB-349. NARA URL: https://catalog.archives.gov/id/6949274. Copyright Status: Unrestricted (Public Domain)

projects in the South-East Asia region of the WHO during the 1950s, the 1960s witnessed a decline in rural health programs.[113] For example, hyper-inflation, political violence, and Soekarno's refusal to accept foreign technical assistance brought rural healthcare to a temporary standstill in Indonesia by 1960. By the 1970s, Indonesia's embrace of international technical assistance was not merely economic. The country viewed it as a strategic move to modernize health infrastructure, aligning domestic priorities with agencies such as UNICEF, the WHO, and USAID (United States Agency for International Development).[114]

"Western Pacific: Region of Contrasts"

Toward his retirement as WPRO Regional Director in 1965, Fang highlighted the heterogeneity of the Western Pacific. He observed:

> Our region, the Western Pacific, is made up of contrasts. In big cities such as Tokyo, Hong Kong or Singapore, millions of people live in close proximity to large urban communities, subject to all the influences of urban life. At the same time, in some remote Pacific islands, scattered, scarce and waning human groups still live according to ancestral patterns dating 2000 years. But the greater part of the region consists of developing countries, a typical example of which is the Philippines. Public health problems and consequent methods of approaching them, are different according to local conditions.[115]

Between 1951 and 1955, WPRO—in conjunction with member states—sought to alleviate the impact of epidemics, famine, civil unrest, and ongoing warfare. Malaria and tuberculosis were widespread. While schistosomiasis was endemic to the Philippines, nearly 30 percent of South Vietnam's population and 65 percent of North Vietnam's population suffered from trachoma.[116] Although the fledgling regional agency assisted countries in combating communicable diseases— as delineated by WHO headquarters—Fang emphasized the need to strengthen the health services of member states.[117] Maternal and Child Health was described as one of the essential functions of any health system.

WPRO partnered with UNICEF to improve nursing and midwifery education in the Western Pacific. Beyond increasing the number of auxiliary midwives, the regional agency also developed training programs for traditional birth attendants, particularly in the Philippines. According to

Fang, these programs served as stopgap measures to provide better care at the time of delivery until adequate numbers of trained midwives were available. Moreover, traditional birth attendants helped bridge the gap between formal health services and the wider community.[118]

In 1951, WPRO exhorted member states to eliminate endemic diseases such as malaria, tuberculosis, and yaws, and epidemic diseases such as diphtheria. Specific WPRO-assisted projects included Malaria and Insect Control Projects in Cambodia and Vietnam, and a rural health training and demonstration center in the Philippines.[119] Following these early priority-setting efforts, WPRO diverted to a pressing health problem: schistosomiasis in the Philippines, a disease that stunts children's growth.

In 1952, US Ambassador to the Philippines R.A. Spruance declared that the primary aim of American technical assistance to the Philippines was to check the advance of the Huks.[120] He observed that ineffective efforts to combat schistosomiasis and other endemic diseases—particularly malaria—stunted development in Mindoro and Mindanao, resulting in poverty and low living standards: conditions congenial for the spread of communism.

The WHO, UNICEF, and the Philippine Health Department jointly instituted a schistosomiasis control project in Leyte, Samar, and Mindoro in the Visayas and on the island of Luzon. Between 1949 and 1950, the WHO conducted a random stool survey in which 39,127 of 39,604 individuals tested positive for schistosomiasis.[121] A control project commenced in Palo, Leyte province, in 1953. Case detection through surveys and treatment using fuadin injections formed the program's core. However, accessibility challenges led many patients to prematurely discontinue therapy. To address these barriers, WPRO introduced mobile treatment units.

As a precaution against schistosomiasis, Filipino health authorities disinfected snail-infested streams. These efforts expanded into three environmental engineering experiments: the removal of weeds, draining of waterlogged areas, and digging fishponds. In each of the three experiments, the snail population declined, and the campaign eventually tripled agricultural yields.[122]

Provincial health officials supervised the implementation of the anti-schistosomiasis campaign. However, administrative changes during the mid-1950s disrupted these efforts, undermining the long-term impact of the otherwise successful environmental interventions.

In 1954, President Ramon Magsaysay enacted the Rural Health Act, mandating the establishment of rural health units across municipal districts.[123] The Philippine Department of Health directed municipal health officers to embed schistosomiasis control within the broader contours of public health programming—encompassing health education, sanitation, and communicable disease management. Yet financial constraints impeded the campaign's reach, limiting national scalability. Filipino planners, however, framed schistosomiasis control as more than a biomedical intervention: the campaign provided an impetus for addressing the structural determinants of health within a community development framework.

The Palo schistosomiasis demonstration and control project exemplified how a narrowly targeted disease control campaign could be informed by—and responsive to—broader community development initiatives across the Western Pacific. Concurrently, the Ministry of Health in Malaya set up the Jitra health demonstration and training center at Kedah with assistance from WPRO and UNICEF.

Attention to rural health in Malaya was concomitant with the onset of the Emergency (1948). Soon after the Pacific War—as the colonial authorities were rebuilding the Malayan economy—the Malayan Communist Party attempted to seize power from the British. By 1950, Harold Briggs, director of anti-communist forces, introduced a resettlement plan to deprive the communists of essential supplies. The Briggs Plan relocated 12 million civilians, particularly the *Orang Asli* [Malay: Indigenous People] and the Chinese, to 600 New Villages.[124] The plan attempted to sever the communists' support base. Lee Tiang Keng, Malaya's Minister of Health between 1951 and 1956, proposed providing state dispensaries in New Villages. However, the colonial government in Malaya—preoccupied with counterinsurgency operations—rejected Keng's proposal. Health problems in the New Villages included widespread prevalence of malaria, even as the disease largely remained under control in urban areas.[125]

The Government of the Federation of Malaya drafted a tentative rural health program for the period from 1954 to 1956. The program incorporated midwife training, establishing one subdistrict health center per 10,000 people, and creating a district health center serving 50,000 individuals.[126] The initiative was supported by the Colonial Development Fund (Image 4.5).

Malaya's plan to expand rural health services was overambitious. In August 1957, as the country achieved independence from the UK, public health underwent an administrative overhaul. The Federal government assumed responsibility for organizing health services in each state of the

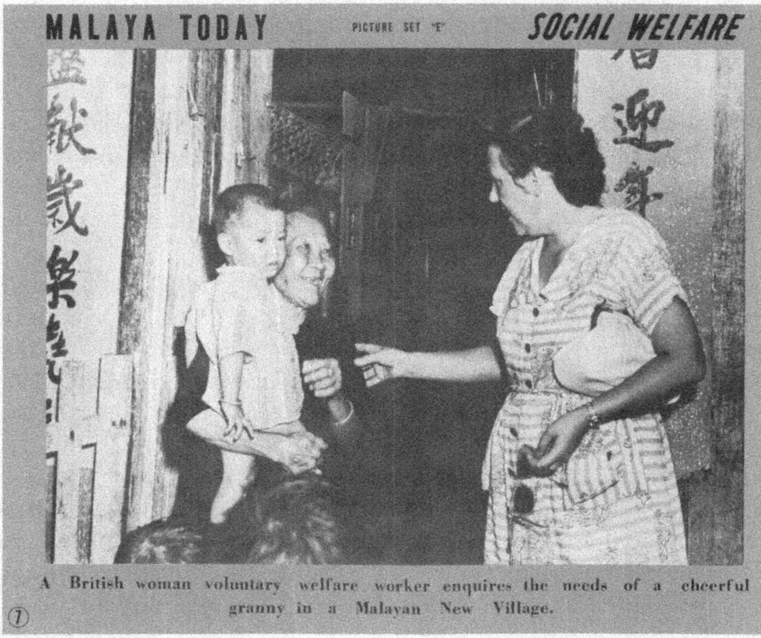

Image 4.5 Malaya Today: Social Welfare. Date Created: November 17, 1953. National Archives Identifier: 5729989. Agency-Assigned Identifier: PO–209–E(7). Local ID: 306–PPA–88. Record Group 306: Records of the US Information Agency. Series: Propaganda Posters Distributed in Asia, 1950–1955. Creator: US Information Agency. NARA. URL: https://catalog.archives.gov/id/5729989. Copyright: Unrestricted (Public Domain)

Malayan federation. As land was a state subject, the Federal government struggled to acquire sites for health centers.[127] Although the rural health training center in Jitra churned out midwives, nurses, and sanitary overseers, Malaya's real need was for doctors willing to serve in rural areas.[128] Another obstacle for post-independence expansion was the lack of morbidity and mortality data for rural areas, which complicated health planning.[129]

For the post-independent state in Malaya, the rural health scheme was an indispensable tool in countervailing the Emergency. In the words of a *Straits Times* article:

> If the rural population is to have any faith in democracy, it must be convinced that democracy can improve their lot. Efficient medical and health services in the rural areas will be more convincing than the discourses on democracy.[130]

The quote underscores that the success of democracy in Malaya hinged upon the government's ability to meet the material needs of rural communities. By demonstrating tangible improvements in health services, the government sought to instill the local population's confidence in democratic governance—making medical care a more persuasive instrument than ideological rhetoric.

Whereas Malayan authorities positioned rural health as an adjunct to democratic governance, the Western Pacific malaria eradication program foregrounded disease control as a tool to maximize economic productivity. Between 1958 and 1966—when the WHO introduced the malaria eradication program to the Republic of Vietnam—infection rates declined from 7.2 percent to 1 percent.[131] The WHO and ICA supported the initiative, though disruptions arose from Việt Minh suspicion that Americans gathered military intelligence under the guise of a malaria eradication program. At the same time, a local rumor gained traction, alleging that "American DDT spray" killed the cats that ate the rats that devastated the crops.[132] The rumor formed the main plank of anti-US resistance in the central lowlands, linking ecological disruption to geopolitical distrust (Image 4.6).

Between 1955 and 1962, Arthur Brown, WHO Area Representative in Vietnam, highlighted additional factors that contributed to failure of the eradication campaign. These included anopheline species developing resistance to DDT.[133] He argued that from the start of malaria eradication in 1955, there was hubris within the WHO and member states about the efficacy of insecticide DDT in eradicating malaria. Consequently, the organization paid little attention to interacting economic, cultural, and logistical problems associated with the disease.[134]

The shortcomings of malaria eradication dislodged the aura of certainty surrounding the proverbial magic bullet approach. The onset of the Seventh Cholera Pandemic in 1961 exposed operational blind spots concerning disease eradication. By 1962—as El Tor cholera spread through the Western Pacific—Fang asserted that the solution to the outbreak was not communicable disease control alone but strengthening environmental sanitation and controlling disease vectors. Fang emphasized the

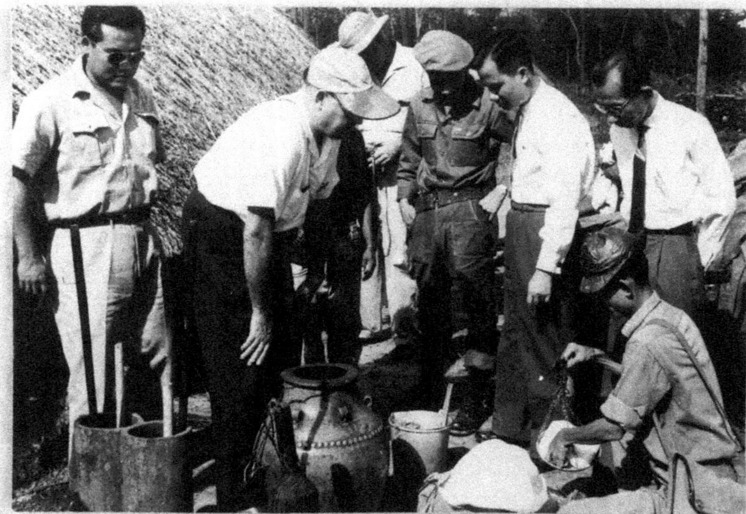

Image 4.6 Malaria Control Program in Vietnam: Rural Health Encounters a Global Program. Local health workers stand outside a grass hut, surrounded by containers for spraying or storing DDT (mid-1950s to early 1960s). These vessels bridge rural tactility with global mandates. Courtesy of the National Library of Medicine. NLM Unique ID: 101446950. NLM Image ID: A018328. Persistent URL: http://resource.nlm.nih.gov/101446950?. Public Domain

interconnection between health and socioeconomic development, urging governments in the Western Pacific to ensure an equilibrium between economic activities and appropriate public health interventions, rather than enforcing stringent quarantines.[135] Fang's skepticism toward the magic bullet approach reflected WPRO's strategic recalibration from 1951 to 1962, as the focus shifted from controlling endemic diseases to the training of auxiliary health personnel.

Many of the regional agency's activities during its formative years were focused on gathering baseline data. Early WPRO documents reflected ambiguity about disease prevalence in member states. For example, one of the regional agency's earliest published documents refers to a malariologist who gathered "considerable data" on malaria and other diseases in Cambodia.[136] The Second WPRO Session mentions that the WHO offered a short-term fellowship to the Director of the Philippines Treponematoses (Yaws) Control Program to study yaws control in Thailand and Indonesia.[137]

During its formative years, WPRO's regional training program operated on an ad hoc basis, responding to member states for technical assistance. In 1953, the agency sponsored eight Laotian students to train at Cambodia's Ecole des Officers de Santé in Phnom Penh, citing shared economic conditions and Cambodia's comparatively lower training costs within the Western Pacific.[138]

Although WPRO facilitated regional medical training programs throughout the 1950s, some states—particularly Singapore—opted for localized workforce development. The British Crown colony not only trained personnel domestically but also recruited doctors from India, the UK, and the Commonwealth to address shortages.[139] Simultaneously, the University of Malaya partnered with WPRO to launch a postgraduate diploma in rural and industrial health.[140]

While Singapore collaborated with WPRO on training health personnel, Fang delineated broader structural challenges that interfered with the effective implementation of regional health programs. He noted that one major obstacle for the regional organization during its early years was the ambiguity among member states regarding the purpose of WHO technical assistance: to assist governments upon request, rather than providing supplementary staff. In resource-constrained WPRO states such as Cambodia, Laos, and Malaya, WHO personnel were frequently misperceived as "extra hands" administering routine public health activities.[141] This misunderstanding not only strained WPRO's resources but also weakened national health systems by fostering a chronic dependence on external aid. The sustainability of WPRO-supported projects was contingent on the country's ability to absorb overseas technical assistance, the availability of trained medical personnel, and political stability.

Conclusion: A Southeast Asian Approach to Health?

Amrith argues that there was a remarkable similarity in the health policies adopted by polities as different as India, Indonesia, and Burma within the broader "Southeast Asian Approach to Health." Each of the three states adopted the WHO's definition of priorities and its definition of health in terms of clearly distinguishable causes of death. Across Southeast Asia, each state had a malaria control organization, undertook mass BCG vaccination campaigns, and followed the lead of the WHO. Yet, in none of these states was public health a priority in government spending.[142] However, it is unclear from Amrith's argument whether the broad Southeast Asian approach to health was identical to the Bandung Spirit. The Bandung Spirit—which emerged in the aftermath of the Asian-African Conference (1955)—advocated an independent foreign policy, solidarity with newly independent nations, and economic self-sufficiency. Alternatively, SEARO and WPRO may have reflected a distinct regional approach to international health.

The trajectory of the WHO in South-East Asia and the Western Pacific suggests that there were few distinctly regional health programs during the 1950s, apart from SEARO and WPRO fellowship schemes for medical officers and undergraduate students. Both regional bodies collated requests from member states for technical assistance. During their early years, they were less concerned about developing a balanced regional program than with representing member states' interest at the WHO headquarters. Until 1953, neither SEARO nor WPRO related health programs to work already undertaken by other agencies or the recipient country's capacity to absorb international technical assistance. Both SEARO and WPRO tailored WHO assistance to align with local requirements.

A conspicuous difference between SEARO's and WPRO's regional health orientation was apparent around 1958, when the WHO launched the Global Program to Eradicate Smallpox at the Eleventh WHA. WPRO played a minimal role in the Smallpox Eradication program because the disease was not of serious health concern to the Western Pacific by the 1950s. Conversely, smallpox remained endemic in South-East Asia, particularly in India and Indonesia. In January 1958, SEARO issued a questionnaire to member states seeking details on vaccination infrastructure. Using comparative data, the agency examined causes of persistent prevalence and instituted pilot eradication initiatives.[143] By 1967, Mani was unalterably opposed to the WHO headquarters' eradication mandate. Given SEARO's challenges in implementing a broad spectrum of projects, Mani found it difficult to mobilize sufficient resources and personnel for smallpox eradication.[144]

Despite operational constraints, regional health organizations in Southeast Asia played a vital role in mediating international aid. SEARO and WPRO aligned WHO prescriptions to local conditions, yet member states of both regional agencies faced challenges in synchronizing national health priorities with WHO prescriptions. Western donors imposed technical assistance on newly independent nations of Southeast Asia, without regard for absorption capacity or sustainability of health projects once aid ceased. Bilateral aid from the Western Bloc to Southeast Asia overshadowed the UN program of technical assistance. Such assistance frequently came with political or economic strings attached.[145] Support for environmental sanitation in SEARO and WPRO suffered due to the vicissitudes of overseas funding. In response, both regional health organizations sought to steer public health priorities toward actionable goals, rather than aligning with the aspirational national agendas of individual postcolonial states.

Notes

1. Socialized medicine is a term for universal healthcare. During the 1950s, in the US, the term had taken on a pejorative connotation in discussing any aspect of government-controlled healthcare. For details see Henry Buchwald, *Healthcare Upside Down: A Critical Examination of Policy and Practice* (Cham: Springer Nature, 2022), 61.
2. Javed Siddiqi, *World Health and World Politics: The World Health Organization and the UN System* (London: Hurst and Company, 1995). See also Elizabeth Fee, Marcos Cueto and Theodore Brown, "At the Roots of the World Health Organization's Challenges: Politics and Regionalization," *American Journal of Public Health* 106, no. 11 (2016): 11–16.
3. Howard Calderwood, "The World Health Organization and its Regional Organizations," *Temple Law Quarterly* 37, no. 1 (1963): 15–27, 16.
4. For an overall understanding of regionalization, see Fee, Brown, and Cueto's "At the Roots of World Health Organization's Challenges." To understand the specific context of regionalization in Latin America, consult Marcos Cueto, *The Value of Health: A History of the Pan American Health Organization* (Washington DC: PAHO, 2006).

   For an insight into how decolonization posed challenges to the WHO's program in Africa, see Jessica Lynn-Pearson, *The Colonial Politics of Global Health: France and the United Nations in Postwar Africa* (Harvard: Harvard University Press, 2018) 3–4. Lynn-Pearson argues that the WHO faced significant challenges in Africa due to hindrances by colonial officials and the establishment of the WHO Regional Office for Africa.

   For South-East Asia, see Monica Saavedra, "Politics and Health in the WHO Regional Office for South East Asia: The Case of Portuguese India, 1949–61," *Medical History* 61, no. 3 (2017): 380–400.

Through the lens of Portuguese Goa's decolonization, Saavedra contends that SEARO priorities from 1949 to 1961 reflected shifting colonial, postcolonial, and international configurations—frequently subordinating health to politics.

5. Amrith, *Decolonizing International Health*, 14.
6. For a SEARO case study, see Vivek Neelakantan, "The Monsoon Asia of Geographers: The Cold War Beginnings of the WHO Regional Office for Southeast Asia (SEARO), 1948–60," in *The Geopolitics of Health in South and Southeast Asia: Perspectives from the Cold War to COVID-19*, Vivek Neelakantan edited (Abingdon, Oxon.: Routledge, 2023), 27–52.
7. For details, see Neville Goodman, "The World Health Organisation and its Interim Commission," *The Lancet* (September 1946): 358–59.
8. Szeming Sze, *The Origins of the World Health Organization: A Personal Memoir* (Boca Raton: L.I.S.Z. Publications, 1982), xiii + 31 pp., Szeming Sze Papers, University of Pittsburgh Digital Collections. Accessed August 19, 2024. https://digital.library.pitt.edu/collection/szeming-sze-papers.

   Szeming Sze Papers, University of Pittsburgh Digital Collections.
9. Amrith, *Decolonizing International Health*, 73–74.
10. See Marcos Cueto, Theodore Brown, and Elizabeth Fee, *The World Health Organization: A History* (Cambridge: Cambridge University Press, 2019), 38.
11. Cueto, Brown, and Fee, *The World Health Organization*, 39.
12. For details, see George Woodbridge, *UNRRA: A History of the United Nations Relief and Rehabilitation Administration* volume I (New York: Columbia University Press, 1950), 304.
13. "Transcript of an Oral Interview with Professor Milton Siegel by Gino Levy and Norman Howard Jones," November 15–19, 1982, WHO Archives, Geneva [hereafter WHOA]. Accessed August 26, 2024. https://cdn.who.int/media/docs/default-source/documents/about-us/milton_siegel_tapes.pdf?sfvrsn=1bb7402_1&download=true.
14. United Nations Economic and Social Council, "Technical Preparatory Committee for the International Health Conference: Summary Record of the Seventh Meeting Held on March 22, 1946," Doc. E/H/PC/17, UN Digital Library, New York. Accessed August 26, 2024. https://digitallibrary.un.org/record/3845241.
15. Theodore Brown, "Andrija Štampar: Charismatic Leader of Social Medicine and Public Health," *American Journal of Public Health* 96, no. 2 (2006): 1382–85. Štampar was the director of public health of Yugoslavia between 1919 and 1931 and was deputed to China as a LNHO expert between 1933 and 1938.

16. "Constitution of the World Health Organization," *Basic Documents* 49th Edition (Geneva: WHO, 2020). Accessed August 27, 2024. https://apps.who.int/gb/bd/pdf_files/BD_49th-en.pdf#page=6.
17. Raymond Gautier, "International Health of the Future," March 15, 1943, Postwar Health Problems: International Health Organization 1943, Doc. R6150/8A/42169/47155, LoN Archives.
18. Andrija Štampar, "Suggestions Related to the Constitution of an International Health Organization," Annex 9, March 20, 1946, *Official Records of the World Health Organization: Minutes of the Technical Preparatory Committee for the International Health Conference Held in Paris from 18 March to April 5, 1946*, no.1 (New York: UN WHO Interim Commission, 1947), WHO Library and Historical Collections, Geneva (hereafter WHOL).
19. Sara Silverstein, "Man with an Impossible Mission? Andrija Štampar's Separation of Politics and Healthcare in Yugoslavia and the World Health Organization," *Rockefeller Archive Center Research Reports* (2013), https://rockarch.issuelab.org/resources/27898/27898.pdf.
20. Christian Burckel, *Who's Who in the United Nations*, Christian Burckel edited (New York: Christian Burckel and Associates, 1951).
21. C. Mani and Szeming Sze, "Proposals on Regional Arrangements," Doc. E/H/PC/W/11, Annex 19, March 27, 1946, *Official Records of the World Health Organization: Minutes of the Technical Preparatory Committee for the International Health Conference Held in Paris from 18 March to April 5, 1946*, no.1 (New York: UN WHO Interim Commission, 1947), WHOL.
22. Sze, *The Origins of the World Health Organization*.
23. Cueto, Brown and Fee, *The World Health Organization*, 45.
24. "Report of the Activities of the Interim Commission of the WHO," January 1947–December 1950, Report E/786 WHO, File 14, Doc. S-1560-0000-0014-00001, UNA.
25. Walter Sharp, "The New World Health Organization," *American Journal of International* Law 41, no. 3 (1947): 409–30, 515.
26. "Summary Report on the Proceedings."
27. Sharp, "The New World Health Organization," 516.
28. Sharp, "The New World Health Organization," 517.
29. "Report of the Activities of the Interim Commission of the WHO."
30. Ibid.
31. "Note on the British Position Regarding the Reopening of the Eastern Bureau," Signed by Yves M. Biraud, April 30, 1946, Eastern Bureau Singapore: Reopening of the Bureau, Transfer of Assets to the World Health Organization, Doc. 6199/8D/43551/347, LoN Archives.

32. Kayo Takuma, "The Far Eastern Bureau of the League of Nations: Linking the Regional and International Orders Through Health Work," in *East Asians in the League of Nations: Actors, Empires, and Regions in Early Global Politics*, Christopher Hughes and Hatsue Shinahora edited (Basingstoke: Palgrave Macmillan, 2023), 61–80, 69.
33. Takuma, "The Far Eastern Bureau," 73.
34. WPRO, *Sixth Annual Report of the Regional Director to the Regional Committee for the Western Pacific: Regional Committee Seventh Session*, July 12, 1956, Doc. WP/RC7/3, WHOL.
35. WHO Interim Commission, "Delimitation of Regional Health Areas on an Epidemiological Basis," March 31, 1947, Doc. WHO IC//61 (Rev.1), Subject 452, Series 1, File 5, *WHO First Generation Files* (*WHO.I*), WHOA.
36. *Report of the Indian Delegate to the First Session of the World Health Assembly Held in Geneva from 24 June to 24 July 1948* (New Delhi: Government of India Press, 1948), 3.
37. "Henry van Zile Hyde Oral History Interview by Richard D. McKinzie," July 16, 1975, Harry S. Truman Presidential Museum and Library. Accessed September 5, 2024. https://www.trumanlibrary.gov/library/oral-histories/hydehvz1#.
38. Neelakantan, "The Monsoon Asia of Geographers," 33.
39. "First World Health Assembly: Definition of Geographical Areas," Doc. A/20, June 28, 1948, Regional Organizations: Definitions of Geographical Areas, Various Correspondence, Subject 900, Series 1, File 1, *WHO.I*, WHOA.
40. "WHO Southeast Asia Regional Office Recommends New Delhi as Headquarters Site for Regional Organization," Office of the United Nations at Geneva Press Release Center, Press Release No. 639, Southeast Asia: Correspondence Concerning General organization of the Regional Office, Subject 902, Series 1, File 1, *WHO.I*, WHOA.
41. Vivek Neelakantan, "Indonesian Health Policy between the Old and the New Orders," in *Public Health and Cold War Politics in Asia*, Liping Bu edited (Abingdon, Oxon: Routledge, 2023), 151–76, 154.
42. "Letter from Johannes Leimena, Minister of Health to the WHO Headquarters, Geneva," March 9, 1950, Member Governments: Indonesia, Doc. WHO2_OD_14 C, *WHO Second Generation Files* (*WHO.II*), WHOA; See also Note from Bahder Djohan, "Chief Indonesian Delegate to the Third World Health Assembly," May 12, 1950, Doc. WHO2_OD_14 C, *WHO.II*, WHOA.
43. "Malaya can Join WHO," *The Straits Times*, September 9, 1948, 4, NLB.

44. "Malaya in New Health Scheme," *The Straits Times*, September 1, 1948, 6, The National Library Board, Singapore (NLB). See also "Malaya and WHO Membership," *The Straits Times*, September 8, 1948, 5, NLB.
45. At the Asian Relations Conference (1947), delegates from Malaya, Burma, and Ceylon drew attention to the economically and demographically exploitative nature of the Indian and Chinese communities in the region. For details see Vineet Thakur, "An Asian Drama: The Asian Relations Conference of 1947," *The International History Review* 41, no. 3 (2019): 673–85, 681.
46. WHA Resolution 3.119, "Temporary Assignment of the State of Vietnam and the Kingdom of Cambodia and Laos to the South-East Asia Region: Resolutions Adopted Without Reference to a Main Committee," *Official Records of the World Health Organization: Third World Health Assembly*, May 8 to May 27, 1950, no. 28 (Geneva: WHO, 1950), WHOL.
47. "Regional Office Agenda 8.19: Proposal of the Delegate of the Philippines for the Establishment of a Regional Office for the Western Pacific," *Official Records of the World Health Organization: Second World Health Assembly*, June 13 to July 2, 1949, no. 21 (Geneva: WHO, 1949), WHOL.
48. Ibid.
49. "Seventeenth Meeting," May 20, 1950, *Official Records of the World Health Organization: Third World Health Assembly*, May 8 to May 27, 1950, no. 28 (Geneva: WHO, 1950), WHOL.
50. Cueto, Brown and Fee, *The World Health Organization*, 75.
51. "Seventeenth Meeting."
52. "Eighth Plenary Meeting," May 27, 1950, *Official Records of the World Health Organization: The Third World Health Assembly*, May 2 to May 27, 1950, no. 28 (Geneva: WHO, 1950), WHOL.
53. Ibid.
54. "Letter from Martha May Eliot to Melville Mackenzie," June 16, 1950, WPRO: Regions and Regional Offices, Western Pacific Regional Office, Doc. WHO 2_OD_20_7, *WHO.II*, WHOA.
55. United Nations Office in Geneva Press Center, "World Health Organization: WHO Office for Western Pacific," July 6, 1950, Press Release WHO/74, WPRO: Regions and Regional Offices, Western Pacific Regional Office, Doc. WHO 2_OD_20_7, *WHO.II*, WHOA.
56. Burckel, *Who's Who*.
57. United Nations Office in Geneva Press Center, "World Health Organization."
58. "Letter from I.C. Fang to Martha May Eliot, Assistant Director General, WHO," July 13, 1950, WPRO: Regions and Regional Offices, Western Pacific Regional Office, Doc. WHO 2_OD_20_7, *WHO.II*, WHOA.
59. Ibid.

60. Ibid.
61. Kelley Lee, *The World Health Organization* (Abingdon, Oxon: Routledge, 2009), 14.
62. "Fifth Plenary Meeting," June 26, 1948, *Official Records of the World Health Organization: The Third World Health Assembly*, June 24 to July 24, 1948, no. 13 (Geneva: WHO, 1948), WHOL.
63. Ibid.
64. Fee, Cueto, and Brown, "At the Roots of the World Health Organization's Challenges," 1912.
65. "Russia Co-operation," *The Singapore Free Press*, July 6, 1951, 4, NLB.
66. Fee, Cueto, and Brown, "At the Roots of the World Health Organization's Challenges," 1913.
67. "Russia Co-operation."
68. Fee, Cueto, and Brown, "At the Roots of the World Health Organization's Challenges," 1913.
69. Ibid., 35.
70. Ibid., 35.
71. "The Second World Health Assembly: Points from Speeches, Andrija Štampar," *Chronicle of the World Health Organization* 3, nos. 8, 9, and 10 (1949): 221, WHOL.
72. Cueto, Brown, and Fee, *The World Health Organization*, 63.
73. Amrith, *Decolonizing International Health*, 86.
74. "Committee on Programme: Second Meeting," June 30, 1948, *Official Records of the World Health Organization: First World Health Assembly*, June 24 to July 24, 1948, no. 13 (Geneva: WHO, 1948), WHOL.
75. Neelakantan, "The Monsoon Asia of Geographers," 35.
76. *The World Health Organization: Twenty Years in South-East Asia, 1948–67* (New Delhi: SEARO, 1967), 33, WHOL.
77. *The World Health Organization*, 70.
78. "WHO Nurse Tells of Two Years' Work in South India," *Indian Daily Mail*, March 3, 1952, 4, NLB.
79. SEARO, *Third Annual Report of the Regional Director to the Regional Committee for South-East Asia: Regional Committee Fourth Session*, September 20 to 25, 1951 (New Delhi: SEARO, 1951), WHOL.
80. "WHO Nurse Tells of Two Years' Work."
81. *Third Annual Report of the Regional Director to the Regional Committee for South-East Asia*.
82. Malaria control operations commenced in June, at the height of the monsoon season that coincides with malaria transmission.
83. *Third Annual Report of the Regional Director to the Regional Committee for South-East Asia*.

84. "Letter from Cora Du Bois to C. Mani," Preliminary Report 12: Comments on Malarial Control, June 6, 1950, File Reports on the Field from Cora Du Bois to SEARO, March to June 1950, Box 7, *Cora Du Bois Papers*, Tozzer Library, Harvard University.
85. Neelakantan, "The Monsoon Asia of Geographers," 37.
86. Ibid.
87. Ernestine S. Thurman, "Asia: A Challenge to Scientists," *AIBS Bulletin* 12, no. 1 (1962): 24–27, 24.
88. G. Sambasivan and Udon Pranith, "Report of Government/ WHO/ UNICEF Malaria Control Demonstration Projects for Period August 1949 to December 1951," Doc. WHO 22/SEARO/THA/60, *WHO Project Files*, WHOA.
89. G. Sambasivan, "Malaria Control Teams: Chiangmai, Thailand: Report of WHO/UNICEF Malaria Control Project for August 9, 1949 to March 31, 1950," Doc. WHO 22/SEARO/THA/60, *WHO Project Files*, WHOA.
90. Letter from Cora Du Bois to E.J. Pampana, "Preliminary Report No. 31: Some Social Resistance to Spraying," WHO Field Reports: Typed Carbon Copy, August to September 1950, Box 67, *Cora Du Bois Papers*, Tozzer Library, Harvard University.
91. Thurman, " Asia," 24.
92. "Letter from C. Mani, SEARO Regional Director to C. Bonne, WHO Headquarters, Geneva," May 11, 1949, Southeast Asia: Program of Activities, Subject 902 Regional Organizations, Series 1, File 1, *WHO.I*, WHOA.
93. For details see Justus van der Kroef, "Point Four in Southeast Asia," *Current History* 22, no. 128 (1952): 193–99.
94. See P.W.E Curtin, "Effect of the Colombo Plan," *Pakistan Horizon* 7, no. 2 (1954): 76–79. The original members of the Colombo Plan from South and Southeast Asia comprised Pakistan, India, and Ceylon, while external members were the UK, Canada, Australia, and New Zealand. Thailand was not a member of the Colombo Plan but was receiving assistance from Colombo Plan members.
95. See also Nicholas Tarling, "The United Kingdom and the Origins of the Colombo Plan," The *Journal of Commonwealth and Comparative Politics* 24, no. 1 (2008):3–34.
96. Neelakantan, "The Monsoon Asia of Geographers," 39.
97. C. Mani, "The Health Problem of South-East Asia: The South-East Asia Region of the World Health Organisation," *The Straits Times*, March 4, 1952, 6, NLB.
98. "Communique of the Bandung Conference," *Current Science* 26, no. 166 (1955): 371–75.

99. "Text of Welcome by Dr. J. Leimena, Minister of Health, Government of the Republic of Indonesia," September 10, 1955, Annex 1, Doc. SEA/RC8/Min.1/ Rev. 1 *Report of the Eighth Session of the World Health Organization Regional Committee for South-East Asia* (New Delhi: SEARO, 1955), WHOL.
100. Neelakantan, "The Monsoon Asia of Geographers," 43.
101. Socrates Litsios, "Cora Du Bois Brief Stint with the World Health Organization, 1950–51): Right Time, Wrong Place," *International Journal for Health Services* 48, no. 4 (2018): 716–34.
102. Vivek Neelakantan, "The Campaign Against the Big Four Endemic Diseases and Indonesia's Engagement with the WHO during the Cold War 1950s," in *Public Health and National Reconstruction in Post-War Asia: International Influences, Local Transformations*, Liping Bu and Ka-che Yip edited (Abingdon, Oxon: Routledge, 2014), 154–74.
103. Randall Packard, *A History of Global Health: Interventions into the Lives of Other Peoples* (Baltimore, MD: Johns Hopkins University Press, 2016), 113.
104. See SEARO, *Fourth Annual Report of the Regional Director to the Regional Committee for South-East Asia,* Doc. SEA/RC 5/2 (New Delhi: SEARO, 1952), WHOL.
105. Neelakantan, "The Monsoon Asia of Geographers," 43.
106. Ibid., 43.
107. See Neelakantan, "The Campaign Against the Big Four Endemic Diseases," 160.
108. Neelakantan, "The Monsoon Asia of Geographers," 44.
109. V.T.H. Gunaratne, *A Voyage to Health* (New Delhi: Tata MacGraw-Hill Publication Company, 1980), WHOL.
110. Neelakantan, "The Monsoon Asia of Geographers," 44.
111. SEARO, *Report of the Thirteenth Session of the Regional Committee for South-East Asia Held in Bandung from August 22 to August 29, 1960*, Doc. SEA/RC13/16/ Rev.1 (New Delhi: SEARO, 1960), WHOL.
112. Ibid.
113. Atsuko Naono, "Rural Health in Modern Southeast Asia," in *Histories of Health in Southeast Asia; Perspectives on the Long Twentieth Century*, Tim Harpe and Sunil Amrith edited (Bloomington: Indiana University Press, 2014), 99–117.
114. Neelakantan, "Indonesian Health Policy," 161–62.
115. I.C. Fang, "Editorial," *World Health: Magazine of the World Health Organization* (April 1965): 3.
116. WPRO, *Fifty Years of the World Health Organization in the Western Pacific Region* (Manila: WPRO, 1998), WHOL.
117. Ibid.

118. Ibid.
119. WPRO, *Report of the Regional Director: Regional Committee Second Session*, September 1952, Doc. WP/RC2/10 (Manila: WPRO, 1952), WHOL.
120. The Hukbalahap were organized in March 1942 to resist the Japanese occupation of the Philippines. In the aftermath of the Pacific War, Huks capitalized on socio-economic issues in central Luzon, which were associated with severe population pressure on land and unequal landlord-tenant relationships. The economic objectives of the Huks—delineated in 1946 and 1950—reflected a distinct communist influence. For a nuanced understanding of the Huk Movement, see Russell H. Fifield, "The Hukbalahap Today," *Far Eastern Survey* 20, no. 2 (1951): 13–18.
121. "Preliminary Proposal for a Program to Control Schistosomiasis and Other Parasitic Diseases in the Philippines," File Philippines 9A: OCD Bilharziasis, Doc. WHO022/WPRO/PHL/109, *Project Files*, WHOA.
122. "Memorandum from I.C. Fang, WPRO Regional Director to N. Ansari," Annex I: Integrated Bilharziasis Control into the Total Health Program of the Local Health Services, File Philippines 9A. OCD Bilharziasis, Doc. WHO022/WPRO/PHL/109, *Project Files*, WHOA.
123. Vivek Neelakantan, "'No Nation Can Go Forward When it is Crippled by Disease': Philippine Science and the Cold War, 1946–65," *Southeast Asian Studies* 10, no. 1 (2021): 53–88, 63.
124. For a detailed account assessing the impact of the Malayan Emergency on public health, see Por Heong Hong, "Tool of Domination and Act of Benevolence: Medicine and Healthcare during the Malayan Emergency, 1948–60," in *Fighting for Health: Medicine in Cold War Southeast Asia*, C. Michele Thompson, Kathryn Sweet, and Michitake Aso (Singapore: NUS Press, 2024), 53–83, 55.
125. Remedios Estrada, "Public Health Administration Rural Health Training Centre: Final Report," November 1954 to 1959," File Malaya 9, Doc. WHO022/WPRO/MAA/105, *Project Files*, WHOA.
126. L.W. Jayesuria, *A Review of the Rural Health Services in West Malaysia* (Kuala Lumpur: Ministry of Health, 1967), 2.
127. Jeyasuriya, *A Review of Rural Health Services*, 4.
128. "Rural Health," *The Straits Times*, November 6, 1957, 8, NLB.
129. "Health in the Kampongs," *The Straits Times*, October 16, 1959, 6, NLB.
130. "Rural Health."
131. Michitake Aso, "Patriotic Hygiene: Tracing New Places of Knowledge Production About Malaria in Vietnam, 1919–75," *Journal of Southeast Asian Studies* 44, no. 3 (2013): 423–43, 433
132. Homer Bigart, "A DDT Tale Aids Reds in Vietnam," *New York Times*, February 2, 1962, 3; See also Patrick O' Shaughnessy, "Parachuting Cats

and Crushed Eggs: The Controversy Over the Use of DDT to Control Malaria," *American Journal of Public Health* 98, no. 11 (2008): 1940–48, 1942.

133. Arthur Brown, "Personal Experiences in the Malaria Eradication Campaign, 1955–1962," *Journal of the Royal Society of Medicine* 95 (March 2002): 154–56. 156.
134. Ibid., 156.
135. WPRO, *Report of the Regional Committee: Minutes of the Plenary Sessions, Minutes of the Sub-Committee, Program and Budget Thirteenth Session*, October 1962, Doc. WP/RC13/p&B/Min/l Rev.l (Manila: WPRO, 1962), WHOL.
136. WPRO, *Report of the Regional Director: Regional Committee Second Session*.
137. Ibid.
138. WPRO, *Report of the Regional Director: Regional Committee Fourth Session*, August 1953, Doc. WP/RC4/2 (Manila: WPRO, 1953), WHOL.
139. E.S. Monteiro, "International Cooperation in Postgraduate Medical Education in Malaya," *The British Medical Journal* 2, no. 5148 (1959): 330–32, 330.
140. Ibid., 330.
141. WPRO, *Sixth Annual Report of the Regional Director to the Regional Committee for the Western Pacific*.
142. Amrith, *Decolonizing International Health*, 102.
143. SEARO, *Twelfth Annual Report of the Regional Director*, August 1959 to August 1960, Doc. SEA/RC13/2 (New Delhi: SEARO, 1960), WHOL.
144. Sanjoy Bhattacharya, *Expunging Variola: The Control and Eradication of Smallpox in India* (Hyderabad: Orient Longman, 2006), 144–45.
145. Neelakantan, "The Monsoon Asia of Geographers," 46.

CHAPTER 5

"Half of the World's Children": History of the UNICEF Regional Office for Asia (ARO), 1948–1961

Introduction

On December 11, 1946, the First Session of the UN General Assembly established UNICEF (United Nations Children's Fund) as a temporary relief agency for children affected by World War II.[1] UNICEF's concern for children across Asia stemmed from its broader mandate to support all war-affected children. While Japan dominated much of Southeast Asia during the Pacific War, the postwar challenges were anything but uniform. During the late 1940s—from the plains of the Punjab to the streets of Saigon—Asia was in a state of political and social flux. While the US conceded independence to the Philippines in 1946, the British extracted themselves from the South Asian subcontinent in 1947. The following year, Burma and Ceylon became independent. Fighting broke out in Indochina in 1946 after the French tried to reassert their control. Between 1945 and 1949, Indonesia was enmeshed in revolutionary struggle against the Dutch. Administering emergency relief across a politically fragmented region with over 450 million children posed a formidable challenge for the nascent UNICEF amid the transition from colonial rule to independence.[2]

International aid agencies could draw a superficial comparison between war-devastated Europe and Asia. However, there was a noticeable difference between the temporary nature of relief in Europe and the more

V. Neelakantan, *The Emergence of International Health Policy in Southeast Asia, India, and Sri Lanka, 1937–1978*,
https://doi.org/10.1007/978-3-032-21233-7_5

permanent nature of relief for those in Asia. In postwar Asia, as over 80 percent of the population inhabited rural areas with limited access to health facilities, millions of mothers and children endured chronic hunger and malnutrition. UNICEF could not discuss an emergency or relief program without addressing the root causes of poverty and deprivation. In the words of Maggie Black, "Asia defied a definition of the word emergency."[3]

This chapter assesses how UNICEF's Regional Office for Asia (ARO) delineated regional health priorities.[4] Between 1948 and 1958—in collaboration with the WHO—the ARO instituted mass campaigns against endemic diseases. In the subsequent decade, the agency prioritized Maternal and Child Health (MCH) across Asia, with a particular emphasis on the Philippines and Indonesia.[5] However, attaining concrete results in reducing maternal and infant mortality was more complicated than implementing mass campaigns against endemic diseases. Maternal and child welfare projects across the region yielded limited outcomes due to the low level of public investments and the dearth of local personnel in health centers. The transition from controlling endemic diseases to strengthening MCH services offers useful insights into how the regional agency negotiated challenges posed by newly decolonized states. Using two case studies—the anti-yaws campaign in Indonesia and the Bacillus Calmette–Guérin (BCG) conundrum in Madras State, southern India—I contend that the ARO was not only a locus to confront different views on international health, but also an actor that realigned international health to local circumstances.[6]

Existential Crises, 1946–1953

In 1946, the UN General Assembly appointed a committee to liquidate the UNRRA (United Nations Relief and Rehabilitation Administration), active during World War II. One of the committee members was Ludwik Rajchman, former director of the League of Nations Health Organization (LNHO) from 1921 to 1939. He proposed to the UN General Assembly that the residual assets of the soon-to-be-liquidated UNRRA be used to create a children's fund. Rajchman suggested setting up the fund as an emergency organization. Concomitant with UNRRA's dissolution, the fund faced competition from the Interim Commission of the World Health Organization (WHO). While the WHO envisioned a long-term program for international health work, UNICEF was preoccupied with meeting the immediate needs of children arising from wartime exigencies. After 1948, UNICEF's initial focus on emergency requirements for children in war-devastated countries of Europe broadened in scope to improve the health, nutrition, and welfare initiatives across Asia. In 1953, UNICEF deleted the word emergency from its name. The name United Nations Children's Fund has remained unaltered ever since.[7]

A staunch advocate of social medicine from Poland, Rajchman was enthusiastic about incorporating MCH into regular medical practice: ideas regarded as revolutionary at the time. In 1943, he articulated his vision for a United Nations Health Service in the magazine *Free World*. In his article, he contended that only freedom from want could ensure adequate health for everybody. Until people were adequately fed, no medicine could keep them healthy. He asserted that health was a purchasable commodity with a price that varied according to changing socioeconomic conditions.[8] The role of the United Nations Health Service would be to assist national health authorities upon request. He suggested the possibility of funding the United Nations Health Organization through a health tax imposed on individual governments. The International Health Conference that convened in New York in July 1946 resulted in the creation of the WHO Interim Commission. The Commission dropped Rajchman's name from the list of invitees, despite his international credentials. Hugh Cumming, director of the Pan American Sanitary Bureau (PASB), was opposed to the creation of a single international health organization. He wrote a 70-page document contending that the participation of delegates from certain East European countries would make the WHO an "instrument of communism."[9] Cumming would have been deeply dissatisfied to see his old foe Rajchman occupying an influential position within the WHO (Image 5.1).

If Rajchman could not put his LNHO expertise at the disposal of the newly founded WHO, he could at least apply his expertise to children's welfare. Rajchman's background in bacteriology predisposed him to advocate for UNICEF's entry into health programs. WHO officials viewed his moves with considerable suspicion. Mandate overlaps between UNICEF and the WHO were apparent in two areas: (a) the coordination of their respective functions and (b) the division of responsibilities, with WHO retaining its health mandate, while UNICEF financed field operations.[10] The original draft of the agreement between WHO and the UN mentioned that the WHO was *a* responsible health organization. At the First World Health Assembly (WHA), the word *a* was changed to *the*.[11] The

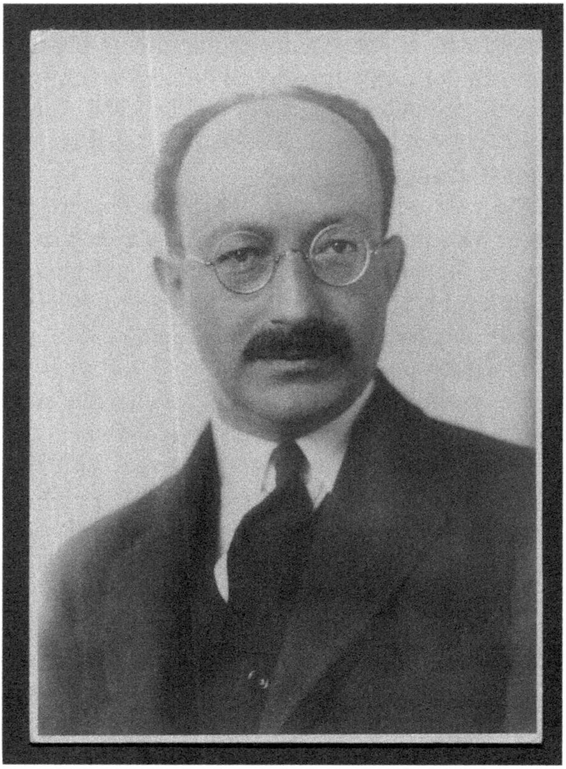

Image 5.1 An Undated Photograph of Ludwik Rajchman, First Founder and Chairperson of UNICEF. Photographer: Saryuoz Wolski. Reference Code P0306. With Permission from United Nations Archives, Geneva

word *a* in the preliminary draft specifying the relationship between the WHO and UNICEF was widely interpreted as Rajchman's ploy to outmaneuver the WHO.[12] Another source of friction between the WHO and UNICEF was the introduction of the BCG (Bacillus Calmette Guérin) vaccine as a prophylactic against TB. Rajchman was willing to take a chance and work with Scandinavian Red Cross Societies. BCG faced resistance within WHO circles, as the vaccine had never been used in mass immunization campaigns across the US.[13]

By 1947—coinciding with heightening Cold War tensions—UNICEF leadership underwent a significant transformation. Rajchman's own experience as the founding chairperson of the fund revealed that geopolitical undercurrents could jeopardize international organizations and their leadership. The best safeguard for the fund's sustainability was appointing leadership that would not provoke political opposition from the US or its Western allies. For the position of UNICEF's Executive Director, Rajchman advocated for an American with established Republican credentials. Such an arrangement reduced the probability of US withdrawal from UNICEF. Among prospective American candidates for the fund's leadership was Maurice Pate, an acquaintance of Rajchman.

Pate—an alumnus of Princeton University—joined the Belgian Relief Commission at the zenith of World War I in 1916 under the supervision of Herbert Hoover, who would later become President of the United States (1929–1933). After World War I, he worked with the American Relief Administration's emergency feeding program for over a million children that transcended political borders, including the new Bolshevik Russia.[14] In 1939, at the onset of World War II—when Germany invaded Poland—Pate became president of the Commission of Polish Relief, a private organization. Pate pursued a non-political approach: negotiating with the Germans and delivering supplies. After the US entered the war in 1941, Pate directed the American Red Cross and organized relief for prisoners of war in Europe and Asia. In the selection of Pate as Executive Director of UNICEF in 1947, Rajchman secured the support of UN Secretary-General Trygve Lie.

Between 1947 and 1950—as founder chairperson of UNICEF—Rajchman left his imprint on UNICEF's management style. He realized that in the immediate aftermath of World War II, organizing relief was beyond the nation-state's capacity and called for human solidarity. He understood the primacy of political means in combating poverty and ill health. He believed that international aid agencies should promote self-help among recipient nations.

The UN General Assembly Resolution 57 (1)—that paved the way for UNICEF, for which Rajchman was a lobbyist—stood the test of time. While the resolution integrated UNICEF into the UN system, it gave the governing body of the fund considerable autonomy. Crucially, the resolution authorized assistance based solely on need, irrespective of race, creed, or political belief.[15] Emergency relief included supplies, materials, and technical assistance. UNICEF's post-World War II mandate was administering relief measures to children. From inception, the fund delegated decision-making authority to field offices, enabling them to align international aid to local contexts.[16]

In the early years of UNICEF, Rajchman and Pate focused their efforts on securing essential medical supplies and the necessary funding to ensure their transportation. The fund inherited US$ 22 million from liquidated UNRRA assets and operated under budgetary limitations.[17] Rajchman positioned the fund not merely as an emergency relief agency but as a catalytic force, demonstrating measurable outcomes, and persuading governments to institutionalize health interventions within national frameworks.[18]

Despite Rajchman's optimism, three challenges plagued the formative period of UNICEF. The first was a structural dependence on Congressional goodwill. The American government could not keep persuading Congress to underwrite the fund once the European emergency ended in 1948–1949. The second challenge was an overlap of the fund's mandate with those of the WHO and FAO (Food and Agricultural Organization). Both organizations regarded UNICEF as a fund-raising and supply agency. The third was the distinction between technical and material assistance. Technical assistance—scientific know-how in health, nutrition, agriculture, employment, and social welfare—was within the purview of specialized agencies. Technical assistance was buoyed by postwar optimism that Western know-how and its hands-on counterpart "show-how" could build a better world.[19] UN agencies regarded material assistance—donated goods that UNICEF provided—as inferior.

However, Pate sought to dispel the misconception that UNICEF functioned merely as a supply agency. To this end, he unsuccessfully lobbied with Eleanor Roosevelt, the chief US delegate to the UN Committee on Social and Humanitarian Affairs. She spearheaded children's causes. Roosevelt asserted that the best way to ensure children's welfare was to eliminate UNICEF.[20] She underestimated the symbolic and material importance UNICEF held for newly decolonized Asian states. However, the fund secured a new lease of life on October 6, 1950, and found a passionate advocate in Ahmed Bokhari, Pakistan's permanent representative to the UN.[21] Delegates from Asia, the Middle East, and Latin America supported Bokhari's appeal to save UNICEF. The question of the agency's continuing existence was not settled until 1953, when the UN General Assembly dropped the words "international" and "emergency" from the name.

"Pinpricks of Assistance": The Beginnings of ARO

Between 1947 and 1948, as Europe's postwar emergency receded, UNICEF redirected its attention to Asia. Whereas Europe retained a skeletal infrastructure that enabled food package distribution, the scale of hunger across Asia undermined the feasibility of mass feeding programs—prompting a strategic pivot toward addressing entrenched socioeconomic inequalities. In response to these constraints, UNICEF commissioned a collaborative study involving Thomas Parran from the United States Public Health Service (USPHS) and C.K. Lakshmanan from the All India Institute of Hygiene and Public Health to ascertain the health needs of Asian children.

Between April and June 1948, Parran and Lakshman visited Burma, the Dutch East Indies, French Indochina, India, Malaya, Pakistan, the Philippines, Singapore, and Thailand.[22] Their collaborative investigation aimed to identify health problems in Asian children that warranted UNICEF's targeted investment. Parran and Lakshmanan advocated maximum budgetary allocation to India, given the sheer size of its population.

However, the Parran-Lakshmanan Report determined that undertaking extensive feeding programs for the region's undernourished children was implausible, as hunger and malnutrition were chronic conditions that required long-term interventions. Instead of focusing on mass feeding, the Parran-Lakshmanan Report recommended that UNICEF prioritize efforts to reduce the high rate of infant mortality.[23] In Burma, the investigators observed a critical shortage of trained medical personnel; notably, Rangoon recorded one death for every three births.[24]

In 1948, the UNICEF Executive Board allocated only US$ 3 million for Asia, which roughly worked out to 1 cent per beneficiary (Table 5.1).[25]

Given the region's rudimentary health infrastructure, Parran and Lakshmanan reiterated that instead of focusing on mass feeding of undernourished children, the fund should prioritize the control of endemic diseases such as malaria, tuberculosis, and yaws that affected mothers and children. Apart from the control of endemic diseases, they emphasized health personnel training. The UNICEF Secretariat accordingly sanctioned US$ 214,000 for a fellowship program that the WHO administered. UNICEF funded the travel of two Thai malariologists to the Malaria Institute of India for training.[26]

Parran and Lakshmanan drew up provisional lists of assistance for all countries that they visited. They emphasized the need for laboratory

Table 5.1 The Parran-Lakshman Report: recommendations for the proposed UNICEF budgetary allocation to Asia (1948)

Territory/ Country	*Recommended allocation in US$*
British Colonial Territories: Malaya, Sabah, Sarawak, Singapore, and British Borneo	3 million
Indonesia (the former Dutch Indies)	800,000
Indochina	500,000
Thailand	105,000
Philippines	150,000
India, Burma and Ceylon	4.23 million

Source: Adapted from the "Diary of Martha May Eliot," July 4, 1948, Folders 711-34, Box 53, MC 229, *Martha May Eliot Papers*, Schlesinger Library, Harvard University

equipment, drugs, vaccines, and programs for endemic disease control. Black characterized the provisional assistance lists as "useful pinpricks" in any UNICEF regional health scheme for Asia.

By 1948, the scope of UNICEF's Asian programs enlarged and covered:

(a) feeding operations in India, Indonesia, the Philippines, Hong Kong, and Japan;
(b) malaria control projects in Pakistan, India, and Thailand;
(c) programs for training pediatricians overseas on behalf of Pakistan, India, Thailand, Indonesia, the Philippines, and Malaya.

With the establishment of WHO regional offices for South-East Asia and the Western Pacific, UNICEF recognized the need for a coordinated approach. In November 1948, Michael Watt, the former director of New Zealand's health services, received a letter from Pate offering him the post of UNICEF Regional Director for Asia.[27] Watt accepted the offer. Between 1949 and 1950, he officiated as the fund's regional director. He was present in Ceylon for inaugurating the mass vaccination campaign against TB in March 1949. In Indonesia—still reeling under the Dutch military action—Watt attempted to persuade the wartime Indonesian Republican authorities to accept a consignment of milk powder from the Dutch. In the Philippines—where UNICEF's school feeding program introduced fish, milk, beans, and shark oil capsules from New Zealand— the authorities were satisfied with the results and introduced school meals as part of government policy (Image 5.2).[28]

UNICEF had initially proposed establishing its regional headquarters for Asia in Manila in 1948. However, the jurisdiction of the regional office stretched from Afghanistan and Korea in the north to the Maldives and Fiji Islands in the south. The UNICEF Executive Board decided that, for effective administrative decentralization, the ARO needed to be near the

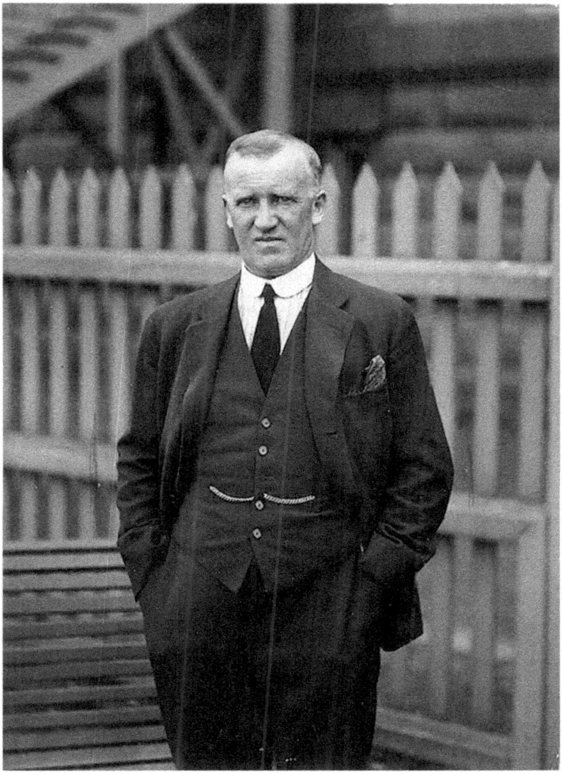

Image 5.2 Michael Herbert Watt. Reference: PACoII-6388-33. Description: Michael Herbert Watt, New Zealand's Director-General of Health, March 18, 1931. He was the founding director of the UNICEF Regional Office for Asia between 1948 and 1949. Photographer unidentified. Published in the *New Zealand Free Lance*, 1931. With permission from Alexander Turnbull Library, Wellington, New Zealand

center of the vast territory and not on the periphery. Bangkok seemed to be a rock of stability in an otherwise geopolitically volatile region. Bangkok's position as the hub in the embryonic regional network of UNICEF in an arc fanning out from Karachi in the west, through Colombo and Manila in the south to Seoul in the northeast, made the city a perfect choice for the site of the regional headquarters since early 1949. However, by 1961, the ARO would lose India, the biggest country within the jurisdiction of the regional agency along with Afghanistan and Ceylon, to the newly constituted South Central Asia Regional Office.[29] The ARO would become the new East Asia and Pakistan Regional Office.

The shift of geopolitical gravity toward Bangkok coincided not only with the Indochina War (1946–1954) but also with leadership transitions within UNICEF that redefined its operational ethos across Asia. Due to ill health, Watt unexpectedly resigned in 1950 and was replaced by Spurgeon Milton Keeny. A homespun philosopher from Pennsylvania—with a Quaker outlook and simplicity—Keeny earned the epithet "Emperor of UNICEF in Asia" during his tenure as regional director (1950–1963).[30] Long before this ascendancy, the YMCA recruited him during World War I to work with British Indian troops in Mesopotamia. After graduating from Oxford, he worked in Poland to repatriate prisoners of war. In 1943, Keeny accepted an offer from the US State Department to work on problems of foreign relief and rehabilitation. Between 1945 and 1948, after officiating as chief of UNRRA in Italy, he joined UNICEF as a supply officer for Europe. Two years later, he became the regional director of ARO.

Keeny had an uncanny ability to bring together representations from the WHO, UNICEF, and FAO alongside national, provincial, and local governments to pursue difficult objectives. He was the architect of the anti-yaws campaign in Southeast Asia, particularly across Indonesia, Thailand, and the Philippines. Keeny's success as ARO regional director stemmed from his direct engagement with ordinary people and his ability to earn the trust of local officials.

Soon after assuming office in 1950, Keeny's first itinerary as regional director of the ARO took him through Indonesia, Thailand, Burma, India, Ceylon, and Pakistan. In his diary, Keeny confessed that he had to "cover the field" and bring back firsthand information to UNICEF headquarters in New York to justify increased budgetary appropriations for Asia and to persuade members of the US Congress to vote for continuing aid to the fund.[31] In Keeny's words:

> To get the money to keep our work going we had to tell about it; for we were an emergency organization—and had to produce or die. I for one did not want to see us that have outlived go on living unless there were very strong reasons for it: the world is full of organizations that have outlived their usefulness but go on living simply out of habit.[32]

Keeny had to walk a tightrope between aligning ARO's work with UNICEF's mission and proving the cost-effectiveness of UNICEF's interventions in child welfare across Asia. As regional director of ARO, he constantly scripted compelling stories to satisfy the expectations of international donors: results.

During his official tours, Keeny noted that the majority of problems that post-World War II Asia encountered were of a less violent but more crippling nature.[33] Diagnostically mapping Asia's poverty and health, he argued that the region's affliction was not merely a consequence of poverty, but a vicious cycle —Asia was poor because it was sick. His vision was to raise living standards through disease control. Keeny argued that, in fighting diseases such as TB and malaria, there was no use in treating a handful of patients with individual doctors. He instead advocated using mass campaigns against disease.[34]

When the Parran-Lakshmanan team visited Asia in 1948, practically all countries of the region recognized TB as a serious health problem and requested UNICEF assistance in launching BCG vaccination campaigns. The Parran-Lakshmanan Report noted:

> Only in Indo-China has BCG vaccine heretofore been done and, there through the use of the dried vaccine administered orally. However, in the Philippines, a small-scale trial of dried vaccire from the Pasteur Institute in Paris is being made. In India plans have been completed for the manufacture of BCG vaccine. In this country, a WHO team is functioning. In Malaya and Singapore the authorities hope to secure a supply of BCG vaccine from Australia and tentatively propose training of field personnel through fellowships. In Indo-China modern drying equipment is requested and, if approved, the government is anxious to supply BCG without cost to neighboring countries.[35]

Of the US$ 2 million that the Executive Board allocated to the BCG vaccination campaigns across Asia, $ 1 million was transferred to India, Pakistan, and Ceylon (Image 5.3).[36]

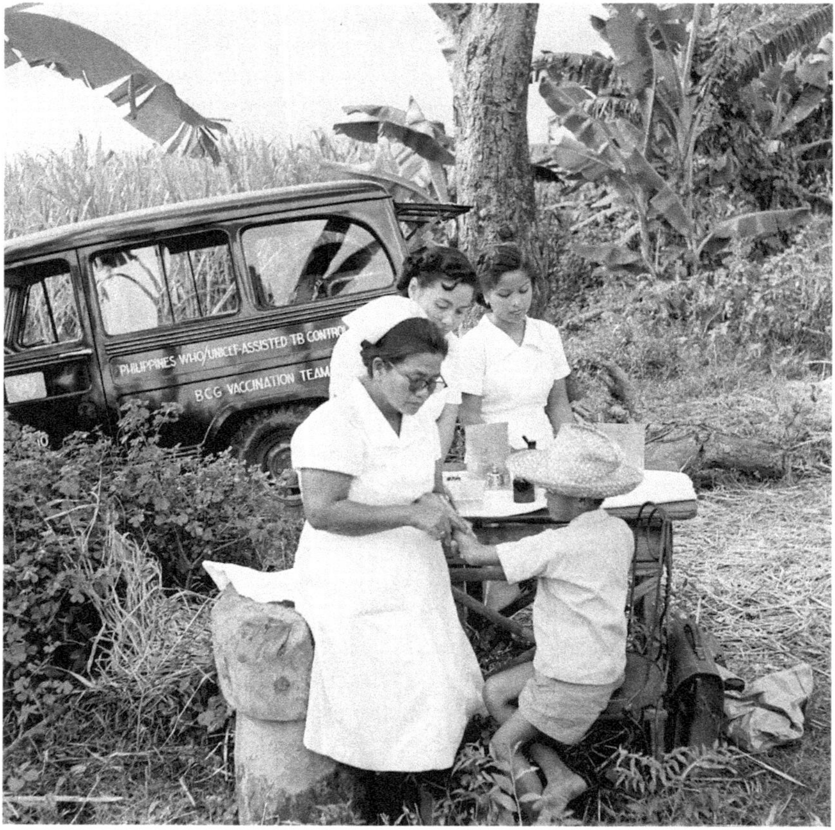

Image 5.3 One of three nurses from a BCG vaccination team tests a boy for tuberculosis at a table set up near a tree where their truck is parked, in the province of Batangas, Philippines (1956). UNICEF Headquarters Unique ID: UNI42503. In-house ID: NYHC 1956-0004. With permission from UNICEF Headquarters, New York

Responding to the findings of the Parran-Lakshmanan Report, UNICEF instituted a collaborative framework for TB control—signing a Joint Enterprise Agreement with the WHO and Scandinavian Red Cross partners. The primary objective of the Joint Enterprise of the International Tuberculosis Campaign (ITC) was to vaccinate children and young adults in afflicted countries. In November 1948, the Government of India and

ITC signed an agreement that initiated a six-month BCG demonstration campaign aimed at protecting children from TB. In India, public response to the BCG campaign varied, ranging from outright vaccine acceptance to passive resistance.[37]

In 1950, UNICEF pledged rupees 33,000 to the Indian government for furthering BCG vaccination in Madras State, southern India.[38] At the time, Rajkumari Amrit Kaur, India's Minister of Health, urged T.S.S. Rajan, the then Madras health minister, to utilize UNICEF funding for undertaking preventive work against TB in rural areas.[39] However, Rajan remained cautious concerning recommending BCG vaccination as a prophylactic measure, citing the severe shortage of skilled medical personnel in Madras State. He warned P.V. Benjamin, TB Advisor to the Indian government, that if any untoward incident occurred in the administration of BCG, it would jeopardize public opinion toward vaccination.[40] Rajan suggested that the Madras government should extend statewide vaccination only after the prophylactic efficacy of BCG was empirically confirmed.[41]

A.V. Raman, a retired sanitary engineer from Madras and editor of *People's Health*, questioned the efficacy of BCG even before the mass vaccination campaign commenced. On February 3, 1949, Raman alleged that the then Madras health minister, A.B. Shetty, steamrolled conflicting opinions of doctors and uncritically followed WHO directives to launch the BCG program.[42] Shetty tried to silence Raman by pointing to the success of the experimental mass vaccination against TB at Madanapalle.[43] He accused Raman of being a hot gospeller on behalf of environmental hygiene.[44] Shetty contended that Raman's opposition to BCG was well-intentioned but had incited fear in people's minds. To assuage public fears, Shetty pointed out that BCG vaccination was purely voluntary and cited the Transactions of the Commonwealth Empire and Tuberculosis Conference to establish vaccine safety.[45]

Raman critiqued the technocratic postwar public health vision, which emphasized the proverbial magic bullet over holistic interventions such as better living conditions for the poor. He specifically targeted the BCG vaccine in the *People's Health* editorials of 1949 and 1950. Emphasizing the vaccine's unproven efficacy, he advocated its restricted use through controlled trials.[46] He published the latest trials on the BCG vaccine in *People's Health*. The February 1950 edition of *People's Health* cited a French publication entitled *La Vie Claire*, which noted that the Soviet Five-Year Plan did not mandate vaccination but attempted to study the efficacy of BCG in relation to other TB control methods.[47] Raman also launched a pointed attack on Amrit Kaur for introducing the BCG vaccine irresponsibly and criticized opposition parties for failing to capitalize on public resistance.[48] In the March 1950 edition of *People's Health*, Raman alleged that the ultimate motive of the BCG campaign was to use Indians as guinea pigs.[49]

In formulating his opposition to BCG, Raman turned to M.K. Gandhi's Constructive Program, which emphasized rural and environmental sanitation, for inspiration. In the January 1950 edition of *People's Health*, Raman criticized the Government of India's adherence to WHO and UNICEF prescriptions concerning disease control:

> Pandit Nehru once declared that, when money can be found for the war against other countries, it must be available for the war against Dirt, Disease, and Death. However, finance has driven the dagger practically into all our health schemes leaving the Health Minister [Rajkumari Amrit Kaur] to seek the aid of well-dollared international bodies, so anxious to foist on us, through her, remedies cheap, even questionable and proportionately ineffective. ... The illiterate feels; he cannot think. All he knows is, a change from the Union Jack to the Tri-colour, a change from Wavell to Rajaji, the substitution of *Raj-Pramukhs* [Governors] for Highnesses, have meant no change in his health, no improvement in his living conditions...
>
> Until the living conditions of the common-man satisfy the accepted minimal requirement of sanitation, discontent will continue to simmer in his breast.[50]

Essentially, Raman warned that poor health and sanitation could fuel public discontent in newly independent India (Image 5.4).

People's Health ceased publication in 1951. A year later, Chakravarti Rajagopalachari became Chief Minister of Madras State, a position he relinquished in 1954. During his tenure, Rajagopalachari opposed Prime Minister Jawaharlal Nehru's centralized planning and later founded the Swatantra Party in 1959. His opposition to BCG should be viewed in the context of the central government's incursion in public health, traditionally regarded as a state responsibility. To address shortfalls in public health spending, he enlisted the support of private philanthropy and established the Maharaja of Bhavnagar Kshayrog Fund (a corpus fund instituted in the name of the former Governor of Madras) to treat indigent tuberculosis patients.[51] In 1954, Rajagopalachari resigned due to his controversial educational reforms. As a fiscal conservative, he sought to reconcile the tension between reducing the cost of primary education, on the one hand,

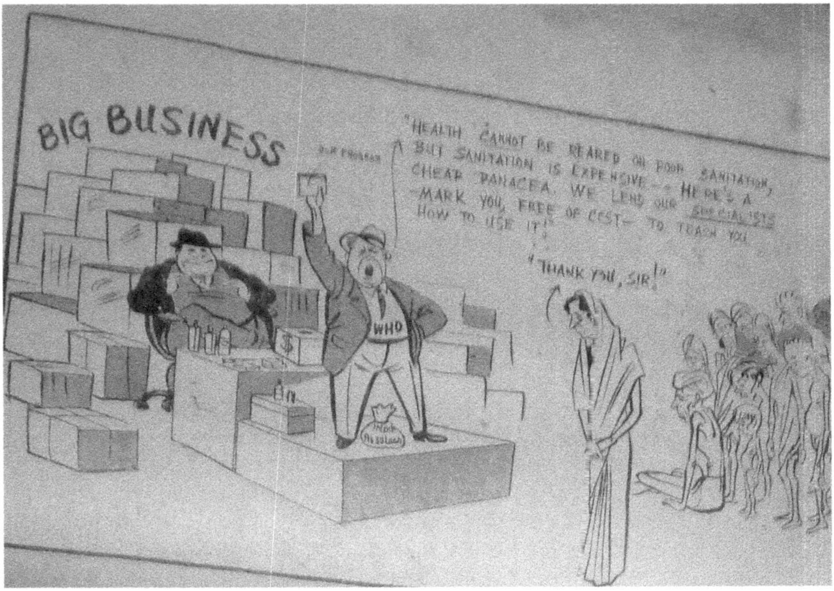

Image 5.4 WHO Renders Service to Poor and Underdeveloped Areas. Text: Health cannot be reared on poor sanitation. But sanitation is expensive. Here's a cheap panacea. We lend our specialists—mark you free of cost—to teach you how to use it. India's Health Minister Rajkumari Amrit Kaur (right) approaching C. Mani (WHO, left) and Sam Keeny (seated) for technical assistance in health. Citation: *People's Health* (April 1950). With permission from Mohan V. Raman, grandson of A.V. Raman, Editor of *People's Health*

and increasing the enrolment of students, on the other.[52] He stressed that children should be trained in their traditional occupations. His policy received much censure from the opposition Dravida Munnetra Kazhagam (DMK) party, which accused Rajagopalachari of perpetuating the Hindu caste-based division of labor. At the time of his resignation, Rajagopalachari developed anti-statist views, partly as a result of disagreements with Nehruvian Big Science and state incursion into the private lives of individuals.[53]

In the summer of 1955, the BCG conundrum in Madras spilled beyond local newspapers as Rajagopalachari published a pamphlet *B. C.G. Vaccination: Why I Oppose It.* He delineated his reservations concerning the vaccine and marshaled critical statements from the latest medical literature and from aggrieved parents to substantiate his arguments. In Rajagopalachari's words, "I cannot resist the feeling that the mass campaign in India is a vast empirical experiment in the supposed interest of scientific progress and that Indian children are being offered for experimentation on the same plan that was put in operation among the people in war-ravaged areas and uncivilised dependent countries."[54] Although Rajagopalachari echoed Raman's concerns about India adopting BCG—a public health intervention of an inferior standard—he lacked Raman's broader vision for systemic reforms.

While claiming to oppose BCG on scientific grounds, Rajaji observed that the wonder drug isoniazid was invaluable in the treatment of tuberculosis.[55] He contended:

> I am not against modern 'western' therapy or modern science. B.C.G. has nothing to do with the principles of modern western therapy. If at all, it is akin to the principles of Homoeopathy. It proceeds on a creed very similar to that of homoeopathy, namely, that diseases are to be dealt with by the administration in mild forms of things that produce identical symptoms. The difference is that the homoeopath does not introduce what multiplies in the human body, but the BCG man introduces a large body of living multiplying organisms, which are intended to remain alive in the body of the patient in order to produce the desired result.[56]

In the booklet, Rajagopalachari assembled arguments from *Current Therapy* to substantiate his claim that BCG vaccination was a form of quackery.[57] International scientists lacked consensus on a satisfactory BCG vaccine. They were uncertain about the vaccine's virulence, the degree of immunity induced, and the best method of administration—whether subcutaneously, orally, or by the puncture method. In his booklet, Rajagopalachari included anecdotal and unverified cases of children developing post-vaccinal complications, ranging from blindness to skin diseases and mental ailments.[58]

Tamil-language newspapers such as *Dina Thanthi* heightened public uneasiness about mass vaccinations in the rural areas of Madras.[59] On September 14, 1955, in the district of Cuddalore, schoolchildren launched a strike against BCG vaccination, alleging that they were "forced" to get vaccinated by the principal.[60] To mollify public anxieties concerning BCG, the Madras government issued a booklet entitled *Truth About BCG: Why the Government Has Launched a Mass Campaign*. The booklet inferred from available statistics that, while 1.5 million individuals in the state were tuberculin tested, only 22 reported post-vaccinal complications.[61]

Niels Brimnes notes that, while Raman's critique of BCG positioned him as a sole crusader when the vaccine barely impacted the lives of most Indians, Rajagopalachari's opposition gathered traction as more Indians encountered vaccination directly. Rajagopalachari used the information he received on BCG to sustain his opposition in ways that breached confidentiality.[62]

Indian parliamentary discussions featured the BCG conundrum. In her defense of BCG, Amrit Kaur emphasized that public doubts in Madras had been dispelled by 1950, enabling India to test 60 million and vaccinate 20 million over the next five years.[63] She asserted that India's Five-year Plans aimed to raise living standards and improve nutrition, though such structural transformations required time.[64] Amrit Kaur's defense of BCG reflected the allure of the proverbial magic bullet—the promise that medical technology could surmount the logistical challenges of a newly decolonized state, particularly shortages of trained medical personnel and financial resources (Image 5.5).

While the mass campaign against TB encountered resistance— efforts to eliminate yaws, a debilitating tropical disease attributed to poor hygiene—were remarkably successful. Unlike BCG, whose therapeutic outcomes are not immediately apparent, penicillin produces rapid results: painful sores disappear, and patients respond positively to treatment.

Mass treatment of yaws became one of Keeny's favorite subjects for seven reasons. First, a single shot of penicillin cures the disease. Second, penicillin was getting cheaper during the 1950s. Third, no doctors were required to administer penicillin injections. Fourth, cured adults could return to work quickly. Fifth, the faster the anti-yaws work progressed, the slower the disease spread. Sixth, curing yaws did not noticeably increase the population: the disease cripples but seldom kills. Seventh, the cure for yaws was dramatic and served as a precursor for strengthening other public health programs.[65]

In the words of Keeny, "You find yaws at the end of the road." In other words, he equated yaws with underdevelopment. The disease is associated with poverty: persons who wear shoes and use soap seldom contract yaws. The anti-yaws campaign reached more remote areas under the jurisdiction of the ARO than any other UNICEF-sponsored program.[66] Endemic regions included the hills of Eastern India, northeast Thailand, most of Laos, Sumatra, Java ("the yaws capital"), Bali, Lombok, Flores, North

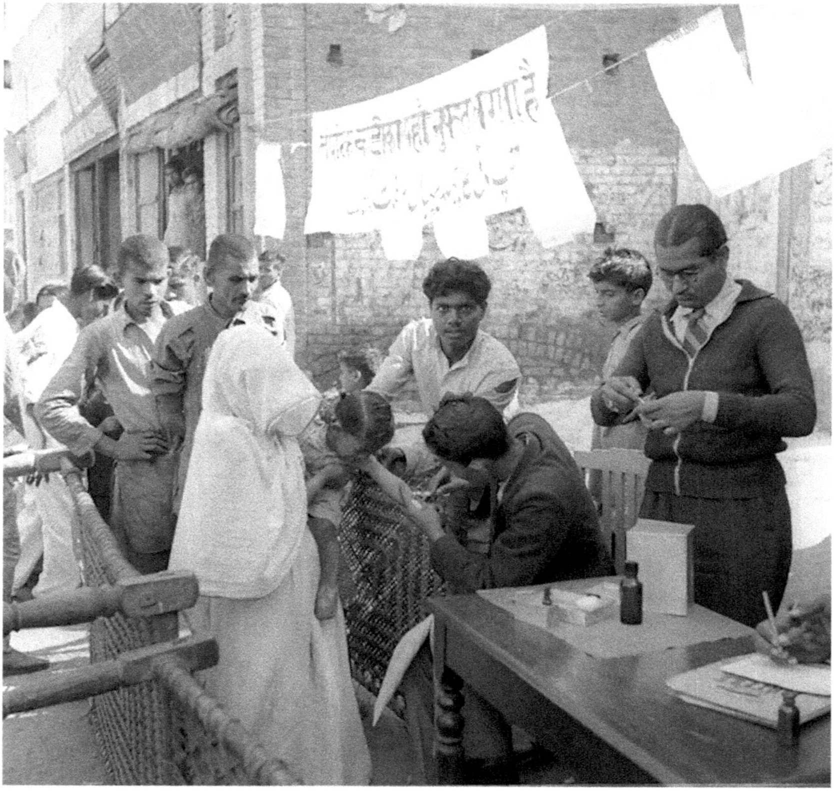

Image 5.5 Mass BCG Vaccination Campaign, Delhi (1953). On BCG Day—February 23, 1953—India, under the stewardship of Rajkumari Amrit Kaur, launched a mass campaign against TB. Source: Photo 32077, Studio/Mar.53, A28(i), Internet Archive. Public Domain. URL: https://archive.org/details/propix.27506850185

Borneo, Mindanao, and the Visayas.[67] During the early 1950s, Indonesia harbored at least ten million yaws cases, probably the world's largest reservoir of the disease at the time.[68]

In 1950—after the transfer of political sovereignty to the Indonesian Republic—the country implemented a Treponematoses Control Project. The focus of the Treponematoses Control Project was the control of yaws and congenital syphilis. Johannes Leimena, the Minister of Health in the Natsir cabinet (1950–1951), noting that most yaws patients in Indonesia were children, enlisted UNICEF's financial support for targeted intervention.[69] The Treponematoses Control Project was initially piloted in Jakarta and Yogyakarta: both on the island of Java. Both yaws and congenital syphilis were treated with an injection of procaine penicillin G (particle size in oil) with 2 percent aluminum monostearate as a one-shot treatment schedule, significantly reducing treatment costs.[70]

M. Soetopo—the Indonesian Minister of Health in Abdul Halim's cabinet between January and June 1950—pursued a policy of mass treatment of entire villagers with penicillin, irrespective of whether or not individuals showed yaws symptoms. However, Raden Kodijat, a retired Javanese regency physician—drawing on his experience treating yaws in Kediri, East Java, between 1930 and 1942—advocated selective treatment of symptomatic cases using penicillin.[71] He opposed the wasteful use of resources. Kodijat's approach, known as the Kodijat Method, tracked down the disease in village populations at intervals of six months and reduced yaws prevalence in Kediri from 10.1 percent in 1934 to 1.7 percent in 1936.[72] Though effective, the Kodijat Method required significant medical personnel and overlooked latent yaws cases, i.e., patients who did not exhibit yaws lesions, prompting Soetopo to design a modified strategy.[73]

The Treponematoses Control Project Simplified (TCPS), developed in 1952, consisted of a two-pronged strategy: (a) the Kodijat Method of selective yaws treatment on the densely populated island of Java; (b) Total Mass Treatment of villagers using penicillin injections on the Outer Islands of the Indonesian archipelago, particularly in Sumatra, Kalimantan, and Flores, where the population was dispersed and distances covered were extensive.

To overcome the shortage of skilled medical personnel, Soetopo appointed yaws scouts with elementary education (Javanese: *djuru patèk*) to detect yaws cases, administer treatment, conduct periodical resurveys of the village population, and follow up on treated patients. Subdistrict polyclinics, aided by regency governments, became the backbone of the anti-yaws campaign.

When the *mantris* [Javanese: male nurses] and *djuru patèks* visited a rural community to undertake yaws control activities, the village headman would summon the people to gather by the traditional method of ringing a gong or sounding on a hollow log a signal. The *mantri* would explain to the villagers the purpose of the anti-yaws campaign. As villagers were already acquainted with smallpox vaccination, they did not fear the penicillin injections. In Keeny's words, "There was magic in the needle."[74] As soon as village volunteers reported yaws symptoms in individual villagers, the *djuru patèk* would reexamine the suspected cases. If they found any lesion, the suspected case would be handed over a card and the *mantri* would treat the infected case with penicillin. If the *djuru patèk* noted that at least 10 percent of villagers were afflicted with the disease, the whole community would be treated.[75] After treating infectious cases, the *djuru patèk* and *mantri* would undertake resurveys of rural communities to assess yaws prevalence and treatment efficacy.

Unlike densely populated Javanese rural settlements—where it was easy to collect villagers for yaws examination—in the Outer Islands, villages were dispersed, and distances covered by the TCPS team were huge. In such cases, Total Mass Treatment emerged as the pragmatic option. This involved administering full penicillin doses to yaws patients with conspicuous lesions, and half-doses to patients' contacts, uninfected individuals, and yaws cases without noticeable symptoms. To offset the shortage of *mantris*, *djuru patèks* were trained not only to diagnose yaws but also to administer penicillin injections. The prevalence of yaws in Indonesia declined from 16 percent in 1949 to 0.58 percent by 1960.[76] Once the prevalence of yaws in a given village dropped below 5 percent, *djuru patèks* were used to detect leprosy. The integration of leprosy surveillance into the TCPS workflow slashed TCPS costs fourfold—translating therapeutic reach into economic efficiency (Images 5.6 and 5.7).[77]

Indonesia's anti-yaws strategy attracted international attention. Modeled on the Kodijat method, the Malayan Federation launched a yaws elimination campaign in the states of Kelantan and Terengganu.[78] In 1953, J.G. Clearkin, Health Officer of West Pahang, was offered a WHO Fellowship to study the organization of the anti-yaws campaign in Indonesia, Thailand, and the Philippines.[79] The same year, health authorities examined over 5000 villagers on the Kelantan-Terengganu border flanking the South China Sea through a house-to-house search, treating infected individuals with penicillin.[80] By 1960, the prevalence of yaws in Kelantan and Terengganu dropped to less than 2 percent.[81]

The USAID commended ARO's efforts in eliminating yaws:

> They [ARO] had found a perfect program. It was a model program for attacking a disease that was a serious health problem and there was a known cure for it, the cure wasn't expensive. And it was done, and was done quickly, and done well, and by the fact that you had shown what penicillin could do.

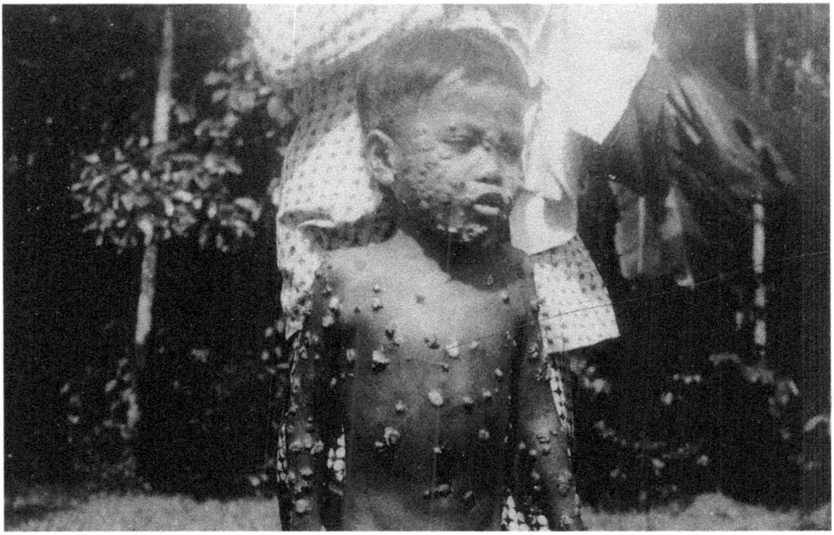

Image 5.6 Yaws Papules in an Indonesian Child (1950s). Source: From the Arnoud H. Klokke Personal Collection. With permission

> There was no problem for the future because clinics in that neighborhood, had stores of penicillin, and people knew what to do if a case came up in their village—they simply went to the mantri, and got a dose of penicillin, and cured it, so the disease was wiped out. It's almost non-existent in Asia now [1960] even in Indonesia.[82]

Despite ARO's preliminary successes in eliminating yaws, eradicating the disease by the mid-1960s was unattainable. Flawed epidemiological strategies contributed to the resurgence of the disease across the Indonesian archipelago. Surveillance was a weak component of the anti-yaws program in Java. *Mantris* were trained to treat only patients with yaws sores, while patients without sores but probably infected were excluded, contributing to a latent reservoir for future infections.[83]

Administrative fractures were no less significant in derailing the progress of yaws elimination across Indonesia. The central government devolved yaws control to the provincial, regency, and village administrations, but these administrations were unable to cover campaign-related expenses. Although the government pledged one-third of the penicillin supplies used to treat yaws, the lack of effective coordination between the

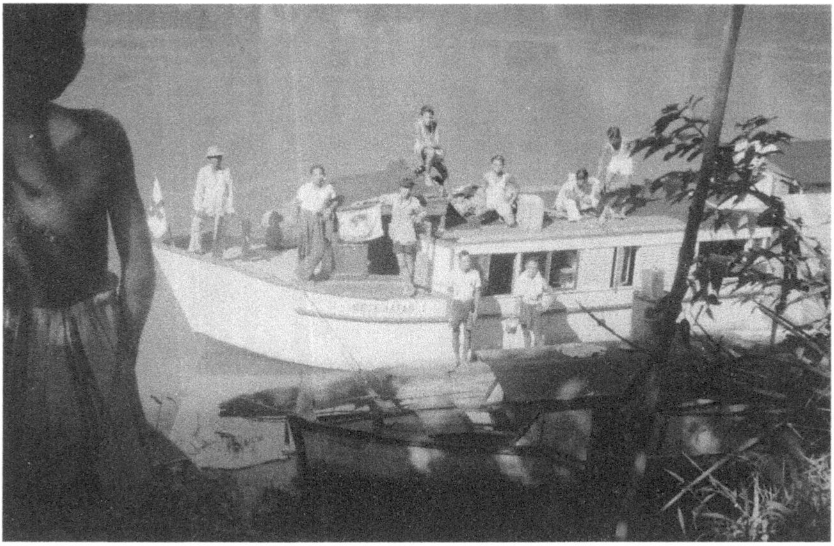

Image 5.7 A mobile polyclinic administering yaws treatment in the Outer Islands of the Indonesian Archipelago: Kalimantan, 1950s. Source: From the Arnoud H. Klokke Personal Collection. With permission

ministries of health and finance resulted in delays in appointing medical personnel. The Indonesian Ministry of Health and aid agencies, UNICEF in particular, had to break administrative protocols to source penicillin supplies or hire *mantri* and *djuru patèk*. In 1965, following the military confrontation with Malaysia, Indonesia announced its decision to withdraw from the UN. UNICEF funding for the campaign was subsequently suspended.[84]

The anti-yaws campaign was, ironically, a victim of its success. Villagers who had witnessed the therapeutic efficacy of penicillin presumed that a single shot of the wonder-drug was a panacea for any disease. The WHO cautioned Indonesian health authorities that penicillin was not public health. Other decisive factors determining the momentum of yaws eradication included strengthening rural sanitation. The realization—that the proverbial magic bullet alone was insufficient—prompted UNICEF and WHO to reframe rural sanitation as the bedrock of disease eradication.

Strengthening rural sanitation in ARO member states was central to UNICEF's strategy to mobilize government, private agencies, voluntary groups, and individuals in advancing child health. The fund aimed to stimulate self-help, using international assistance to leverage local resources. UNICEF and WHO supported large-scale campaigns against endemic diseases, simultaneously igniting rural engagement with modern public health principles. Nearly 45 percent of UNICEF Asian aid by the late 1950s targeted endemic diseases.[85] The organization framed disease eradication as a necessary precursor to building a network of primary health services for MCH.

Lack of supporting public health infrastructure inhibited the development of MCH across Indonesia and the Philippines during the 1950s. UNICEF emphasized the training of paramedical personnel to overcome the lack of trained nurses and midwives. During her official trip to the Philippines, Thailand, India, and Indonesia in October 1956, WHO Assistant Director Martha May Eliot observed the organization of MCH services. She noted that during the Magsaysay administration's reorganization of health services, the Philippine Health Department constituted an MCH division. A specialist in maternal and child health staffed the division. However, provinces suffered from a dearth of specialists. In Eliot's words, "In the rural health centers one finds health officers floundering in a sea of children for which they are unprepared."[86] Underlying the poor delivery of MCH services across the Philippines was the neglect of pediatrics in medical education. Eliot noted instances of health authorities pressurizing UNICEF staff to provide specialized equipment such as oxygen tents in pediatric wards lacking adequate sanitation.[87] In such unsanitary surroundings, the implementation of health education was not merely challenging—it was structurally impossible.

In most countries that Eliot visited, MCH services prioritized obstetrics. Midwives showed limited interest in children beyond early infancy. MCH workers in the region expressed serious reservations that UNICEF's emphasis on pediatric care could undermine the emphasis on maternal health.

This tension between maternal and child health priorities also surfaced in Indonesia, where the Parran-Lakshmanan survey (1948) investigated how the country could optimize the utilization of UNICEF aid. The Republican government requested fund support for yaws control and for strengthening MCH. The agency responded to the second request by introducing a milk distribution program in Indonesia in 1950 to combat malnutrition among children. In 1951, the government invited the fund to establish a dairy farm to ensure continued production.[88] Although top

Indonesian health officials welcomed the use of milk and educated the public about its nutritive value, Leimena was unsure if Indonesia had the wherewithal to establish dairy herds at sufficient scale to transform the country into a milk-drinking nation.[89] However, health officials perceived the milk distribution program as the beginning of further largesse from UNICEF. During his official visit to Jakarta, Pate heard a rumor that Indonesian doctors resisted the program, as the country could not afford to spare money and scarce medical personnel for milk distribution.[90]

MCH initiatives failed in Southeast Asia, most notably in the Philippines and Indonesia. Stumbling blocks for the ARO included logistical challenges, opposition from local medical personnel concerned about resource allocation, and cultural resistance toward milk consumption in Indonesia. WHO officials mistakenly perceived MCH programs as country-specific rather than UNICEF-assisted.[91] UNICEF staff in the field were reluctant to permit WHO staff to enter MCH projects due to concerns that UNICEF headquarters might stymie the collaboration. Within the WHO, there was a general apprehension that the agency might rubber-stamp proposals agreed upon by UNICEF. The main disagreement between the WHO and UNICEF in MCH stemmed from UNICEF's perceived role as a supply agency—a portrayal that affected both institutional dynamics and field-level implementation. Yet this perception misrepresented the fund's core mission—UNICEF's programs were about people, not equipment.

Conclusion

By 1950, the ARO began mass campaigns against TB, yaws, and malaria. At the same time, health centers were established across the Philippines and Indonesia, allowing for the synchronization of mass campaigns into routine public health activities once the initial surge subsided. The anti-yaws campaign proved particularly successful, aided by the postwar decline in penicillin prices and the drug's dramatic therapeutic efficacy. Keeny, at the 1953 session of the UNICEF Executive Board, reflected on public health challenges facing the region:

> We shall all look forward to the happy day when the village, to which our thoughts constantly return, will, as a matter of course, be protected from disease by prevention wherever possible, but by cure when necessary; when they will be free from malaria, from yaws and from trachoma and tuberculosis; and when their water and food will be protected from contamination.

> For some diseases, such as with malaria and yaws, this step will be a matter of a few years; at other times it will involve a plan that is nearer 50 years than 5—but the plan will have to be-made and we shall have to stick to the job.[92]

Keeny's reflections implied the need for a long-term strategy to tackle diseases, such as TB, which are associated with unsanitary living conditions.

During the 1950s, as rural health centers in the Philippines and Indonesia were in a formative state, prospects for developing MCH activities were dim. Outside puericulture clinics and vaccination centers, mothers might line up with their infants under a tree or a veranda expecting health promotion therapy. But the similarity ended there. Every mother and child merited individualized treatment. Only fully trained medical staff could make such a judgment. The only reliable MCH service auxiliary staff could provide was handing milk powder to nursing mothers. Across the Philippines and Indonesia, UNICEF and the WHO equipped health centers in peri-urban areas. Yet, the real demand for MCH services was in rural areas, where over 80 percent of the population lived.[93] UNICEF's MCH trajectory in these countries highlighted the organization's evolving priorities in resource-constrained contexts.

Angela Villani observes that by 1959, the protection of children was not merely a matter of addressing humanitarian crises, but a fundamental element of human capital, congruent with post-World War II development discourse.[94] This discourse shaped the inclusion of child welfare into national plans.[95]

The emphasis on optimal resource utilization and long-term health planning was the cornerstone of UNICEF's operational strategy. As Keeny's assertion demonstrates:

> We can do much with little. Thirty cents from UNICEF will cure a case of yaws. A nickel's worth of DDT will protect a person for a year if we provide all—and usually, we provide only half.[96]

Keeny's statement exemplified UNICEF's pragmatic philosophy: maximizing impact with minimal resources, an underlining feature of postwar health interventions.

Notes

1. UN General Assembly Resolution, "Establishment of an International Children's Emergency Fund," 56th Plenary Meeting: UN Assembly First Session, 1946, Doc. A/RES/57/I, UN Digital Library, New York.
2. Maggie Black, *The Children and the Nations: The Story of UNICEF* (New York: UNICEF, 1986).
3. Black, *The Children and the* Nations, 71.
4. For an overall understanding of priority setting in health in the context of the WHO's Regional Office for South-East Asia, see Vivek Neelakantan, "The Monsoon Asia of Geographers: The Cold War Beginnings of the WHO Regional Office for Southeast Asia (SEARO), 1948–60," in *The Geopolitics of Health in South and Southeast Asia: Perspectives from the Cold War to COVID-19*, Vivek Neelakantan edited (Abingdon, Oxon: Routledge, 2023), 27–51.
5. Maurice Pate, "UNICEF Goals in Maternal and Child Welfare: Statement by Maurice Pate at the Annual Meeting of the American Public Health Association," October 22, 1959, Doc. CF/HST/034/anx.02/05, UNICEF Archives.
6. On these perspectives, see Sunil Amrith and Glenda Sluga, "New Histories of the United Nations," *Journal of World History* 19, no. 3 (2008): 251–74, 265; See also Angela Villani, "Children in the Development Debate: The Role of UNICEF from 1947 to the First UN Development Decade," *Journal of World History* 32, no. 3 (2021): 405–38.
7. "Undated UNICEF Draft, 1961," Box 17, Folder 13, MC 103, *Maurice Pate Papers*, Seeley G. Mudd Manuscript Library, Princeton University (hereafter SGMML).
8. Marta A. Balińska, *For the Good of Humanity: Ludwik Rajchman, Medical Statesman,* trans. Rebecca Howell (Budapest: Central European University Press, 1998), 201.
9. Balińska, *For the Good of Humanity*, 202.
10. "Excerpts of Interview with Milton Siegel by John Charnow," Interviewed May 11, 1984, Doc. CF/NYH/USAA/DB01/HS/1996-0067, UNICEF Archives.
11. Ibid.
12. Ibid.
13. Ibid.
14. Richard Jolly, *UNICEF (United Nations Children's Fund): Global Governance that Works* (Abingdon, Oxon: Routledge, 2014).
15. John Charnow, "Reflections on Dr Ludwik Rajchman's Contribution to UNICEF: A Personal Memoir," September 3, 1985, Doc. CF/HST/1985-044, UNICEF Archives.

16. Ibid.
17. "Interview with E.J.R. Heyward Conducted by Mrs. Margaret Catley-Carlson," July 14, 1983, Doc. CF/HST/INT/HEY-001/M, UNICEF Archives.
18. "Interview with Lord Noel-Baker Concerning Ludwig Rajchman, Considered as Founder of UNICEF," July 1, 1982, Doc. CF/RAI/USAA/DPP/RAM/2010/00091, UNICEF Archives.
19. See also David Webster, "Development Advisors in a Time of Cold War and Decolonization: The United Nations Technical Assistance Administration, 1950–59," *Journal of Global History* 6, no. 2 (2011): 249–72.
20. Black, *The Children and the Nations*, 82.
21. Ibid., 82.
22. "Letter from Maurice Pate to Thomas Parran," March 30, 1948, Correspondence, Notes, Etc., Folders 711–24, Box 53, MC 229, *Martha May Eliot Papers*, Schlesinger Library, Harvard University (hereafter Schlesinger).
23. Black, *Children and the Nations*, 71.
24. "Plight of Children in Far East More Desperate than in Europe," *Morning Tribune*, September 24, 1948, 12, National Library Board, Singapore (hereafter NLB).
25. Wah Wong, "UNICEF in Asia: A Historical Perspective," *UNICEF History Series Monograph X* (New York: UNICEF, 1988), 15, Doc. CF/HST/MON/1988-010, UNICEF Archives.
26. Wong, "UNICEF in Asia," 16.
27. Black, *Children and the Nations*, 73.
28. Ibid., 73.
29. Wong, "UNICEF in Asia," 31.
30. Paul M. Limbert, "Dateline 1933: Sam Keeny Makes Association Press a Winner!", *Perspective* (May 1989): 50–53, YMCA Biographical Files: S.M. Keeny, Box 110, Folder 3, Y-USA-12, Kautz Family Papers, Elmer L. Anderson Library, University of Minnesota Libraries (hereafter UMN).
31. S.M. Keeny, *Half of the World's Children: A Diary of UNICEF at Work in Asia* (Association Press: New York, 1957), xx.
32. Keeny, *Half of the World's Children*, xix.
33. Howard Lewis, "Asia's Best Friend," *Collier's*, April 29, 1955, YMCA Biographical Files, Box 110, Folder 3, Y-USA-12, Kautz Family Papers, UMN.
34. Ibid.
35. Wong," UNICEF in Asia," 28.
36. Ibid., 28.

37. Vivek Neelakantan, "Tuberculosis Control in Postcolonial South India and Southeast Asia: Fractured Sovereignties in International Health,1948–60," *Wellcome Open Research* 2, no. 4 (2018), https://doi.org/10.12688/wellcomeopenres.10544.2,
38. Ibid.
39. "Letter from Rajkumari Amrit Kaur to T.S.S. Rajan," September 18, 1949, Government Order (GO) 1313, Health Department MS Series, April 15, 1950, Tamil Nadu State Archives, Chennai (hereafter TNSA).
40. "Draft of Letter from T.S.S. Rajan to P.V. Benjamin on Tuberculosis Vaccination," September 14, 1949, GO 1313, Health Department MS Series, April 15, 1950, TNSA.
41. Ibid.
42. A.V. Raman, "BCG: What About It," *People's Health* 3, no. 3 (1949).
43. Ibid.
44. "Address Delivered by the Hon. Sri A.B. Shetty, M.L.A, Minister of Public Health, Govt. of Madras, at the Inauguration of B.C.G. Vaccination Campaign, by His Excellency the Maharaja of Bhavanagar Governor of Madras on 15-2-1949 at the Medical College, Madras," The *Miscellany: Monthly Journal of the South Indian Branch of the Indian Medical Association* 15, No. 8 (1949): 2–4, TNSA Library Annex.
45. Shetty, "Address."
46. Niels Brimnes, *Languished Hopes: Tuberculosis, the State and International Assistance in Twentieth Century India* (Hyderabad: Orient Blackswan, 2015), 150.
47. Lionel Dole, "French Doctors Doubt Efficacy of BCG," *People's Heath* 4, no. 4 (1950).
48. A.V. Raman, "Editorial," *People's Health* 4, no. 4 (1950).
49. A.V. Raman, "American Citizen's View on BCG," *People's Health*, 4, no.4 (1950)
50. Raman, "Editorial."
51. Neelakantan, "Tuberculosis in Postcolonial South India and Southeast Asia."
52. Ibid.
53. Ibid. For a foundational understating of Nehruvian Science, see David Arnold, "Nehruvian Science and Postcolonial India," *ISIS* 104, no. 2 (2013): 360–70.
54. C. Rajagopalachari, *B.C.G. Vaccination: Why I Oppose It* (Madras: K.J. Ramanujam, 1955), 2.
55. Rajagopalachari, *B.C.G.*, 3.
56. Rajagopalachari, *B.C.G.*, 6.
57. Rajagopalachari, *B.C.G.*, 8.
58. Rajagopalachari, *B.C.G. Vaccination*, 33–41.
59. Neelakantan, "Tuberculosis in Postcolonial South India and Southeast Asia."

60. "Tuberculosis: BCG Vaccination in Cuddalore, Alleged Complications: Press Note Issued by the Government," September 15, 1955, GO 3069, MS Series, TNSA.
61. TB: BCG Vaccination, Issue of a Booklet entitled *Truth about BCG: Why Government has launched a Mass-Campaign, Papers Recorded*, August 26, 1955, GO 2682, MS Series, TNSA.
62. Brimnes, *Languished Hopes*, 159.
63. Rajkumari Amrit Kaur, "BCG Vaccination Campaign," August 31, 1955, Debate: Calling Attention (Rule 197), Part II: Other Than Questions and Answers, Session 10, *Lok Sabha Debates*, Parliament of India Digital Library. Accessed November 22, 2024. https://eparlib.nic.in/bitstream/123456789/896040/1/01_X_31-08-1955_p31_p33_PII.pdf#search=BCG%20vaccination.
64. Ibid.
65. Keeny, *Half of the World's Children*, 83.
66. Keeny, *Half of the World's Children*, 84.
67. Ibid., 84.
68. S.M. Keeny, *Twenty Years Together: Written for WHO Review*, August 8, 1967, YMCA Biographical Files: S.M. Keeny, Folder 10, Box 110, Kautz Family Papers, UMN.
69. Vivek Neelakantan, "The Campaign Against Yaws in Postcolonial Indonesia: Forgotten Disease, Unfinished Victories," *IIAS Newsletter* 61, no. 4 (2014): 10–11, 10.
70. Ibid., 11.
71. The Kodijat Method restricted penicillin injections exclusively to patients displaying active yaws lesions.
72. Neelakantan, "The Campaign Against Yaws," 11.
73. M. Soetopo, R. Wasito, H. Soedarsono, and D. Tjokrodipo, "The Indonesian Treponematoses Control Project," *Bulletin of the World Health Organization* 15, no. 6 (1956): 937–58.
74. "Interview with Spurgeon Milton Keeny Conducted by Peter Jessup," November 27, 1980, Doc. CF/HST/INT/KEE-009/M, UNICEF Archives.
75. Ibid.
76. Neelakantan, "The Campaign Against Yaws," 11.
77. Ibid., 11.
78. Neelakantan, "The Campaign Against Yaws," 10.
79. "Big Fight Against Yaws," *The Straits Times*, December 10, 1953, 6, NLB.
80. "Major Anti-Yaws Drive Starts," *Singapore Standard*, May 22, 1954, 2, NLB.
81. "Campaign to Beat Rural Area Disease," *The Straits Times*, February 12, 1960, 11, NLB.

82. "Interview with Spurgeon Milton Keeny."
83. Neelakantan, "The Campaign Against Yaws," 11.
84. Ibid, 11.
85. Maurice Pate, "UNICEF Goals in Maternal and Child Welfare: Statement at the Annual Meeting of American Public Health Association," October 22, 1959, CF/HST/1985/034/anx.02/05, UNICEF Archives. The Executive Board set forth the following three criteria for UNICEF regional offices while emphasizing campaigns against endemic disease: (a) the disease should have a high incidence in children; (b) effective treatment for the disease is possible; and (c) per capita treatment costs are low.
86. Dr Eliot's Trip, "Report on Trip to Observe MCH Services Aided by UNICEF in Lebanon, Jordan, Syria, Iran, Philippine Islands, Thailand, Indonesia and India," UNICEF 1956, Folder 723, Box 53, MC 229, *Martha May Eliot Papers*, Schlesinger.
87. Ibid.
88. "Letter from Professor Kenneth Hill to Joe," February 14, 1951, Correspondence, Reports, Etc, Folder 756, Box 53, MC 229, *Martha May Elliot Papers*, Schlesinger.
89. Ibid.
90. Ibid.
91. Ibid.
92. Wong, "UNICEF in Asia," 44.
93. Black, *Children and the Nations*, 170.
94. Angela Villani, "Children in the Development Debate," 433.
95. Angela Villani, "Planning the Needs of Children in the Global South: UNICEF's Contribution to the Development Debate during the 1960s," *Histoire Politique* no. 41 (2020). Accessed November 27, 2024. https://journals.openedition.org/histoirepolitique/356.
96. Wong, "UNICEF in Asia," 33.

CHAPTER 6

The ILO's Health Mandate in Newly Decolonizing Asia, 1947–1978

Introduction

Founded in 1919 under the auspices of the League of Nations, the International Labor Organization (ILO) acquired the status of a UN agency by 1946. What distinguishes the ILO from other specialized UN agencies, such as the World Health Organization (WHO), is tripartism, which ensures representation from governments, labor unions, and workers in decision-making process.

The ILO, the only League vestige to have survived World War II, initially focused on workers' rights but broadened its mandate after the 1944 Declaration of Philadelphia.[1] The Declaration advocated for a significant shift toward economic and social policies aimed at ensuring full employment, raising living standards, expanding social security, and improving housing, child welfare, and maternity protection. It pledged the ILO's full cooperation with UN bodies entrusted with measures to promote socio-economic advancement of less-developed regions. It asserted that all human beings, irrespective of race, creed, or sex, have the right to pursue their well-being and spiritual development. Soon after, the ILO became a forum where demands for equality could be formulated in the new language of social rights. Labor standards drafted during the interwar years were reincarnated in the postwar era as human rights, offering newly decolonized Asian states a universal yardstick for social progress.[2]

V. Neelakantan, *The Emergence of International Health Policy in Southeast Asia, India, and Sri Lanka, 1937–1978*,
https://doi.org/10.1007/978-3-032-21233-7_6

After World War II, Asian nations exhorted the ILO to abandon its Eurocentric framework centered around industrial labor. Across Asia, agricultural labor—largely informal—formed the backbone of national economies. Yet agricultural workers remained outside the ambit of formal labor protections and faced seasonal unemployment, inadequate wages, and economic precarity. The year 1947—coinciding with Indian independence—marked the onset of ILO's postcolonial engagements. India's economic potential and the confidence of the Nehruvian administration, which aimed to position the country as Asia's leading power, compelled the ILO to reorient its priorities toward regionalization.[3] Asia's political decolonization necessitates revisiting the ILO's engagement with community development, spanning comprehensive socioeconomic initiatives in public health, rural welfare, and infrastructure.

Early ILO histories paid attention to the ideological and institutional roots of the organization dating from the nineteenth century.[4] Unsurprisingly, Eurocentric perspectives dominated historiography during the interwar years, even though Asian countries—notably China, Japan, Siam (Thailand since 1939), and British India—had joined the organization. Historian Jasmien van Daele observes that in the postwar decades, particularly the 1950s and 1960s, scholarship shifted from institutional architecture to decision-making processes.[5] These historiographical turns were driven by tensions between the ILO's constitutional design and its operational realities—gaps that became conspicuous under Cold War pressures.[6] Amid escalating North-South divide, the ILO's role in promoting universal human rights—especially rights at work, freedom of association, social security, and non-discrimination—gained scholarly traction. These evolving lines of inquiry mirrored the ILO's practical challenge: recalibrating global mandates to local conditions.

Between the 1950s and the 1970s, the ILO faced the challenge of reconciling its worldwide membership with regional needs in postcolonial Asian states such as India, Ceylon, Burma, Indonesia, and the Philippines. The ILO's Technical Assistance Program (TAP) in Asia further heightened this challenge.[7] To make the TAP an effective tool in the fight against communism, the ILO supported modernization efforts in newly independent countries. In 1948, American David Morse, a New Dealer, took over as Director-General of the ILO, a position he held for 22 years. The communist victory in mainland China pushed Morse to ensure that Asian countries remained aligned with the Western democratic sphere through an integrated approach to community development.[8] Starting in

1952, India was the first country to implement ILO-directed community development projects. However, the benefits of community development were limited and unevenly realized.[9] At the local level, community development plans were limited in scope, prioritizing the construction of wells, community centers, roads, and markets, which disproportionately benefited the village elite. Consequently, dominant caste groups resisted the ILO's and Indian government's attempts to redress socioeconomic inequalities, such as unequal land holdings.

In this chapter, I argue that during the post-World War II era, the ILO was both the *de facto and de jure* advisory agency scaffolding postcolonial Asian nations in their efforts to implement Universal Health Coverage (UHC). However, geopolitical constraints—most notably the Cold War and inter-agency friction between the WHO and the ILO—complicated and, in certain contexts, constrained these initiatives.

"Infectious Disease Somewhere Might be a Danger to Healthy Conditions Elsewhere": ILO and Regionalization

The post-World War II era posed significant challenges for the participation of newly independent Asian states in ILO deliberations due to their geographical distance from Geneva. The distance hindered meaningful engagement for states such as the Philippines, Indonesia, Burma, and Ceylon, which joined the ILO between 1947 and 1957. Recognizing these difficulties, the ILO disembarked on administrative decentralization to address regional specificities.

The Preparatory Asian Regional Conference of the ILO, held in New Delhi in 1947, highlighted the symbolic and territorial asymmetries of decolonization, with Burma, Ceylon, Malaya, and French Indochina still under colonial rule. Conference delegates urged the establishment of direct liaison with Asian constituents. In response, the ILO inaugurated an Asian field office for technical training in Bangalore in 1949. However, geopolitical conflicts between India and Pakistan postponed plans for a full-fledged Asian Regional Office.[10]

In 1963, the Asian field office was provisionally transferred to Colombo before its merger with the UN's regional Economic Commission for Asia and the Far East, headquartered in Bangkok in 1966. The consolidation highlighted ILO's attempts to liaise with other UN agencies to ensure the coordinated delivery of regionally benchmarked development initiatives.

Building on British India's precedent-setting labor diplomacy at the International Labor Congress in 1930, the proposal to hold a regional ILO conference gained institutional traction in Montreal (99th Session, 1946). At this session, Director-General Edward Phelan (1941–1948)—mindful of wartime disruptions and postcolonial transitions—advocated sustained and regionally embedded engagement with Asia.[11] The ILO's Mission visits to China, India, Siam, Burma, Ceylon, Indochina, Malaya, the Philippines, and Singapore (1946) catalyzed the Preparatory Asian Regional Conference, which addressed social protection frameworks, general labor concerns, and a programmatic framework for implementing international labor standards.[12]

Social security topped the agenda of the Preparatory Asian Regional Conference. Since the Great Depression (1929), the ILO has advocated protection of workers against involuntary unemployment and incapacity to work due to accident, illness, or maternity. Sir William Beveridge's proposals to reorganize social security in the UK in 1943—amid World War II—galvanized similar demands across postwar Asia. This surge stemmed from multiple forces. A nationalist awakening—rooted in postcolonial dignity—fueled aspirations to elevate living standards. These aspirations converged with US national interests in opening new markets for domestic manufacturers. In the Asian context, economic development shaped how social security measures could contribute to national reconstruction. Yet implementation was contingent on international collaboration.[13] The Declaration of Philadelphia—which asserted that poverty anywhere threatened prosperity everywhere—affirmed the international basis of development. The ILO adopted the Declaration as a cornerstone for postwar reconstruction across Asia.

At the Preparatory Asian Regional Conference, the ILO recommended to its Asian members:

> In view of the extreme poverty, the wide prevalence of disease and epidemics, the high incidence of infant and maternal mortality, the low expectation of life, and the misery and destitution caused by unemployment and underemployment among the working peoples of most Asian countries, the establishment of social security services, which are an essential condition of building up a genuine democratic society, has become an urgent task.[14]

Delegates emphasized that public health was foundational to any welfare state. For raising the overall living standards, the Conference urged governments to ensure access to essential foodstuffs, a living wage, decent housing, and a healthy environment.

Recognizing the tangible benefits that social security conferred, the ILO cautioned newly independent Asian states against perceiving such measures as a panacea for their social problems.[15] While the disbursement of social security benefits was typically linked to income loss due to illness, such frameworks presumed that individuals earned a subsistence wage and enjoyed baseline health. Instead, the ILO advised member states to focus on endemic diseases that sapped the population's vitality. Nonetheless, the organization warned against postponing the introduction of social security until disease eradication was complete. The ILO recommended that the risks covered by such services remain manageable and that contributions not encumber individuals below the poverty line.[16] To improve living standards, the ILO advised Asian governments to prioritize essential needs such as nutrition, shelter, and basic health services.

Building on ILO's earlier caution against overreliance on social insurance, the Preparatory Asian Regional Conference recognized the predominantly rural character of most Asian countries. Delegates were unanimous that, given the low standard of living and the widespread prevalence of preventable diseases, it was essential to provide medical care to the entire population rather than depend exclusively on social insurance. The Conference invited the ILO to conduct detailed studies of social insurance schemes, liaise with the Food and Agricultural Organization (FAO) on crop insurance in Asian countries, and communicate with the WHO regarding the resolution of the ILO Subcommittee on Medical Care.[17]

Emphasizing its focus on health and social welfare, the Conference investigated factors affecting the productivity of Asian labor. Delegates identified key impediments to labor productivity, notably poor health resulting from undernutrition, malnutrition, disease, poor working conditions, and low wages.[18] Furthermore, labor productivity was impeded by three interlinked factors:

(1) Pressure of population on land, which through the law of diminishing returns, resulted in low average output per unit of agricultural labor;
(2) Low level of capital stock available for production;

(3) Inefficiency in production due to the absence of industrial tradition.[19]

Consequently, delegates resolved to strengthen healthcare by integrating curative and preventive health services to enhance delivery effectiveness.

Recognizing the communitarian structure of Asian societies, the ILO Preparatory Asian Regional Conference supported the universalization of healthcare.[20] Public health, in the view of the ILO, was part of a broader push toward a welfare state, transforming beneficiaries from the status of a recipient of a charity or a pauper subjected to means-testing into citizens entitled to medical care as a right.[21] The Conference's resolutions and recommendations embodied a utopian vision. The dilemma, then, facing the ILO and Asian member states was how the right to health could be effectively implemented.

In grappling with how to operationalize the right to health, the Conference turned its focus to the demographic realities of the region. Among countries represented at the Preparatory Asian Regional Conference, the percentage of the population residing in rural areas was notably high and ranged from 87.2 percent in India to 92.5 percent in Indonesia.[22] The densely populated rural areas of Asia offered organizational advantages often absent in sparsely populated districts. Sanitary engineering on a small scale in Asian villages was cost-effective and benefited the closely-knit rural populations. At the conference, the ILO recommended establishing primary health units centered on the village community, drawing on three examples: the Rockefeller-funded Kalutara rural health unit in Ceylon, founded in 1926; the organization of health services in French Indochina; and the recommendations of the Health Survey and Development (Bhore) Committee (1946). For India, the Bhore Committee recommended a network of rural health centers connected to referral hospitals in larger towns.

Based on the ILO Mission to Asia's (1946) conclusions, the conference deliberations noted:

> In the Indian villages, the standard of sanitation is shown by the Bhore Committee's report to be very low; water supplies are not everywhere protected from contamination in most villages no system of collection and disposal of night soil exists; and no attempt has, on the whole, been made for the collection and disposal of household refuse. Similar conditions are found in China and certain other Asiatic countries.[23]

At the conference, the ILO exhorted Asian member states to focus on strengthening environmental hygiene.

Furthermore, the ILO cautioned Asian states that the organization of health services would be illusory without integrating maternal and child welfare services.[24] However, the organization's stance toward family planning remained ambiguous. At the Preparatory Asian Regional Conference, the ILO adopted an equivocal position on birth control. While infectious disease control contributed to population growth, the agency urged a shift in public attitudes. Notably, the ILO made an unsubstantiated claim that the birth rates declined in areas where living standards were improving.[25] The ILO emphasized that recognizing health as integral to individual and family well-being was a prerequisite for socioeconomic development.

Extending its diagnostic scope, the Conference also acknowledged structural impediments in mobilizing public health as an instrument of national reconstruction. Yet, optimistically, the ILO asserted, "Thus, community structure, health conditions and general lack of health facilities in rural Asia would seem to create a strong presumption in favour of a public medical care service."[26]

The Preparatory Asian Regional Conference refashioned the Bhore Committee recommendations to the exigencies of the postcolonial state in Asia. The conference's Subcommittee on Medical Care reiterated the Bhore Committee recommendations:

(1) No individual should fail to secure medical care because of inability to pay for it.
(2) In view of the complexity of modern medical practice, the health services should provide, when fully developed, all the consultant, laboratory, and institutional facilities necessary for proper diagnosis and treatment.
(3) The health program must, from the beginning, lay special emphasis on preventive work. The creation of as healthy an environment as possible in the homes, workplaces, and recreation areas is essential. The lack of attention to environmental hygiene, faulty modes of life, and disease susceptibility factors must be rectified; otherwise, villages and towns will continue to supply cases to hospitals.[27]

Yet in the light of fiscal constraints grappling newly decolonized Asian states, the Subcommittee on Medical Care allowed considerable flexibility in implementing Bhore Committee's recommendations on preventive health. It recommended devolving schemes concerning environmental hygiene to local bodies and financing them through taxpayer contributions. For plantation-dominated economies such as Ceylon, the Subcommittee proposed assigning responsibility to employers for providing adequate housing and sanitation to workers. While offering comprehensive recommendations for organizing preventive health services, the Subcommittee left key ambiguities in other areas of healthcare provision: a case of balancing between pragmatism and shared responsibility.

The Subcommittee's recommendations relating to the provision of maternal and child health benefits to workers across Asia were notably ambiguous:

> Variation must be allowed for also in dealing with women of different races and customs, and according to the type of work they have to do. In some places, a total of three months' abstinence from work is often longer than is strictly necessary. In considering the period of benefit after confinement, it must be remembered that from the point of view of the infant's chance of survival, the longer that period can be, the better. On the other hand, from the viewpoint of costs, the rate of benefit or sick pay must be considered, as well as the duration. Two months' benefit on full pay costs the employer or the fund the same as three months on two thirds' pay, and in some cases the shorter period with the higher pay may be better for the mother. Some women, because of their poor physique or because of the nature of their work, would require a longer period. Others, who are robust, will suffer no harm if the time is shortened. From a medical point of view, under the conditions at present prevailing in Asia, a fair average period is two months' benefit, but there must be provision to extend this by at least another month where the woman's health is unsatisfactory.

The discussion on maternity benefits revealed a disjuncture between universal labor standards and the socio-cultural heterogeneity underpinning Asian labor regimes—a principled negotiation between fiscal realism and the physiological imperatives of postnatal care.

Indian Premier Jawaharlal Nehru's welcome address to the Preparatory Asian Regional Conference delegates emphasized the urgency of regional action on part of the ILO. Nehru noted:

> Somewhat inevitably, perhaps, the attention of the Organisation has been concentrated—probably more than the facts of geography warranted —on problems other than Asian problems. I do not wish to minimise the work

> which is done in Asia; nevertheless, the perspective was largely—if I may say so—European. Again, political factors also came in, that is to say, a number of Asian countries were under colonial domination, and politics and economics are interlaced so that one cannot separate them. One effect of this political domination in various Asian countries was to turn the minds of men in those countries towards the achievement of political freedom. The economic issues were somewhat hidden by this political struggle for freedom, although the economic issues of course can never be ignored and are apt to produce catastrophic consequences if you seek to ignore them. There was this difficulty in Asia, and now, when most of the countries in Asia are politically free or, I hope, on the verge of freedom, these economic questions are coming very much to the fore.[28]

Nehru asserted that even affluent nations could be pulled into an economic vortex arising from Asian poverty. Therefore, the ILO should elevate living standards—not as charity but as strategic foresight in a decolonizing world (Image 6.1).

During the interwar years, the ILO had prioritized the concerns of industrial over agricultural labor. However, as India and other newly independent Asian countries were primarily agricultural, Nehru urged the organization to assist member states in increasing food production.[29] He asserted that the solution to agricultural and industrial questions was interrelated. Excessive population pressure on land, according to Nehru, was the root cause of poverty in India. Since the turn of the nineteenth century, India's rural population grew disproportionately compared to the urban population. While Nehru perceived industrialization as the key to harnessing the population surplus engaged in agriculture, he also recognized that industrialization could not be separated from broader social progress. As Nehru noted, "Again, if we think of the industrial aspect, we have to think of the development of the social services, sanitation, health, education, etc."[30] Nehru's holistic perspective aligned with ILO's emphasis on integrating public health within socioeconomic development—recalibrating universal standards to local contexts, ensuring that economic development did not override social welfare.

India's engagement with the ILO was not driven by economic imperatives, but by broader geopolitical ambitions to assert its leadership in post-colonial Asia. The Nehruvian administration challenged the agency's Eurocentric labor policies, arguing that the Philadelphia Declaration's

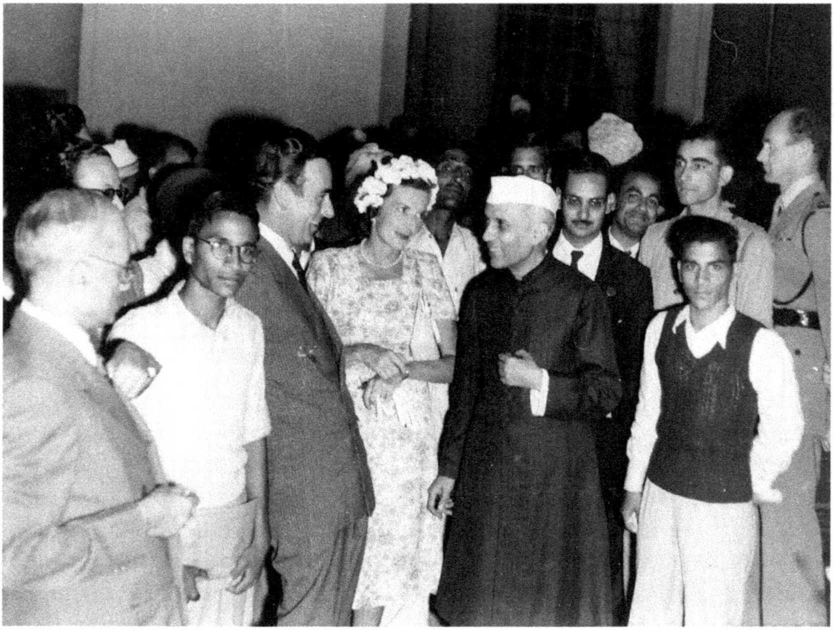

Image 6.1 ILO Preparatory Asian Regional Conference, New Delhi (1947). Mr Zahid Hussain (Pakistan, extreme left) with Lord and Lady Mountbatten and Jawaharlal Nehru at Pakistani delegation's party to Conference delegates. Source: With permission from the ILO Historical Archives, Geneva

normative framework required contextual reinterpretation to reflect the socioeconomic structures of newly independent states.[31]

Historically, the ILO maintained limited engagement with Asia, with only two contact bureaus in New Delhi and Nanking operating during the interwar period.[32] The Pacific War witnessed a significant contraction of ILO's Asian footprint. Recognizing the need for a robust regional structure, Asian states represented at the Preparatory Asian Regional Conference wanted a guarantee from Geneva against a reversion to skeletal branch offices. Instead, they advocated for a comprehensive regional network equipped to relay Asia-specific concerns to ILO headquarters. For newly independent Asian states, regionalization ensured continued technical assistance for postwar reconstruction.

At the ILO's Asian Regional Conference convened in Nuwara Eliya, Ceylon, in January 1950, Director-General Morse observed:

> Great principles had been proclaimed in the ILO Constitution and the Declaration of Philadelphia; the ILO decided upon the positive and rapid implementation of their principles, and would set out to the extent of the resources in the interest of positive social and economic action in Asia.[33]

In the postwar era, the notion of development—highlighted in the 1944 ILO Declaration of Philadelphia—became a rallying point for newly decolonized Asian states. These states demanded that the ILO transform the new mandate into concrete action. Conversely, several European states were apprehensive about a dilution of ILO's classical standard-setting activities and treated the demands from developing countries with noticeable skepticism. ILO's European delegates feared that any shift toward technical assistance would result in the erosion of international labor standards and consequently unregulated competition from low-cost Asian workers.[34] Faced with these competing demands, the ILO sought a middle ground: balancing the needs of newly independent Asian states with the concerns of European delegates. A key step in the process was regionalization, exemplified by the establishment of the ILO Field Office in Bangalore, India, that Morse announced at Nuwara Eliya. This move signified the ILO's efforts to reconcile broader tensions between development mandates and preservation of labor standards.

The Bangalore Field Office identified the absence of trained manpower in Asian countries as a significant obstacle to development. Responding to the demands from Asian countries, the TAP during the 1950s promoted industrialization.[35] Development theorists of the time, particularly W. Arthur Lewis asserted that the panacea to the problems of underdeveloped countries lay in rapid industrialization.[36] A central development dynamic was the linear progression from the agricultural to the industrial sector. Only industrialization could substantially improve living standards.[37] The Technical Manpower Program of the Bangalore Field Office was congruent with Lewis' viewpoint. Morse contended that human resources equate to wealth. In Morse's perspective, for a country to generate wealth, the country must have production, and to produce, people must be trained. The net result of all this was the generation of national wealth.[38] Consequently, what Asian member states needed from the ILO was concerted assistance for economic reconstruction.

The ILO's emphasis on technical assistance and the subordination of social goals to economic growth resonated with the political elite of newly decolonized Asian states. By the end of the 1940s, there was a concerted effort toward state-building. Economic growth during the 1950s was treated as a tool to mask contradictions within Asia's modern economies—forestalling communist advance, reducing poverty, cementing national bonds, and securing domestic capitalist support for state-led development.[39]

Building on the question of national reconstruction, the ILO's regional initiatives in Asia during the early 1950s began to translate developmental rhetoric into operational reality. By 1951, India commenced its First Five-Year Plan. Political Economist Francine Frankel notes that the Plan Frame intended to achieve the economic and social goals delineated by Nehru: (1) expand the scope of the public sector; (2) develop heavy industry and further economic self-sufficiency; (3) promote labor-intensive small-scale industries; (4) eliminate unemployment; (5) increase agricultural productivity; (6) improve the quality of social services including housing, health, and education for the poorer sections of the population. These measures were calculated to increase the national income by 25 percent and achieve an equitable income distribution.[40] Underlying all programs was a single metric: the economic goal of increasing production. The Planning Commission asserted that public health was an instrumental tool in advancing the goal of national development.[41]

Burma embarked on its own vision toward a planned economy in 1952—ideologically distinct yet rooted in the same postcolonial context as India's First Five-Year Plan. The initiative, known by the appellation of *Pyidawtha* [Burmese: Prosperous Royal Country], attempted to blend Burma's rich cultural traditions with modern aspirations.[42] The Plan comprised ten grand schemes covering: (1) transfer of power to regional governments, (2) public health, (3) education, (4) economy, (5) nationalization of arable lands, (6) transportation, (7) sufficiency (welfare), (8) democratic local councils, (9) development in frontier and non-developed areas, and (10) rebuilding.[43]

When Burmese Premier U Nu inaugurated the *Pyidawtha* Conference in 1952, he outlined that the goal of the administration was to transform lives through comprehensive development, emphasizing the five pillars: physique, intellect, economy, morality, and society.[44] In his speech, U Nu pledged to work hard so that the citizens could be as healthy as the legendary heroes Kyan-is thà and Tha-main-ba-yan, who could singlehandedly fight tigers, gorillas, and crocodiles.[45] U Nu's speeches evoked nostalgia more than they outlined concrete development plans. Although health was a central ingredient in postcolonial Burma's national reconstruction, social insurance struggled to gain traction due to ethnic unrest and financial instability. The Constitution stipulated, "The State shall protect workers ... as soon as circumstances permit by promoting schemes for housing and social insurance."[46] The ILO's Report to the Government of Burma on Social Security noted that Burma's low per capita income—estimated at US$ 33 in 1949—significantly constrained public spending on social security.[47] As a solution to limited public spending on social security, the Report recommended a tripartite approach for the urban areas of Burma, involving contributions from employers, workers, and the government.

Encountering domestic constraints and the ambition of decolonized states in Asia, American experts saw social reform as integral to curbing communist influence.[48] Raising Burmese living standards was seen as crucial to establishing the economic foundation of a welfare state modeled along Western lines. American strategists attempted to narrow the divide between the employed and the rest of the population through this transformation. In Burma, numerous government reports highlighted strong reservations about acceptance of overseas aid, fearing such measures would compromise the country's hard-won political sovereignty. In November 1947, the US charge in Rangoon noted that given the anti-US sentiments in Burma, the best counteroffensive for the Americans might be to channel US technical assistance on maternal and child health, strategically winning the hearts and minds of the masses.[49]

Against this backdrop of America's recalibration of international aid in newly decolonized Asia, India intensified its efforts to decolonize the ILO and reorient its focus toward the needs of newly decolonized countries. India's move reflected a broader push for equitable representation and regionalization within international organizations, long dominated by Europe and North America.[50] India and Burma—advocating for the continuation of the ILO's technical assistance—framed modernization not merely as a policy imperative, but as a key driver of postwar recovery.

However, Pakistan contested India's quest for regional leadership. Between 1949 and 1951, Pakistan attempted to relocate the ILO Field Office out of India but received lukewarm support. At the Asian Manpower Conference in Bangkok (1951), rather than insisting on removing the ILO Field Office from India, Pakistan pressed for the establishment of more field offices in all Asian member states.[51] During the conference, Indian delegate Subramanian cautioned that a second field office for Asia risked duplicating efforts.[52]

Coinciding with the Bangkok Conference (1951), the ILO deputed TAP Field Missions to each country in the region. The TAP Field Mission Reports highlighted considerable disparities in the implementation of social insurance.[53] Burma's Social Security Act (1954) established a contributory social insurance scheme that covered workers against sickness, maternity, and death, but financial difficulties restricted implementation to urban areas.[54] In India, the report noted that the Employees State Insurance Scheme (1948)—piloted in Delhi and Kanpur in 1952—was expected to cover the entire country progressively. The program was financed through joint contributions from employees, and employers, and subsidies from central and state governments concerning the disbursement of medical benefits. The scheme faltered due to unclear lines of responsibility between the central and provincial governments concerning hospitalization and the inclusion of families into medical insurance.[55] The ILO's recommendations concerning social security were largely normative in nature.

Following the Bangkok Conference, ILO reoriented its mandate from setting prescriptive labor standards toward technical assistance. This transformation aimed to redress the colonial labor legacies of decolonized Asian states, which had prioritized extractive plantation economies over worker protection. The region's structural challenges—seasonal agricultural unemployment, low living standards, and demographic pressure—collectively militated against integrating postcolonial Asian states into the world economy. Consequently, Cold War undercurrents steered the ILO toward social security and community development, reflecting the organization's efforts to counter ideological polarization. The agency's regional strategy sought to reconcile international labor norms with postcolonial Asia's distinct socioeconomic realities.

Rural Underdevelopment in India: Insights from ILO-Commissioned Surveys, 1950s

On October 2, 1952, commemorating the birth anniversary of M.K. Gandhi, Nehru launched India's community development program. Nehru announced:

> The scheme of community development projects, a direct result of the Indo-American technical cooperation agreements signed in the beginning of 1952, have been spelled out in the draft of the First Five-Year Plan in July 1951. The 500 community centres, contemplated in the Plan, were to undertake home building, road-making, canal digging, school construction, medical and health units, cooperative farming, multipurpose cooperative societies, cottage industries and a host of other projects.[56]

Nehru invoked Gandhi's legacy to frame community development as a continuation of the ideals espoused by the anti-colonial movement.

Community development projects in India could be traced to a lineage of model village experiments carried out by late colonial bureaucrats, Gandhian rural reconstruction, and American missionary programs from the early twentieth century.[57] However, American involvement in Indian rural development remained limited until the 1950s. With the advent of Cold War-era development initiatives, US engagement grew, emphasizing the localization of technical expertise for rural application. Community development in India was embedded within a broader matrix of international development institutions, including the Colombo Plan, UNICEF (United Nations Children's Fund), the FAO (Food and Agricultural Organization), the WHO, and the ILO.

Since 1947, the ILO has promoted technical assistance across Asia, construed as the starting point of a modernization process marked by economic growth, increased productivity, and industrialization. In 1949, Morse framed technical assistance as a mechanism to build institutional and economic foundations required to implement ILO standards.

In the context of the Cold War, Morse argued that the ILO could precipitate social change by focusing on the advancement of newly decolonized nations.[58] He envisioned the TAP as a Cold War instrument—supporting the global struggle between capitalist and communist systems. This integrated strategy positioned the TAP as a vehicle for aligning pro-Western initiatives with postwar national reconstruction in Asia.[59]

Notwithstanding Morse's leadership in steering the ILO toward technical assistance, his advocacy of an integrated approach to development for Asia did not go unchallenged. Morse's universal TAP unsettled colonial powers by erasing the distinction between colonial and independent states, destabilizing the performative exceptionalism undergirding imperial governance.[60]

Amid geopolitical tensions ascribed to decolonization and the Cold War, the International Labor Office advanced its agenda through quieter means. Its promotion of the "ILO Way" was subtle.[61] Rather than overt intervention, the organization provided information, advisory services, and practical support in domains aligned with labor standards. ILO staff periodically produced Mission Reports diagnosing impediments to labor productivity but their utility remained diagnostic—more prescriptive than transformative. By comparison, postcolonial India took a hands-on approach to community development, privileging local agency and participatory engagement over abstract externally driven technical expertise.

In postcolonial India, community development was conceived as a coordinated effort to uplift villages by enhancing productivity, living standards, expanding access to health and education, and reshaping rural attitudes toward work and life. V.T. Krishnamachari, vice-chairman of the Planning Commission, argued that democracy in India had to be built bottom-up from the rural areas. Consequently, he envisioned every Indian family working collaboratively to combat poverty and elevate living standards thereby strengthening moral and social cohesion.[62] Yet, development economist Gunnar Myrdal captured the irony: despite the program's optimistic launch and promises of rapid transformation, conditions in Indian villages remained largely unchanged.[63]

Other Asian nations adopted a similar approach to community development but with far less zeal. During the 1950s, the Philippine community development landscape was punctuated by siloed institutional structures, despite efforts to project coordination.[64] Although the Philippine program emphasized the *barrio* [Tagalog: village] and self-help projects for implementing community development at grassroots level, barrio community development workers were only one of several state agencies contacting villagers. These multiple points of contact led to administrative overlaps. Furthermore, personnel from state agencies lacked orientation to rural conditions. Indonesia, on the other hand, began with greater potential for village cooperatives during the early 1950s.[65] However, these efforts waned as vice-president Mohammed Hatta abdicated the political scene in 1956. In essence, both the Philippines and Indonesia had the right ingredients for community development—cooperatives, self-help, and political participation. Despite initial promise, implementing community development in both countries faltered as administrative and political changes disrupted momentum, leaving community development adrift in bureaucratic inertia. The Philippines and Indonesia reflected a broader

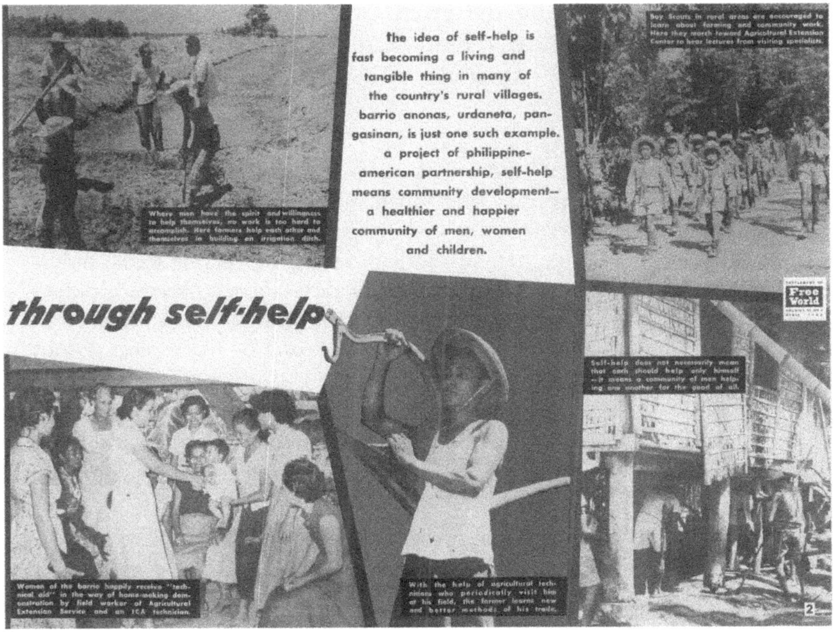
the idea of self-help is fast becoming a living and tangible thing in many of the country's rural villages. barrio anonas, urdaneta, pangasinan, is just one such example. a project of philippine-american partnership, self-help means community development—a healthier and happier community of men, women and children.
through self-help
Boy Scouts in rural areas are encouraged to learn about farming and community work. Here they march toward Agricultural Extension Center to hear lectures from visiting specialists.
Where men have the spirit and willingness to help themselves, no work is too hard to accomplish. Here farmers help each other and themselves in building an irrigation ditch.
Self-help does not necessarily mean that each should help only himself—it means a community of men helping one another for the good of all.
Women of the barrio happily receive "technical aid" in the way of home-making demonstration by field worker of Agricultural Extension Service and an ICA technician.
With the help of agricultural technicians who periodically visit him at his field, the farmer learns new and better methods of his trade.
Free World

Image 6.2 Philippines: Community development through self-help. Date created: March 20, 1957. National Archives Identifier: 6949000. Local ID: 306-PPB-128. Record Group 306: Records of the US Information Agency. Series: Propaganda Posters Distributed in Asia, 1950–1965. Creator: US Information Agency. NARA. URL: https://catalog.archives.gov/id/6949000. Unrestricted (Public Domain)

regional pattern where siloed governance and political volatility trumped the postcolonial state's symbolic commitment to grassroots empowerment (Image 6.2).

While several postcolonial nations faced challenges in implementing community development, India's rural transformation was a bold experiment in Asia that attempted to transform the socioeconomic landscape. One such notable example was the Etawah pilot community development program in the northern state of Uttar Pradesh that began in 1948. The Etawah project was the brainchild of US architect Albert Mayer, who served as a soldier in British India during World War II. Mayer was moved by the poverty of Indian villagers and their remarkable resilience. The Etawah project was an experiment that blended the Gandhian village development program with the extension service techniques of the US Department of Agriculture.[66] Remarkably, Indians funded the project themselves. In 1952, American Ambassador to India, Chester B. Bowles noted:

> When we first visited Etawah the work was being carried out in ninety-seven villages with some sixty thousand inhabitants. Village workers had been carefully trained, first to win the confidence of the villagers and then to introduce in each village new methods of fertilizing, better seeds, public health measures, primary education and literacy courses. We were deeply impressed by the nearly 50-per-cent increase which had been achieved in food production, by the clean, healthier villages and by the earnest groups of villagers learning to read and write.[67]

Initial results of the Etawah experiment appeared promising and the US pledged $54 million to the Indian government to further community development across the country.[68]

The Indian government's approach to community development was the subject of considerable debate during the 1950s. Advocates of a perfectionist model contended that every community development project should strive to be a self-sufficient utopia, encompassing impressive schools, hospitals, roads, and robust industries alongside improvised agriculture and health services. The second group argued that implementing a feasible community development program in every Indian village would require compromising some aspects of quality. They warned that focusing on showcase projects might impress foreign journalists but overlook broader rural needs. They advocated for a comprehensive community development program that aimed at ameliorating the lives of rural populations.[69] Nehru endorsed the viewpoint of the second group.

Nehru's preference for scalable development—that entailed administrative reach and replicability—over showcase community development projects aligned with the broader diplomatic choreography of the 1950s, where India navigated foreign aid without signifying ideological commitments to either superpower bloc. Even modest American aid could be tactically leveraged to underscore India's commitment to grassroots mobilization, without deviating from its non-alignment principle. On October 2, 1952—Gandhi's birth anniversary—India's strategic deployment of non-alignment found resonance in the joint inauguration of 55 community development projects, fusing Indian symbolism with international partnership.

By 1956, the Nehru administration introduced 400 community development projects that covered over 100 million people, or one-third of rural India, and considerably more than the combined populations of France, Italy, Belgium, and Holland.[70] These projects necessitated training at least 30,000 multipurpose village workers and hundreds of specialists in soil conservation, irrigation, agricultural engineering, public health, and malaria control.

The aim of Albert Mayer—when he was deputed to Etawah in 1952—was to transform villagers' habits, aligning with the broader objectives of community development. He argued:

> Poor drainage is not only unhealthy and troublesome for bullock carts but it is ugly, sloppy, and should be considered disgusting. A continued effort in lifting the habits of villagers accelerates the crystallization of village leadership. If the village can see more and more of these needs, the emerging leadership can keep getting its teeth into things, will have something to do, and, as it were, something to keep practicing itself on. And as we have undoubtedly increased village incomes by improving crop yields, villagers can afford to do more things. Already a large number of brick houses have replaced mud houses. We already [1952] have a target of fourteen villages which are raising money to improve drainage by paving ditches and lanes.[71]

Mayer intended to awaken a sanitary conscience amidst villagers that would mobilize them to act as a pressure group on the *gram panchayat* [Hindi: a village council] to introduce sanitary bylaws. Mayer contended that agricultural enhancement was the linchpin of Etawah's success. By creating a solid economic base, agriculture would create a demand for improved housing and sanitation, both of which required expenditure by people individually and collectively.[72]

Public health and environmental sanitation were the second item on the agenda of the Etawah project. Sanitation outcomes—unlike agricultural enhancements—remained symbolically muted and operationally uneven. In his Mission Report, Surendra Kumar Jain—member of the ILO Technical Assistance Division—pointed out that while villagers embraced agricultural improvements with zeal, sanitation efforts in the project area stalled due to civic inertia. Jain noted that between 1948 and 1952, the major accomplishment of the Etawah project was agricultural:

an increase in crop yields from 800 to 2190 lbs. per acre.[73] Villagers were willing to experiment with new agricultural techniques and were no longer skeptical of government officials. The multipurpose village worker successfully created enthusiasm in rural communities for development work. Although Indian authorities incorporated environmental sanitation into the Etawah project in 1952, results were less discernible than agricultural enhancements (Images 6.3, 6.4, 6.5, and 6.6).[74]

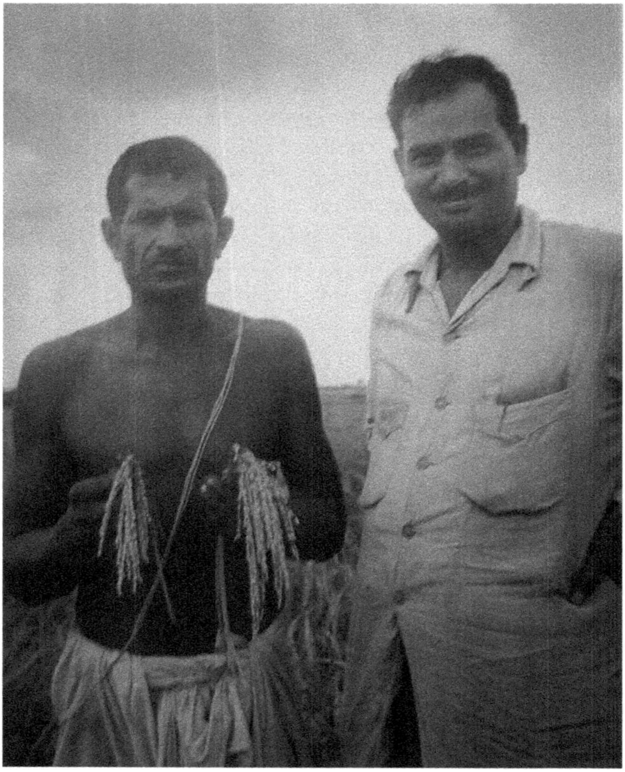

Image 6.3 Rudra Bhal Tiwari (left) and L.R. Bajpai (right). Mr Tiwari holds samples of rice grown by regular method and the Japanese paddy method, c. 1952. Photographer: W.W. McIlroy. Source: Mission: Surendra Kumar Jain, File 177, Jacket 1, September 1951 to December 1958, MI Series, Registry 1159775, ILO Archives. With permission

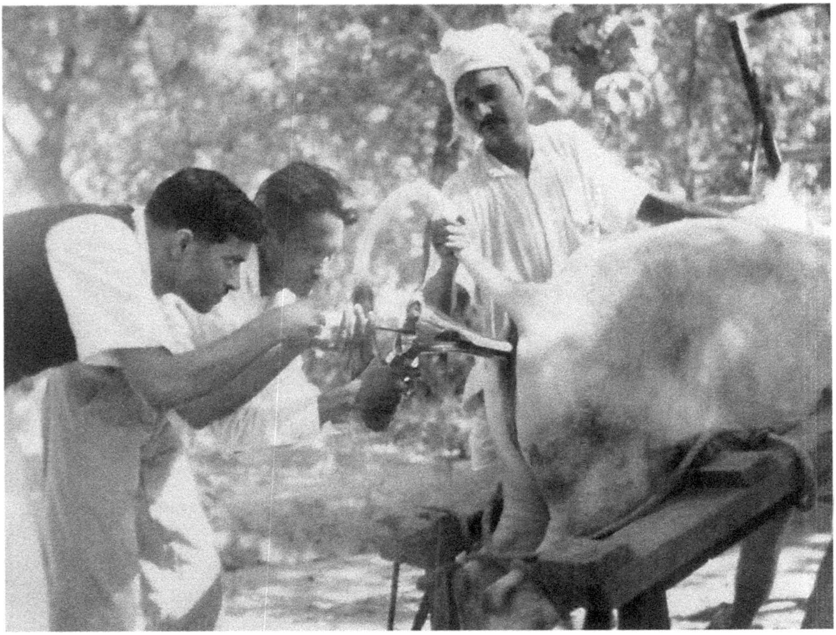

Image 6.4 A cow getting the careful attention of a veterinary doctor, c. 1952. Photographer unknown. Source: Mission: Surendra Kumar Jain, File 177, Jacket 1, September 1951 to December 1958, MI Series, Registry 1159775, ILO Archives. With permission

During the formative years of the Etawah project, prophylactic measures against malaria and cholera were offered in a relatively deprived section of the project area. Given Etawah's low incidence of malaria and cholera, the rural public was unable to appreciate the urgency of preventive hygiene. Consequently, the project staff aborted the campaigns. In 1953, multipurpose workers liaised with public health personnel from the Uttar Pradesh state health department to implement smallpox vaccination across areas under the jurisdiction of the Etawah project.[75] The diversion of personnel to Etawah left the state health department ill-equipped to manage broader smallpox outbreaks.

Scholarly assessments of community development have diverged sharply. In 1959, Harvard Economist William H. Nicholls observed on a cautious note:

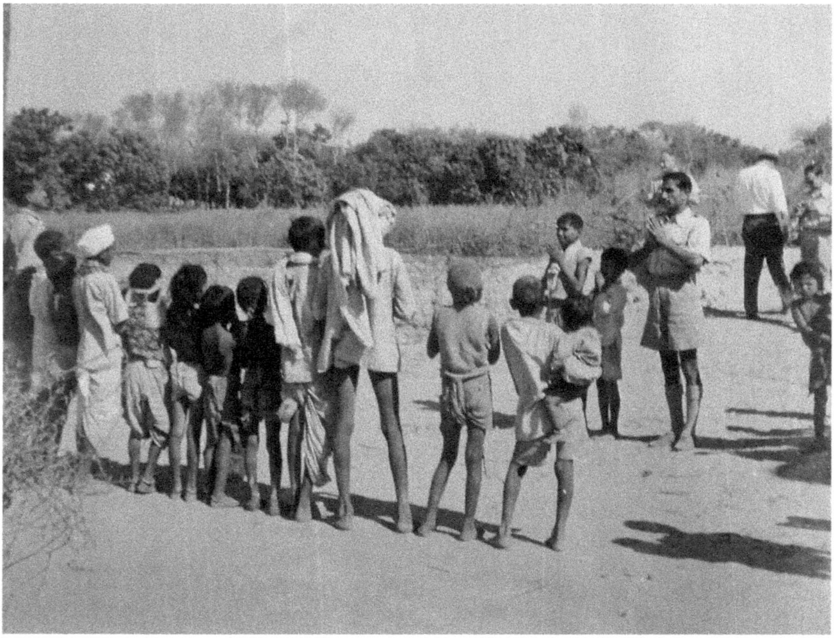

Image 6.5 Youth work being carried out by trainees at Bakshi ka Talab in a nearby village. Many community development trainees found that they could gain entrance to the village by working with the youth of the village first, c.1952. Photo Credit: W.W. McIlroy, on behalf of the TCA (Technical Cooperation Administration). Source: Mission: Surendra Kumar Jain, File 177, Jacket 1, September 1951 to December 1958, MI Series, Registry 1159775, ILO Archives. With permission

> While much too ambitious and diffuse for its present resources, India's community development program is sound in its objectives and, over a generation or two if not during the present five year plan, holds much promise in developing effective community leadership. In these and other programs, however, local government representatives must be imbued with a spirit of service, a belief in the dignity of labor, and a zeal for successful communication by demonstration, example, and persuasion if they are to succeed in overcoming the traditional conservatism and suspicion of the rural masses.[76]

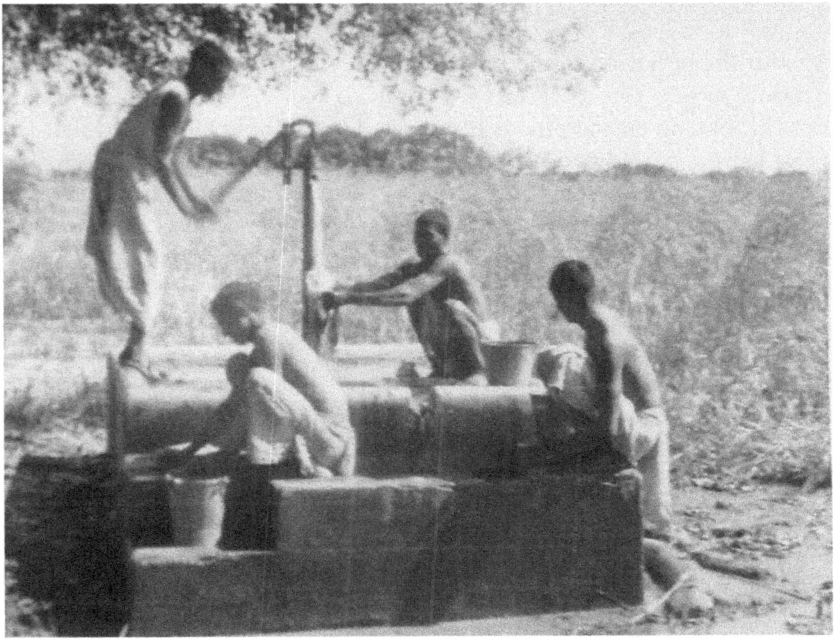

Image 6.6 Sanitary Well: A Handpump, c. 1952. Source: Mission: Surendra Kumar Jain, File 177, Jacket 1, September 1951 to December 1958, MI Series, Registry 1159775, ILO Archives. With permission

The momentum of community development was contingent on the initiative of the *gram panchayat* leadership that was lacking in many parts of India. Consequently, community development tended to favor dominant castes in the village. Myrdal alluded to a caste-like discrimination prevalent among the elite Indian Administrative Service cadre deputed to work in rural areas. They regarded village workers as subordinates, not collaborators.[77] The caste-like discrimination hindered effective grassroots leadership, pivotal to the success of the community development program across India.

The benefits of community development were elusive. Although villagers were willing to compose local development plans when nudged by the government, these plans were strikingly modest in their scope: the construction of wells, market roads, or community centers that benefited well-off members of the rural community.[78]

The Eclipse of UHC

Against the backdrop of the Philadelphia Declaration (1944) and postwar national reconstruction, the ILO sought to codify its vision of social justice through an enforceable convention. The ILO initially hoped that the WHO would endorse the Philadelphia Declaration. Although the Preamble to the WHO Constitution proclaimed the human right to the highest attainable standard of health, the article on strengthening national health services pledged technical assistance only upon request.[79] In 1951, the ILO invited the WHO to cooperate in the formulation of its proposed Convention on Social Security. While social medicine stalwarts such as Henry Sigerist and René Sand endorsed the ILO's position favoring universal coverage, the WHO's Executive Board quickly distanced itself from this.[80] By the early 1950s, the WHO had embraced the proverbial magic bullet. However, national interests influenced by US Cold War concerns trumped UHC, particularly in newly independent Asian states such as the Philippines.

Convening in Mysore, India (December 1949–January 1950), the ILO resolved to revisit the Philadelphia mandate by scheduling "Objectives and Minimum Standards of Social Security" for formal discussion in 1951.[81] The Philadelphia Recommendations on Income Security and Medical Care provided cash benefits to workers in case of maternity, sickness, old age, death of breadwinner, unemployment, or workplace injury, accompanied by medical care. These recommendations encouraged governments to provide comprehensive healthcare to all community members regardless of their employment status. However, a coalition of interests—that included medical professionals, employers, and governments—overshadowed the wartime euphoria concerning social security. Against intensifying Cold War tensions, these interests equated comprehensive medical care to socialized medicine: the provision of medical care for all using taxation.[82] The organization whittled its proposal concerning comprehensive medical care to accommodate political sensitivities.

Against the backdrop of postwar reconstruction, the ILO pursued a convention to implement the Philadelphia recommendations.[83] Following a protracted debate, the agency introduced a dual-track model—permitting member states to ratify either minimum or universal standards. Dilution intensified at the 1952 International Labor Conference, where the final convention permitted ratification of just three of nine branches of social security, with no obligation to include social insurance.[84] In place of these recommendations, the ILO recommended a voluntary insurance system.[85] Low-income countries were granted temporary exemptions, and the ILO ultimately recommended a voluntary health insurance instead of comprehensive guarantees.

The ILO's rollback of comprehensive guarantees unfolded amid mounting Cold War anxieties within the US. During the early 1950s, strengthened hostility toward the USSR colored the US debate about international organizations. The USSR had played a limited role in the founding of the WHO and had refused to join the ILO until 1956. The American Medical Association's opposition to Truman's health insurance developed into attacks on intergovernmental agencies seen as sympathetic to the agenda. The American employer report of the 1951 International Labor Conference warned that the effort of the present ILO government-labor majority—alluding to the Truman administration—to impose centralized government control was being allowed to take precedence over its primary goal of raising standards of living.[86] The tension between government control and individual welfare was a recurring theme in debates concerning social welfare, particularly in the Philippines.

The question of social insurance was a contentious issue in Filipino politics during the presidencies of Elpidio Quirino (1948–1953) and Ramon Magsaysay (1953–1957). The Philippine Medical Association (PMA), founded in 1939, was an affiliate of the American Medical Association. Consequently, PMA physicians were conditioned to be skeptical of a state-centered approach to public health.[87] During the 1950s, the PMA faced the dilemma of meeting the goals of the Philippines' rapidly expanding health programs without diluting professional standards.

The year 1949 was significant for the Philippine working class as President Quirino recommended before Congress the passage of legislation providing prepaid medical services to rural populations.[88] At the time, a faction within the PMA expressed apprehension that Quirino's proposal would lead to the growth of socialized medicine. One such PMA member—also affiliated with the Philippine Federation of Private Medical Practitioners—who vehemently opposed Quirino's proposed legislation was Luis Torres.[89] Torres argued that socialized medicine promised too much, made unreasonable demands on doctors' time, and disrupted the doctor-patient relationship. He warned that socialized medicine spelled the death knell for democracy in the Philippines.

However, PMA members—particularly the incoming president Rodolfo Gonzalez (1950)—did not subscribe to Torres' views. His logic was that minimum state intervention in public health would constrain people's ability to engage in productive work. This would lower the national productivity resulting in a drastic reduction in state income and making it nearly impossible for the Quirino administration to implement its social amelioration program.[90] However, at the inaugural session of the First Southeast Asian Medical Conference in Manila on May 8, 1951, the then incoming PMA President Eugenio Alonso criticized the Quirino administration's shortcomings in providing prepaid medical services to the rural population. He pointed out that no variety of want was more individualized than illness. The illness of a wage earner due to TB or the poor health of a child attributed to malnutrition required the treatment of individual patients.[91]

In 1952, despite opposition from sections of the PMA, President Quirino succeeded in passing Republic Act 747. The Act had two objectives: (1) regulate user fees in government and charity hospitals; (2) determine the eligibility of individuals for free treatment in government hospitals using a classification system.[92] A year later, Quirino liberalized the classification system such that Filipino families with incomes less than 100 pesos were classified as indigents and were eligible for free hospitalization.[93] As a result, nearly 90 percent of Filipinos qualified as indigents under the Act.[94] Following the passage of the Act, there was a rapid construction boom of public hospitals. Government doctors could not staff such hospitals acquired through pork-barrel funds.

Public spending on health acquired a new lease of life under the Magsaysay administration. During his election campaign, Magsaysay promised a better quality of life and exhorted the PMA about extending healthcare to rural communities. In line with his preelection promises, Magsaysay was forced to increase public spending on health and, consequently, taxation. When the Social Security Act (1954) was on the brink of being implemented in 1955, influential segments of management and organized labor revolted.

The political deadlocks underpinning the introduction of social security in the Philippines signaled that the idealism of the 1944 Philadelphia Declaration receded by the 1950s. Despite the ILO's push for broad ratification of the 1952 Convention, few developing countries committed. Newly independent countries such as India hesitated, citing the predominance of unorganized labor sectors.[95] The 1952 Convention—premised on organized labor relations—implicitly embodied the interests of the Global North.[96] In privileging contributory models over universal guarantees, the ILO missed a critical opportunity to embed UHC within the architecture of international development.

During the 1950s and the 1960s, the ILO's approach to health planning was divorced from the WHO. The global spread of social security programs motivated the ILO to launch a study program on medical care in 1966.[97] The study compared the costs, benefits, and healthcare outcomes of distinct social security models. The study selected eight countries based on their representativeness of the most specific types of medical care under social security: Belgium, Canada, Ecuador, the Federal Republic of Germany, India, Poland, Tunisia, and the UK.[98] The ILO's final report on medical care recommended that UHC was beneficial from an administrative perspective and avoided the need for complex eligibility criteria. Christopher Sirrs notes that since the 1950s, the ILO's activities in the Global South were hamstrung due to political, economic, and administrative constraints. The ILO's reliance on European health models—untested in the Global South—further impinged UHC adoption.[99]

By 1970, a paradigmatic shift was underway in the ILO's strategy to health protection in the Global South. The organization had begun to recognize the shortcomings of superimposing Western models of health protection on developing countries. This recognition ultimately led to a change in the organization's approach: strengthening coordination with the WHO. One area of WHO-ILO collaboration was the Joint Committee on Personal Healthcare and Social Security that convened in Geneva between November 10 and 16, 1970. In his opening remarks, the then Assistant Director-General of the WHO, Halfdan Mahler emphasized the discrepancy between states' aspirations to provide the best possible personal healthcare to rapidly growing populations and escalating costs.[100] In striving to provide the best possible care, most countries at the time relied on social security mechanisms to finance individualized care provision. The structural disconnect between financial mechanisms and national health strategies impeded the realization of equitable care.

While the ILO moved toward strategic coordination, the WHO, for its part, remained non-committal regarding the optimal pathway toward UHC. Sirrs notes that barred from promoting particular models of UHC, the WHO's approach was pluralistic: whatever worked, depending on the economic or political situation of the country in question.[101]

By 1975, the WHO—thinking alongside UNICEF—promoted basic health services such as maternal and child health. The evolution of the Basic Needs Approach owed partly to the growing clout of newly decolonized countries which called for the establishment of a new international economic order. Additionally, the success of China's Barefoot Doctors inspired its conceptualization.[102] Framed as a central development priority, the Basic Needs Approach aimed to ensure a certain minimum standard of essentials—safe drinking water, sanitation, health, education, public transport, and cultural facilities—for all.[103] Proponents of this approach noted that the underprivileged comprised at least 80 percent of the population in several less-developed countries.

The ILO's interest in the Basic Needs Approach emerged from the agenda of the World Employment Program (WEP), initiated by Morse in 1969.[104] ILO missions to nations such as the Philippines in the early 1970s revealed that economic growth through conventional developmental frameworks failed to generate rural employment and prosperity.[105] In response, the WEP advanced an employment-centric agenda—youth training, international trade, and rural development—as tools to combat poverty.[106] The Basic Needs Approach reached its apex at the 1976 World Employment Conference which called for a fundamental reorientation of international development toward poverty alleviation.[107] At the conference, basic needs were synonymous with the minimum essentials: adequate food, clothing, shelter, essential health services, and rudimentary education—including knowledge of contraception. Some of the basic needs dovetailed with the agenda of the WHO. Sirrs notes that despite the ILO's adoption of an ambitious action program, the organization struggled to translate the Basic Needs approach into operational outcomes.[108]

During the late 1960s and the 1970s, the ILO struggled to articulate a coherent strategy for UHC amid the global ascendance of the Primary Health Care (PHC) paradigm. Ahead of the Alma-Ata Conference (1978), the directors of UNICEF and the WHO in their joint report noted that financing for healthcare might come from taxation, a social security system with contributions from employers, employees, or both, from philanthropic sources, or out-of-pocket payments.[109] However, they cautioned that relying on national taxation to cover healthcare costs was impracticable for developing countries dependent on agriculture. Replicating social insurance models from industrialized countries risked privileging limited population groups in developing contexts. The joint report, in effect, undermined the ILO's attempts to use social insurance schemes to further UHC.[110] Unsurprisingly, the ILO's approach toward PHC remained ambivalent.[111]

ILO officials—particularly Richard J. Szal from the Employment and Development Department—contended that PHC and basic needs were primarily social endeavors. Both endeavors required an equitable redistribution of income, particularly in the Global South context.[112] Furthermore, he observed that low-income levels, often attributed to unemployment or underemployment, were correlated to ill health. An improvement in the general health situation in any country required a "total approach encompassing improvements in nutrition, housing, household technology, education, water and sanitation and even transportation."[113] His arguments were congruent with those of Jain, who was now the ILO Assistant Director-General.[114] However, not all ILO officials endorsed Szal's views.

While some ILO officials were disengaged with PHC, Jain had heard about the Alma-Ata Conference from personal contacts. Despite this, the file related to PHC was not circulated to the Social Security department of the ILO.[115] The ILO initially declined the WHO-UNICEF offer to address the Alma-Ata Conference, assuming that receipt of relevant documents was sufficient.[116] The organization's initial indecisiveness in addressing the Alma-Ata Conference illustrates that the organization was not a monolithic entity. Departments failed to liaise with each other. While PHC had direct relevance for the departments of Social Security and Employment and Development, it was far removed from others. The primary focus of the ILO's mandate was to advance social and economic justice, with healthcare being a secondary concern.

For Jacques Lemoine of the ILO's International Liaison Office, the agency's participation in Alma-Ata was significant for the political capital that conference attendance would bring. Lemoine was hopeful that Alma-Ata would allow the ILO to link PHC not only to the implementation of social security but with the broader concern about basic needs.[117] However, G. Tambouri, from the ILO's Social Section highlighted ILO's underlying reservations toward PHC, a WHO-led initiative. He contended:

> Primary Health Care is provided in many developing countries by social security programmes and the ILO has been instrumental in the planning and organisation of such services. ... However, WHO has shown a tendency to underestimate and even to oppose the development of health services through social security, an attitude that many developing countries have criticized and rejected.[118]

The reservations of Tambouri indicated that the ILO suffered an existential threat from the WHO and its PHC agenda. However, ILO officials such as consultant Derrick Fulcher attempted to leverage the Alma-Ata agenda favoring social health insurance.[119] Fulcher claimed that the emergence of PHC increased the viability of social insurance as a sustainable instrument for financing health systems in resource-constrained settings. The pressure to find new financial solutions to extend "Health for All" became more acute after Alma-Ata.

By the early 1980s, due to mounting sovereign debts in the Global South and the International Monetary Fund's Structural Adjustment Programs, several countries were forced to scale back on public health spending. Under such circumstances, developing countries regarded social health insurance as an attractive extra-budgetary solution for governments to finance healthcare.[120]

Conclusion

Sandrine Kott and Joëlle Droux observed that the birth of the ILO and the subsequent production of conventions and recommendations stimulated epistemic communities that had developed around knowledge sharing.[121] A quarter of a century after it was set up, the organization's landmark Philadelphia Declaration asserted that labor was not a commodity. Guy Standing observes, "By spreading labour standards around the world, lauding 'tripartism' and helping the so-called 'backward' nations to introduce legislation along lines developed in 'advanced' countries, the ILO embodied a systematic attempt to circumvent the labour market, an institutional device to reduce the commodity character of labour relationships."[122]

The development of these international norms hinged not only on epistemic communities and the sharing of global expert knowledge but also on the interchanges between local, and various influential groupings, and the ILO. Information gathering for ILO conventions and recommendations depended on the good offices of the postcolonial state through surveys sent to national civil services. Intermediate reports, drawn up by ILO officials with the help of the expert committee, were validated by national committees before deliberations at the International Labor Conference. In this critical interchange, national and international officials, for example, Jain, played an intermediary role. Between 1946 and 1949, Jain served the Government of India's Department of Handicrafts and Cooperatives before being deputed to the ILO.[123]

Among the conventions shaped through an iterative process of norm development—linking postcolonial state bureaucracies and expert committees—the Social Security Convention No. 102 (1952) most clearly reflected the ILO ethos. The Convention exhorted governments to introduce benefits for nine contingencies that included medical care, sickness, unemployment, old age, employment-related injury, family, maternity, disability, and survivor benefits, all linked to formal employment. If the Philadelphia Declaration ushered in a paradigmatic shift—from enforcing universal labor norms to advancing economic and social policies—then the 1950s marked the ILO's metamorphosis into a development agency.

In the aftermath of the Pacific War, the ILO responded to the exigencies of Asian decolonization and the emergence of independent states. Constrained by Cold War geopolitics and the need to balance regional priorities with international standards, the ILO promoted community development and social security, positioning them as elements of holistic development.

Between 1947 and the early 1950s, the organization's standard-setting encountered criticisms from the Global South, particularly India. Developing countries found it challenging to allocate resources to meet the ILO standards. Asia was a geopolitical prize for the superpowers during the early years of the Cold War between 1945 and 1960. The region's structural challenges—rooted in agricultural volatility and demographic pressure—obstructed the enforcement of universal labor standards.

The Cold War provides the backdrop for contextualizing the timing of social reforms in India, Burma, and the Philippines. While India and Burma pursued non-alignment, the Philippines remained an American ally in the struggle against communism. In each of the three countries, distinct actors were involved in remolding social security programs: international aid agencies, such as the ILO; superpowers such as the US; and the domestic non-communist establishments. Western actors, including the ILO, designed community development and social security as Cold War instrumentalities to buttress newly decolonized Asia against communist incursion.

However, the ILO faced significant challenges in implementing its flagship projects in Asia—most notably community development and social health insurance—in countries such as India and the Philippines. By emphasizing public works such as the construction of wells or village roads that primarily benefited the rural elite, community development projects steamrolled socioeconomic determinants of community well-being. Additionally, the lack of coordination with the WHO stymied the implementation of UHC. These setbacks reveal the fault lines of technocratic internationalism when divorced from local conditions and inter-agency coordination. These limitations underscore inner tensions within the ILO: between normative internationalism and the instrumentalization of social reform as an adjunct to the Cold War. These contradictions expose fault lines in the postwar order, where the ILO's normative aspirations clashed with Cold War exigencies—revealing how international social reform was simultaneously shaped by and subordinated to geopolitical interests.[124]

Notes

1. Eddy Lee, "The Declaration of Philadelphia: Retrospect and Prospect," *International Labour Review* 133, no. 4 (1994): 467–84, ILO Library, Geneva (hereafter ILOL).
2. Daniel Maul, *Human Rights, Development and Decolonization: The International Labour Organisation, 1940–70* (Basingstoke: Palgrave Macmillan, 2012), 86.
3. Maul, *Human Rights, Development and Decolonisation*, 112.
4. André de Maday, *Le Charte International du Travail* (Neuchâtel: F. Ridier et cie, 1921); see also G.A. Johnston, *International Social Progress: The Work of the International Labour Organization* (London: George Allen and Unwin Ltd., 1924).
5. Jasmien Van Daele, "The International Labor Organization (ILO) in Past and Present Research," *International Review of Social History* 53, no. 3 (December 2008): 485–511, 498; see also Ernst Haas, *Functionalism and International Organization* (Stanford, CA: Stanford University Press, 1964).
6. Van Daele, "ILO," 501.
7. See Daniel Maul, "The ILO in Asia and the Beginnings of Technical Assistance," in *The ILO from Geneva to the Pacific Rim: East Meets West*, edited by Jill M. Jensen and Nelson Lichtenstein (Basingstoke: Palgrave Macmillan, 2016), 110–34.
8. Maul, *Human Rights, Development and Decolonization*, 138.
9. Daniel Immerwahr, *Thinking Small: United States and the Lure of Community Development* (Cambridge, MA: Harvard University Press, 2015), 10.
10. See "Letter from V.K.R. Menon, Ministry of Labor, Government of India to K.P.S. Menon, Foreign Secretary," February 20, 1952, Doc. P.S.54,

118th Session of the Governing Body of the ILO, March 1952, Identifier PR_000005014113, File No. UI/52/2711/10003, Ministry of External Affairs, National Archives of India (hereafter NAI). Accessed December 18, 2024. https://www.abhilekh-patal.in/jspui/handle/123456789/2753909?searchWord=&backquery=[query=&filter_field_1=subjectCollection&filter_type_1=equals&filter_value_1=External+Affairs&originalquery=&sort_by=dc.date.accessioned_dt&order=asc&rpp=10&etal=0&start=790], Confidential.

11. "Preparatory Asian Regional Conference of the International Labour Organisation, New Delhi, October 21 to November 8, 1947," *International Labour Review* LVII, no. 5 (1948): 425–37, ILOL.
12. *Preparatory Asian Regional Conference of the International Labour Organisation: Record of Proceedings, October to November 1947* (Geneva: ILO, 1948), ILOL.
13. Report of the Director General, *Preparatory Asiatic Regional Conference of the International Labour Organisation, New Delhi, 1947* (New Delhi: ILO, 1947), 3, ILOL.
14. *Preparatory Asian Regional Conference of the International Labour Organisation*, 273.
15. Ibid., 273.
16. "Preparatory Asian Regional Conference," 3.
17. *Preparatory Asian Regional Conference of the International Labour Organisation*, 276.
18. "The Economic Background of Social Policy Including Problems of Industrialization," *Preparatory Asiatic Regional Conference of the International Labour Organisation*, Report IV (New Delhi: ILO, 1947), ILOL.
19. Ibid.
20. Sunil Amrith, *Decolonizing International Health: India and Southeast Asia, 1930–65* (Basingstoke: Palgrave Macmillan, 2006), 78.
21. "Preparatory Asiatic Regional Conference of the International Labour Organisation, New Delhi 1947," *Problems of Social Security: First Item on the Agenda*, Report I (New Delhi: ILO, 1947), 111, ILOL.
22. "Preparatory Asiatic Regional Conference," 73.
23. Ibid., 73.
24. "Preparatory Asiatic Regional Conference," 74.
25. "Preparatory Asiatic Regional Conference," 79.
26. "Preparatory Asiatic Regional Conference," 80.
27. *Preparatory Asian Regional Conference of the International Labour Organisation*, 216.
28. *Preparatory Asian Regional Conference of the International Labour Organisation*, 2.

29. *Preparatory Asian Regional Conference of the International Labour Organisation*, 4.
30. Ibid., 4.
31. Maul, *Human Rights, Development and Decolonization*, 112.
32. Maul, *Human Rights, Development and Decolonization*, 114.
33. "Second Item on the Agenda: Record of the Asian Regional Conference in Nuwara Eliya, Ceylon," January 16 to 27, 1950, 111th Session of the Governing Body of ILO, Geneva, 1950, Ministry of External Affairs UN-II, Identifier PR 000005014106, File No. 8 (18) UND-50, Ministry of External Affairs (Volume II), NAI. Accessed January 2, 2025. https://www.abhilekh-patal.in/jspui/handle/123456789/2753901?searchWord=ILO&backquery=[query=ILO&originalquery=&sort_by=dc.date.accessioned_dt&order=desc&rpp=20&etal=0&start=100].
34. Maul, "The ILO in Asia," 112.
35. Maul, "The ILO in Asia," 115.
36. Ibid., 115.
37. Ibid., 115.
38. Maul, "The ILO in Asia," 116.
39. Amrith, *Decolonizing International Health*, 86.
40. Francine Frankel, *India's Political Economy: The Gradual Revolution, 1947–1977* (Princeton: Princeton University Press, 1977), 122.
41. Government of India Planning Commission, *The First Five-Year Plan: Draft Outline* (New Delhi, 1951), 194.
42. Tharaphi Than, "The Languages of Pyidawtha and the Burmese Approach to National Development," *Southeast Asia Research* 21, no. 4 (2013): 639–54, 639.
43. Than, "The Languages of Pyidawtha," 646.
44. Than, "The Languages of Pyidawtha," 648.
45. Ibid., 648.
46. International Labour Office, "Expanded Program of Technical Assistance Report to the Government of Burma on Social Security," Doc. ILO/TAP/Burma/R.l (Geneva: ILO, 1952), ILOL.
47. Ibid.
48. Michele Moni and Klaus Peterson, "Cold War and Social Security in Burma and Malaysia," in *From Colonialism to International Aid: External Actors and Social Protection in the Global South*, Carina Smith edited (Basingstoke: Palgrave Macmillan, 2020), 45–78, 55.
49. Ibid., 56.
50. Maul, "The ILO in Asia," 117.
51. Letter from V.K.R. Menon, Ministry of Labour to K.P.S. Menon, February 20, 1952, 118th Session of the Governing Body of the ILO, March 1952, Identifier PR_000005014113, File No.

UI/52/2711/10003, Ministry of External Affairs, NAI. Accessed January 5, 2025. https://www.abhilekh-patal.in/jspui/handle/123456789/2753909?searchWord=&backquery=[query=&filter_field_1=subjectCollection&filter_type_1=equals&filter_value_1=External+Affairs&originalquery=&sort_by=dc.date.accessioned_dt&order=asc&rpp=10&etal=0&start=790. Secret.

52. "Undated Draft Speech of Subramanian," Identifier PR_000005014113, File No. UI/52/2711/10003, Ministry of External Affairs, NAI. Accessed January 5, 2025. https://www.abhilekh-patal.in/jspui/handle/123456789/2753909?searchWord=&backquery=[query=&filter_field_1=subjectCollection&filter_type_1=equals&filter_value_1=External+Affairs&originalquery=&sort_by=dc.date.accessioned_dt&order=asc&rpp=10&etal=0&start=790.
53. International Labour Office, "Social Security in Asia: I," *International Labour Review* 82, no. 1 (1960): 72–78.
54. Mya Maung, "The Burmese Way to Socialism beyond the Welfare State," *Asian Survey* 10, no. 6 (1970): 533–51.
55. Usha Mehta, "The Working of the Employees' State Insurance Scheme in India: An Aspect of Centre-State Relations," *Indian Journal of Political Science* 22, no. 3 (1961): 205–13.
56. Jawaharlal Nehru, "The Development of the Nation," September 14, 1952, in *Selected Works of Jawaharlal Nehru* 19 (July 19, 1952, to October 18, 1952), Second Series (New Delhi: Jawaharlal Nehru Memorial Fund, 1996), 8–9.
57. Subir Sinha, "Lineages of the Developmentalist State: Transnationality and Village India, 1900–1965," *Comparative Studies in Society and History* (2008): 57–90.
58. Maul, *Human Rights, Development and Decolonization*, 121.
59. Maul, *Human Rights, Development and Decolonization*, 125. For the overarching Cold War context see "David Morse Oral History Interview by James R. Fuchs," August 3, 1977, Harry Truman Presidential Museum and Library. Accessed January 16, 2025. https://www.trumanlibrary.gov/library/oral-histories/morse.
60. Maul, "ILO, Asia and the Beginnings of Technical Assistance," 123.
61. Maul, "ILO, Asia and the Beginnings of Technical Assistance," 122.
62. Gunnar Myrdal, *Asian Drama: An Inquiry into the Poverty of Nations* volume 2 (New York: Pantheon, 1968), 870.
63. Ibid., 870.
64. Robert A. Polson, "Community Development in the Philippines: Observations and Comments," *Philippine Sociological Review* 4, no. 4 (1956): 7–14.
65. Ibid., 873.

66. Chester Bowles, *Ambassador's Report* (New York: Harper and Brothers, 1954), 197.
67. Bowles, *Ambassador's Report*, 198.
68. Bowles, *Ambassador's Report*, 199.
69. Bowles, *The Ambassador's Report*, 201.
70. Bowles, *The Ambassador's Report*, 202.
71. Albert Mayer, *The Story of Rural Development at Etawah, Uttar Pradesh: Pilot Project, India* (Berkeley: University of California Press, 1958), 232.
72. Mayer, *The Story of Rural Development at Etawah*, 237.
73. S.K. Jain, "The Etawah Pilot Development Project," File No. 177, Jacket 1, September 1951 to December 1958, Registry 159775, ILO Archives, Geneva.
74. Mayer, *The Story of Rural Development at Etawah*, 263.
75. Mayer, *The Story of Rural Development at Etawah*, 268.
76. William H. Nicholls, "Accommodating Economic Change in Underdeveloped Countries," *The American Economic Review* 49, no. 2 (1959): 156–68, 164.
77. Myrdal, *Asian Drama* volume 2, 888.
78. Immerwahr, *Thinking Small*, 10.
79. Martin Gorsky and Christopher Sirrs, "The Rise and Fall of 'Universal Health Coverage' as a Goal of International Politics, 1925–52," *American Journal of Public Health* 108, no. 3 (2018): 334–42, 339.
80. Gorsky and Sirrs, "The Rise and Fall of 'Universal Health Coverage'," 340.
81. International Labour Conference, "34th Session: Objectives and Minimum Standards of Social Security," Report IV (I) Fourth Item on the Agenda (Geneva: ILO, 1950), ILOL.
82. Christopher Sirrs, "Promoting Health Protection Worldwide: The International Labour Organisation and Health Systems Financing, 1952–2012," *International History Review* 42, no. 2 (2020): 371–90, 371.
83. International Labour Conference, "34th Session."
84. Gorsky and Sirrs, "The Rise and Fall of 'Universal Health Coverage'," 339.
85. Ibid., 339.
86. James A. Gillespie, "Social Medicine, Social Security and International Health, 1940–60," in *The Politics of Healthy Life: An International Perspective*, Esteban Rodrìguez Ocaña edited (Manchester: Manchester University Press, 2002), 219–40, 226–27.
87. Vivek Neelakantan, "'No Nation Can Go Forward when it is Crippled by Disease': Philippine Science and the Cold War, 1946–65," 53–87, 78.

88. Philippine Government, "President's Month in Review: February 1949," *Messages of the President Elpidio Quirino*, Proclamations Book 6, vol. 3 (Manila: Bureau of Printing, 1949).
89. Neelakantan, "'No Nation Can Go Forward when it is Crippled by Disease,'" 78.
90. Neelakantan, "'No Nation Can Go Forward when it is Crippled by Disease,'" 79.
91. Ibid., 79.
92. Republic Act No. 747, "An Act to Regulate Fees to be Charged Against Patients in Government Hospitals and Charity Clinics Classifying Patients According to Their Financial Condition," House Bill No. 1859, 2nd Congress of the Republic, *Official Gazette* 48, no. 7, 2582, Senate of the Philippine Legislative Digital Resources. Accessed January 25, 2025. https://issuances-library.senate.gov.ph/legislative-issuance/republic-act-no-747.
93. Neelakantan, "'No Nation Can Go Forward when it is Crippled by Disease,'" 80.
94. Ibid., 80.
95. Sirrs, "Promoting Health Protection Worldwide," 375.
96. Ibid., 375.
97. Sirrs, "Promoting Health Protection Worldwide," 378.
98. Ibid., 378.
99. Ibid., 378.
100. International Labour Office, "Report of a Joint WHO-ILO Committee on Personal Health and Social Security," November 10 to 16, 1970, Doc. D.2.1971 (Geneva: ILO, 1971), ILOL.
101. Sirrs, "Promoting Health Protection Worldwide," 379.
102. V. Djukanovic and E.P. Mach, "Alternative Approaches to Meeting Basic Needs in Developing Countries" (Geneva: WHO, 1975), WHOL.
103. J. Stephen Hoadley, "The Rise and Fall of the Basic Needs Approach," *Cooperation and Conflict* 16, no. 3 (1981): 149–64, 150.
104. Sirrs, "Promoting Health Protection Worldwide," 380.
105. Gustav Ranis, "Employment, Equity and Growth: Lessons from the Philippine Employment Mission," *International Labour Review* 110, no. 1 (1974): 17–27, ILOL.
106. Sirrs, "Promoting Health Protection Worldwide," 380.
107. M.J.D. Hopkins, "Basic Needs Approach to Development Planning: A View," *World Employment Program Research Papers*, Doc. WEP-32/WP3 (Geneva: ILO, 1977), ILOL.
108. Sirrs, "Promoting Health Protection Worldwide," 380.

109. *Primary Health Care: A Joint Report by the Director-General of the World Health Organization and the Executive Director of the United Nations Children's Fund* (Geneva: WHO, 1978), 42, WHOL.
110. Minute Sheet from Jacques Lemoine entitled "International Conference on Primary Health Care, USSR, September 1978," July 17, 1978, WHO International Conference on Primary Health Care: Alma-Ata, USSR, September 6 to 11, 1978, File No. 1110-1, File Series WHO, Registry 177769, ILO Archives.
111. Sirrs, "Promoting Health Protection Worldwide," 380.
112. Richard J. Szal, "Health, Employment and Development," Paper Presented at the WHO International Conference on Primary Health Care, Alma-Ata, USSR, September 6 to 12, 1978 (Geneva: ILO, 1978), 1, ILOL.
113. Szal, "Health, Employment and Development," 2.
114. S.K. Jain, "Notes on Mission to Alma-Ata," September 2 to 13, 1978, Mission: Surendra Kumar Jain (August 1976 to November 1986), File No. 177, Jacket 2, File Series MI, ILO Archives.
115. Minute Sheet from Lemoine.
116. Sirrs, "Promoting Health Protection Worldwide," 380.
117. Minute Sheet from Lemoine.
118. G. Tambouri, Social Section, "Minute Sheet," July 17, 1978, Ref. WHO-1119-1, WHO International Conference on Primary Health Care, World Health Organization File 1119-1, Registry 177769, ILO Archives.
119. Sirrs, "Promoting Health Protection Worldwide," 381.
120. Aviva Ron, Brian-Abel Smith, and Giovanni Tambouri, *Health Insurance in Developing Countries: The Social Security Approach* (Geneva: ILO, 1990), v, ILOL.
121. Sandrine Kott and Joëlle Droux, "Introduction," in *Global Social Rights: The International Labour Organization and Beyond*, Sandrine Kott and Joëlle Droux edited (Basingstoke: Palgrave Macmillan, 2013), 1–16, 4.
122. Guy Standing, "The ILO: An Agency for Globalization?," *Development and Change* 39, no. 8 (2008): 355–84, 355.
123. Gerry Rodgers, "Surendra Kumar Jain: Interview for the ILO Century Project," March 2008, ILO Century Project. Accessed February 2, 2025. https://www.ilo.org/resource/surendra-kumar-jain.
124. For a parallel with the WHO, consult Marcos Cueto, Theodore Brown, and Elizabeth Fee, *The WHO: A History* (Cambridge: Cambridge University Press, 2019).

CHAPTER 7

Reconciling Barefoot Aspirations and Cold War Realities: Alma-Ata and the Regional Quest for Primary Healthcare Across Southeast Asia

Introduction

In 1957, President Dwight D. Eisenhower pledged US support for the Global Malaria Eradication Program, arguing that improved health alleviated poverty and misery—the breeding grounds of communism. He declared:

Of all diseases, malaria which attacked 200 million people last year and killed two million, is probably the world's worst remaining source of poverty and misery.

> We are now about to undertake, in cooperation with the World Health Organization and the countries affected, a project to abolish malaria once for all from the face of the earth. We are willing to cooperate with Soviet Union and Communist China in this work of peace if they will agree.[1]

Eisenhower's speech, inspired by the 1955 WHO's launch of the Global Malaria Eradication Program, strengthened worldwide momentum toward eradication. Yet within a decade technical setback—particularly the resistance of the anopheline vector to DDT—cast doubts on the program's sustainability.[2] At the same time, skepticism grew within sections of the World Health Assembly (WHA) about the feasibility of disease

V. Neelakantan, *The Emergence of International Health Policy in Southeast Asia, India, and Sri Lanka, 1937–1978*,
https://doi.org/10.1007/978-3-032-21233-7_7

eradication programs as a quick fix for poverty.[3] The skepticism highlighted the need for deeper health system reforms—premised on equity, rights, and community participation—core tenets of Primary Health Care (PHC).

Between 1955 and 1978, significant global events shaped the trajectory of PHC across Southeast Asia. These included the worldwide campaigns against malaria and smallpox. This chapter delves into three interrelated themes:

1. The US-sponsored Global Malaria Eradication Program (1955–1969), challenged by technical and political setbacks, contrasted with the Soviet-supported Global Smallpox Eradication Program, which succeeded by tailoring interventions to local epidemiological and infrastructural conditions (1967–1980);
2. The export of Communist China's Barefoot Doctors' model to the Global South, including Southeast Asia;
3. The Soviet initiative to host the Alma-Ata Conference on PHC.

The three interrelated themes underscore the centrality of political ideologies in the quest for PHC.

In this chapter, I argue that although Cold War rivalries foreshadowed the formative years of PHC, its trajectory across Southeast Asia reflected attunement to local needs rather than bold geopolitical imperatives. Additionally, this chapter traces the local antecedents of PHC in Indonesia, India, Thailand, and Sri Lanka, examining how socioeconomic and political conditions, national health systems, and the influence of non-governmental agencies collectively influenced the development of PHC. By analyzing Southeast Asia's trajectory, this chapter seeks to decenter the PHC narrative from the dominant institutional histories of the WHO by emphasizing the strategic role of local actors in defining the meaning and implementation of PHC.[4]

International Influences: Cold War and the Evolution of PHC

PHC did not emerge overnight but reflected intellectual and ideological shifts within and beyond the WHO between 1955 and 1978. Historians differ about the significance of the Alma-Ata Conference: Marcos Cueto sees it as a small Soviet victory in the Cold War.[5] Similarly, Socrates Litsios contends that the Conference reflected Soviet pressure to "kidnap" the WHO's PHC agenda.[6] Through extensive research on unpublished USSR and Kazakh sources, Anne-Emanuelle Birn and Nikolai Krementsov observe that although Soviet delegates to the WHO were enthusiastic about PHC, Soviet authorities did not initially seek to host the conference. The highest echelons of the Soviet leadership did not view Alma-Ata as a diplomatic milestone even as they used it to showcase domestic health achievements. The Conference thus held different meanings for USSR and WHO actors, shaped by ideologically distinct visions of PHC.

Even before the Alma-Ata Conference, Cold War tensions underlined international health initiatives. The failure of the Global Malaria Eradication Program by 1969 exposed the limits of quick technical fixes and reignited calls for health system reform. Randall Packard observes that the WHO approved the program in 1955 despite opposition within the World Health Assembly (WHA), whose members felt that the WHO should concentrate its resources on strengthening health services.[7] The USSR and its allies withdrew from the WHO (1949–1956) over ideological differences with the US regarding socialized medicine. In 1958, the Soviet delegate to the Eleventh WHA at Minneapolis, Viktor Zhdanov—echoing Soviet premier Nikita Khruschev's policy of Peaceful Coexistence—exhorted the WHO to launch a global smallpox eradication campaign, drawing on methods developed in the USSR during the 1930s. While the practical logic of smallpox eradication was unimpeachable, the geopolitical context complicated the American response.[8] The US, having championed the malaria campaign since 1955, remained fixated on technical solutions over structural reform. The Soviet initiative thus doubled as a strategic bid for leadership in international health—one met with strategic hesitation by the US, the WHO's largest donor.

By 1959, although smallpox was an official WHO priority, without American initiative, the campaign remained on paper for several years. Each year at the WHA, the Soviets expressed disappointment at the WHO's institutional inertia toward smallpox eradication and contrasted it with massive investment in the malaria eradication program. Despite absorbing a significant proportion of the WHO's budget, malaria eradication's prospects waned by the mid-1960s as the anopheline vector developed resistance to DDT, thwarting eradication efforts.[9] By 1967, the US

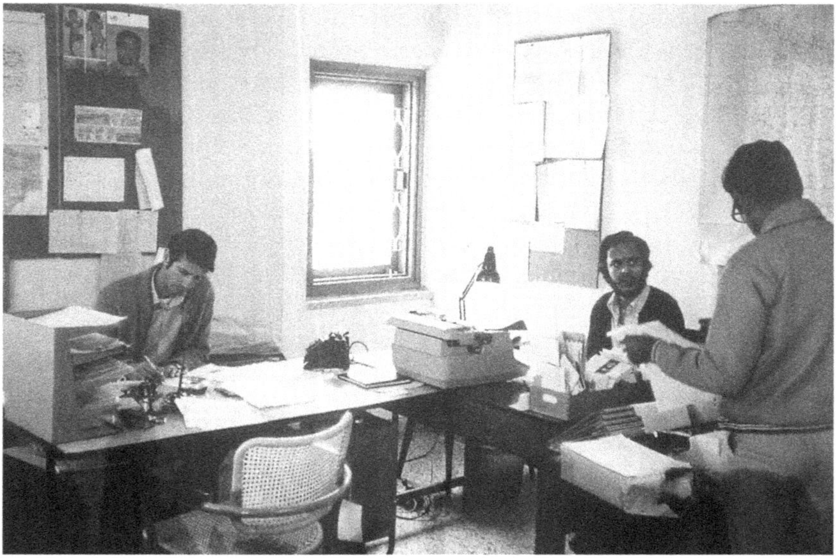

Image 7.1 Smallpox eradication: Cold War diplomacy meets field-level coordination in Patna, India (1975). Former Centers for Disease Control and Prevention (CDC) staffer and WHO operations officer Jay Freedman (seated left) analyzing epidemiological data at the field level alongside Sushant K. Sharda, during a field operation in Bihar. Founded in 1946 at the dawn of the Cold War, the CDC evolved into a global actor in disease surveillance and eradiation. Image ID: 19070. Courtesy of the CDC/Dr. J.C. Millar. URL: https://phil.cdc.gov/Details.aspx?pid=19070. Public Domain

reversed its position and threw its weight behind smallpox eradication (Image 7.1).

By 1969, the Soviets urged a reappraisal of the Global Malaria Eradication Program at the Twenty-Second WHA. The reassessment highlighted socioeconomic, financial, administrative, and operational factors in explaining the program's technical and institutional failure.[10] The WHA resolution urged member states to strengthen basic health services.

PHC, or the notion that health services development should focus on providing basic care at the village or neighborhood level, was not a novel idea for the 1970s.[11] In 1953, the WHO's Expert Committee on Public Health Administration had set out a model of basic health services. The Committee's report included many elements later incorporated into the

PHC model: maternal and child health, communicable disease control, environmental sanitation, maintenance of health records, health education, public health nursing, provision of medical care, and, where needed, access to larger medical centers.[12] Yet, there was implementation lag until the late 1960s in operationalizing the basic health services model.[13]

UNICEF's engagement with the basic health services model between 1971 and 1979 drew on lessons from the disease eradication campaigns of the 1950s. Moving beyond narrow single-disease interventions, the organization's Executive Director Henry Labouise (1965–1979) spearheaded a holistic approach that linked child development to broader socioeconomic development.[14] The basic services model integrated health, potable water, nutrition, education, and women's programs, marking a shift from vertical campaigns to community-driven strategies.

While UNICEF under Labouise's leadership connected health to broader developmental concerns, Cold War priorities favored short-term high-impact public health programs such as the campaigns against malaria, tuberculosis, and yaws. Disease eradication campaigns, with their clear metrics, were congruent with US Cold War rhetoric, making mass campaigns targeting endemic disease more appealing than the expansion of basic health services. In Southeast Asia, American and Soviet aid, despite rhetorical support for basic health services, channeled resources into hospital-based systems, rather than the decentralized community-driven approach that UNICEF espoused.

The tension between rhetorical endorsement of basic health services and infrastructural investment in hospitals was especially apparent in Laos. The United States Agency for International Development (USAID) launched its Maternal and Child Health (MCH) and family planning project in 1969. This initiative, however, lacked strategic coordination with the Royal Lao Ministry of Health and the WHO.[15] The Americans classified the USAID-supported MCH initiative as a technical assistance project, though the agency's focus remained on construction. Key infrastructural undertakings included a 200-bed MCH facility in Vientiane, 4 provincial MCH centers, renovation of 11 rural facilities, and the expansion of the USAID medical warehouse.[16] USAID auditors expressed reservations about the Lao government's capacity to maintain these facilities once aid was withdrawn.

The fragmented nature of American aid in Laos reflected a wider challenge: international health assistance in Southeast Asia during the Cold War was punctuated by a multitude of aid agencies that lacked coordination. Consequently, PHC developed in a piecemeal manner across the region.

A decade before USAID's stopgap engagement with maternal and child health in Laos, the Soviets strategically positioned public health as a tool to extend their influence in newly decolonized nations. In Indonesia, Soviet health initiatives functioned as instruments of soft power, operating through technical assistance and symbolic solidarity. Following the Asian-African Conference convened at Bandung in 1955, the Soviets pursued technical cooperation with Indonesia. Although Indonesia did not fit the strict definition of a socialist state, its condemnation of colonialism at Bandung made it a prospective partner for Soviet engagement in Southeast Asia.[17] The interest materialized in 1956 when the USSR signed an agreement to assist Indonesia in implementing its Five-Year Plan. In a bid to curtail America's growing geopolitical clout in Southeast Asia, the Soviets framed Indonesia's poverty as both a legacy of colonial exploitation and a result of growing American intervention.[18] Indonesian leaders weighed Soviet overtures against American aid, navigating both with caution to ensure that their health programs remained autonomous from superpower intervention.

The Soviets used public health as an instrument of ideological projection. In 1960, the Soviet Embassy in Jakarta translated Deputy Health Minister D.D. Venediktov's vision for international health to Bahasa Indonesia for domestic dissemination. Venediktov argued that public health was primarily a socioeconomic question, particularly in newly decolonized nations of Asia and Africa.[19] These countries lacked an adequate health infrastructure to deal with the burden of infectious diseases such as smallpox, cholera, or plague. The USSR was keen to share its technical expertise in public health with newly decolonized Asian and African nations and assisted in organizing mass campaigns against smallpox.[20] In Indonesia, the Soviets sponsored the visit of the then Minister of Health, Satrio, to Moscow in 1961 to study the organization of the Soviet health system.[21] Between 1959 and 1965, Indonesia was arguably the largest recipient of Soviet technical assistance across Asia. Despite considerable Soviet investment, Indonesia realized only one health infrastructure outcome: The Soviet-Indonesian Hospital of Friendship (Bahasa Indonesia: *Rumah Sakit Persahabatan*).[22] At the time, the Soekarno administration diverted 90 percent of USSR's aid into the war-front—against Malaysia and to press for Indonesia's claims to West Irian.[23]

Beyond Indonesia, Cambodia became a key site of Soviet health diplomacy between 1955 and 1970—welcoming technical assistance in strategically framed yet nominally apolitical fields such as biomedicine while resisting overt ideological entanglements.[24] The Khmer-Soviet Friendship Hospital was constructed in 1960, equipped with advanced technology and staffed by USSR physicians. Soviet medical aid to Indonesia and Cambodia reflected a post-Bandung strategy of technical cooperation where medical diplomacy transcended ideological binaries without demanding political alignment.

Following their withdrawal from the WHO (1949–1956), the Soviets institutionalized annual meetings of health ministers from the communist bloc. From 1961, the USSR offered fellowships to medical students from Asia, Africa, and Latin America—hosted at Patrice Lumumba Moscow People's University, named in honor of the assassinated Congolese leader.[25] Between 1969 and 1975, the Soviets pursued bilateral ties with the West, enabling access to technologies such as the artificial heart. In sum, the Soviets distrusted WHO interventions, seeing the agency as misaligned with their national interests.

Despite the Soviet incredulity of WHO initiatives, significant changes were underway in international health during the early 1970s. In 1973, Halfdan Mahler, the Danish TB specialist, was appointed WHO Director-General. Mahler's experience in India between 1951 and 1961 as a WHO officer for TB control shaped his thinking on healthcare. Animated by the doctrine of social medicine, he was skeptical of clinical specialism. Mahler embraced community participation in health and accommodated indigenous medical traditions such as Ayurveda and Unani, core aspects of PHC.[26] Mahler's antipathy toward centralized biomedical models made him distrustful of the USSR's approach to healthcare.[27] His PHC vision and efforts to steer the WHO away from disease eradication campaigns were instrumental in shaping the "Health for All" trajectory.

Amid divergent approaches toward health system organization, at the 1974 WHA, Venediktov proposed that the WHO organize a special conference on the exchange of experiences on developing national health services.[28] At the January 1975 WHO Executive Board meeting, Venediktov's renewed proposal for holding an international conference mirroring the scale of the 1974 World Population Council in Bucharest was rejected.[29] Also, in 1975, the WHO, in collaboration with UNICEF, issued a report entitled "Alternative Approaches to Meeting Basic Needs in Developing Countries." The report recommended that health systems should proactively anticipate and respond to the needs of the underprivileged, who constituted at least 80 percent of the population of less-developed countries.[30]

By the early 1970s, developing countries created sophisticated health services, often modeled on industrialized infrastructures but concentrated in urban areas. However, the WHO-UNICEF collaborative study noted that the vertical disease control programs implemented in developing countries during the 1950s lost momentum, largely because rural health infrastructures remained underdeveloped.[31]

As alternative frameworks for health system development gained traction by the mid-1970s, Kenneth Newell of New Zealand was instrumental in advancing global support for PHC through his publications.[32] In 1967, the WHO appointed Newell as the Director of the newly created division for Research in Epidemiology and Communication Sciences. The division's interest in health planning prompted a Soviet invitation for Newell to send a team to examine their health service organization. Newell opposed the USSR's centralized, specialist-driven infrastructure, which contrasted with his vision of community-based care.[33]

In 1975, Newell edited *Health by the People*. The volume proffered detailed models of effective PHC for "some of the poorest rural populations of the world."[34] Newell avoided overt ideological framing, attributing PHC momentum to administrative resolve and national will.[35] However, the imprint of China's Barefoot Doctors was discernible in the events leading to Alma-Ata in 1978.

By 1971, the quest for alternative healthcare models had attracted WHO attention. During this period, the Chinese Medical Association invited Victor Sidel from the Department of Social Medicine at Montefiore Hospital and Medical Center in New York City to visit the People's Republic of China (PRC) and observe the delivery of healthcare through the mobilization of village-level health workers, known as Barefoot Doctors.[36]

Cold War hostilities between the PRC and the US made American citizens' travel to China rare. Sidel served to stimulate his American colleagues about PHC developments and critique the shortcomings of the US health system. He also professed the Barefoot Doctors' approach, framing it as a viable alternative to Western clinical paradigms. Two events catalyzed international interest in the Barefoot Doctors' Model: American President Richard Nixon's one-week visit to the PRC between February

21 and 28, 1972, and the PRC's accession to the WHO on February 26, 1972.

The Barefoot Doctors' antecedents trace back to the 1930s Nationalist-led Rural Reconstruction spearheaded by C.C. Chen in Ding County, northern China.[37] James Yen's Ting Hsien movement (Chinese: Mass Education), also rooted in Ding County, blended public health with rural reconstruction. Mao Zedong's involvement in Ting Hsien informed his later promotion of the Barefoot Doctors model.[38]

Village health workers constituted the cornerstone of Rural Reconstruction, inspiring later community health initiatives. The Communist regime adapted this legacy, but it was only in the post-Cultural Revolution period that the Barefoot Doctors became institutionalized within PRC's health policy implementation.

During Mao's victory over the Nationalist forces in 1949, Communist China had one of the world's most impoverished health systems. In 1950, the PRC possessed only 40,000 Western-educated physicians, grossly inadequate to serve a population of 540 million.[39] In practice, the only medical personnel accessible to the urban poor and the countryside were practitioners of Traditional Chinese Medicine (TCM). To provide medical care after Liberation (1949), the PRC prioritized medical training, modeled on Soviet lines. Between 1949 and 1965, 150,000 doctors were trained in Western medicine, a staggering increase of almost 300 percent in less than 20 years.[40] Efforts were made concurrently to train assistant doctors along the lines of the Soviet *feldshers*. Yet these newly trained medical personnel were concentrated in the cities. Recognizing the rural-urban disparities, the PRC authorities integrated TCM into rural health.

Liping Bu observes that the socialist reconstruction of China was shaped by superpower rivalry in the post-World War II international order.[41] America's diplomatic isolation of China pushed it into the Soviet orbit. Despite adopting the Soviet model of economic development during the 1950s, the PRC maintained a strong emphasis on self-reliance.

Building on earlier efforts to integrate public health into socialist planning, the mid-1960s marked a decisive shift toward rural healthcare reform that culminated in Mao's directive to reorient medical care to the countryside. On June 26, 1965, before the start of the Great Proletarian Cultural Revolution, Chairman Mao issued a directive, "In health and medical work, put the stress on the rural areas."[42] Starting in 1965, the PRC launched the Socialist Education Campaign that targeted the inequitable distribution of healthcare. The communes selected youths with primary or

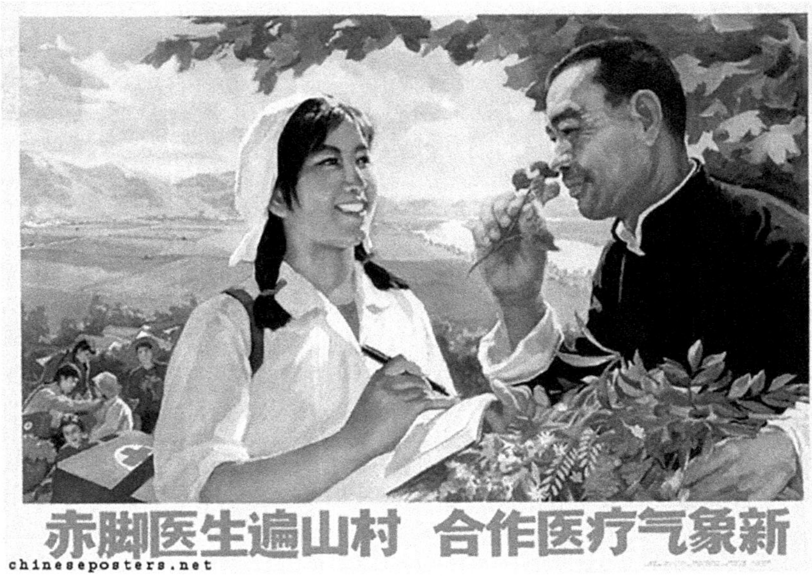

Image 7.2 Barefoot doctors in mountain villages: cooperation fosters a new medical environment, September 1974. By Wang Linkun, Shanghai People's Publishing House. BG E13/659 (chineseposters.net, Landsberger Collection). With permission

middle-school education, good family origins, "correct" political thoughts, and love for the countryside for medical training. In Shanghai's suburbs, locals colloquially referred to these young health workers as Barefoot Doctors (Chinese: *chijiao yisheng*) (Image 7.2).

In 1974, Lucien Bernard, WHO Assistant Director-General, led the WHO's first Study Mission to the PRC. The team noted that in the rural areas they visited, Barefoot Doctors were members of production brigades. Each commune had its own health facility and a referral system to refer patients to higher-level services. Preventive medicine and family planning were freely provided and considered a human right.[43]

"Prevention First," central to Mao's health doctrine, was regarded as a cardinal principle of care.[44] The rural health network across the PRC vigorously applied Mao's directive, launching recurring hygiene campaigns that included the destruction of the four pests, that is, rats, flies, mosquitos, and bedbugs.[45] The WHO's Study Mission concluded that with the mobilization of available resources, most countries could attain an acceptable level of health at an affordable cost.[46] In conformity with Mao's Prevention First Directive, the PRC's rural health network mobilized mass movements—reinforcing the notion that public health was a community responsibility.

Mao was responsible for defining China's domestic and foreign policy trajectory toward the Third World. The origins of Chinese policy toward Asia and Africa can be traced to the Sino-Soviet Treaty of Friendship in 1950, coinciding with the Korean War and communist containment. During the 1950s, China aimed to forestall US political and military encirclement by participating in the Asian-African Conference at Bandung in 1955. China sought to engage its Southeast Asian neighbors through a policy of peaceful coexistence. The early 1960s was marked by the Sino-Soviet conflict. Soviet social-imperialism began to rival US imperialism as China's principal enemy.[47]

Despite China's efforts to engage its Southeast Asian neighbors, the 1950s ended without significant success. However, the early 1960s brought new challenges and opportunities for cementing China's relations with the Third World, following the Sino-Soviet tensions. During the 1960s, China actively supported African anti-colonial movements. The PRC's friendship with Tanzania symbolized the viability of China as a developmental model. China argued that Sino-Tanzania economic interaction represented a "new type" of cooperation and that the Third World could achieve genuine development through mutual cooperation.[48] The PRC's ability to redress health disparities, particularly through its incorporation of TCM into national health services, inspired Asian, African, and Latin American governments where traditional medicine formed an integral component of national identity.

In Southeast Asia, Cambodia's Pol Pot regime (1975–1979) adapted elements of the Barefoot Doctors' model. Healthcare in the countryside was delivered by appointed cadres (Khmer: *pet padewat*).[49] Medical training was rudimentary: experiential learning, revolutionary zeal, and loyalty to the Khmer Rouge were considered adequate. To address the scarcity of hospitals, the Khmer Rouge repurposed suitable buildings as makeshift infirmaries. Medication primarily consisted of herbal pills—drawn from traditional Khmer medicine and designed to resemble western pharmaceuticals.[50]

Recognizing the potential of health projects to promote a new international order against colonialism, the PRC embarked on initiatives aligned with its ideological commitment toward non-aligned socialism. This stance attracted interest from African states and socialist countries in Southeast Asia, which sought Chinese medical aid and training. On June 5, 1971, Chinese Premier Zhou Enlai met his Somalian counterpart and emphasized that health collaboration between both nations was tailored to suit local conditions.[51]

The transnational interchange of health ideas was not without friction: Newell, a long-term nemesis of Venediktov, stymied the latter's 1975 initiative to convene a WHO conference in the USSR.[52] Concurrently, the PRC—citing its Barefoot Doctor experiment—endorsed the exchange of experiences and recommended convening the conference in a developing country such as Egypt.[53] However, between January and March 1976, the Soviets exerted diplomatic pressure, leading Egypt to withdraw its offer.[54] The USSR ultimately hosted the conference, and China did not object.

Despite this favorable outcome, Mahler's views on the medical profession as an obstacle to PHC delayed the conference in the Soviet Union. However, he misunderstood the role of Soviet doctors: they were not a profession and did not control the health system. As salaried state employees, they championed public health but lacked authority over the system's orientation—a domain firmly controlled by the Communist party.[55]

Underlying the clash between the Soviet and Western medical systems were differing political philosophies. For the Soviets, showcasing their technological prowess took precedence over achievements in social well-being, such as pensions, housing, sanitation, and maternal and child protection.[56] This emphasis shaped the Kazakh Soviet Socialist Republic Health Minister Turgel'dy Sharmanov, who focused on medical services infrastructure, detailing the number of hospitals, beds, sanitary stations, and research establishments of the republic.[57] In a related development, although Mahler was initially reluctant to proceed with the Alma-Ata Conference, it eventually became his signature achievement, while the Soviets downplayed its significance.[58] Domestically, even though the Alma-Ata meeting yielded limited impact, it allowed Soviet health administrators to lobby Politburo patrons for health ministry budgets.[59] Cold War orthodoxy prevented Soviet recognition of divergent PHC interpretations.

Mahler, Newell, and other Western advocates of PHC criticized the Soviet health system's clinical orientation and its neglect of community participation.[60] For Newell, PHC had to respond to resource-constrained settings and advance local agency. Soviet officials, by contrast, did not showcase achievements such as universal and equitable access to care, or the elimination of poverty—regarding these dimensions as axiomatic outcomes of socialism. The USSR's tepid engagement with Alma-Ata also underscored the WHO's peripherality in Soviet international health diplomacy.

The Local Antecedents of PHC in Southeast Asia

This section investigates the local antecedents of PHC in four disparate contexts: Indonesia, India, Thailand, and Sri Lanka. In 1963, Indonesian physician Gunawan Nugroho, a public health graduate from the University of Toronto—affiliated with the World Council of Churches (WCC)—pioneered a community health program that emphasized health promotion over curative care in Solo, Central Java. Similarly, in 1970, Indian physicians Rajanikant and Mabelle Arole, also affiliated with the WCC, launched a socio-medical initiative to improve health outcomes in Jamkhed, central India. The common denominator in both experiments was that public health—rooted in equity, access, and community participation—could be operationalized outside state-led frameworks.

In contrast, the demand for PHC in Thailand was strongly influenced by Cold War exigencies. At the time, Thai and US authorities were concerned that neglecting rural health would invite communist influx across Southeast Asia. Meanwhile, the Vietnam War exacerbated Thailand's medical challenges, as newly minted Thai physicians emigrated to the US. To stem the exodus of Thai physicians, in 1967, the then Minister of Health Phra Bamradnaradura instituted a bond requiring medical students to serve in rural areas for two years. The first cohort of government-bonded Thai physicians suffered several logistical problems such as inadequate equipment, a dearth of health staff, and a huge backlog of clinical cases. The need for PHC workers to improve health conditions across the Thai countryside became acute after 1968. That year, China introduced a rural medical program under the directive of Mao that redefined community-based care. In response to regional sifts, Thailand commissioned a PHC project at Saraphi in Chiang Mai province. Saraphi's success affirmed that recruiting basic-trained volunteers at subdistrict stations was key to expand rural healthcare. Inspired by the PRC's Barefoot Doctors' model, the Rural Doctor Society was established in 1978. The mandate for the Society was the betterment of Thai society, teamwork, and a holistic approach to health.

While Thailand grappled with physician exodus to the US and rural shortages, Sri Lanka confronted distinct health challenges associated with the procurement and affordability of essential medicines. Emerging from the Bandung aftermath, the Non-Aligned Movement (NAM) sought to engender solidarity among developing countries and reduce reliance on external aid. International health became a key forum for such cooperation. At the Fifth NAM summit in Colombo (1976), Sri Lanka shared its pharmaceutical regulatory experiences with other developing countries. This effort was championed by Sri Lankan pharmacologist Senaka Bibile.

Despite the diverse geopolitical and local factors at play, the common denominator underlying the evolution of PHC in the four countries was the struggle to improve accessibility to health services. The four case studies underscore the importance of local context in the appropriation and transformation of PHC.

Indonesia

Johannes Leimena served as Indonesia's health minister between 1947 and 1956, with a brief interlude (1953–1955) when Lie Kiat Teng held the position.[61] He inspired Nugroho's community health experiments in 1960s Central Java. Leimena introduced the Bandung Plan (1951), which formalized community health initiatives by integrating preventive and curative care. The Plan established a blueprint for subsequent health reforms. Although Leimena conceptualized the ideological framework, G. Siwabessy, Indonesian Minister of Health (1966–1978), operationalized PHC by establishing Puskesmas [Bahasa Indonesia: *Pusat Kesehatan Masyarakat* or community health centers]. Together, Leimena's and Siwabessy's contributions established the institutional bedrock for Nugroho's experiments.

Leimena's political philosophy—an eclectic blend of Christianity, nationalist ideology, and internationalism—influenced his public health outlook. Invoking biblical metaphors, he championed peace, economic development, the urgency of raising living standards, and the need to confront four goliaths: poverty, ignorance, disease, and unemployment.[62]

Leimena's thinking on public health was congruent with that of the US bacteriologist C.E.A. Winslow who published the treatise *The Cost of Sickness and the Price of Health*.[63] Winslow's poverty-disease cycle—where sickness led to poverty, which in turn exacerbated disease, creating a self-perpetuating cycle—shaped Leimena's argument. Echoing this logic,

Leimena asserted, "Health activities carried out without improving socio-economic conditions could create an unbalanced situation in the community."[64] John B. Grant's 1930s rural reconstruction in China inspired Leimena's call to integrate preventive and curative medicine in community settings.[65] He also benefited from collateral Rockefeller funding during the interwar years.[66]

Leimena's utopian thinking on public health crystallized into the Bandung Plan. Bandung, home to curative facilities—particularly the missionary-run Immanuel Hospital, where Leimena served as a physician for a decade in the 1930s—provided the backdrop for his early interventions. During his tenure, Leimena noted that the local Sundanese Muslim population was hesitant to access missionary hospitals due to concerns over Christian proselytization.[67] In response, he devised a referral system under the leadership of *djuru rawat* [Bahasa Indonesia: female nurse] and *mantri* [Bahasa Indonesia: male nurse] to integrate preventive and curative care during the mid-1930s.[68] This proto-PHC experiment of the interwar years became the fulcrum of the Bandung Plan.

The Indonesian health ministry implemented the Bandung Plan as a pilot project in Bandung regency in 1951. The plan was subsequently extended across the Indonesian archipelago by 1954. The plan emphasized strengthening rural health services and established a referral system for curative care focused on the *desa* [Bahasa Indonesia: village] and *kecamatan* [Bahasa Indonesia: subdistrict]. To achieve this vision, the plan envisioned one health center per subdistrict, and constructed auxiliary hospitals at district headquarters.[69]

To enhance implementation, the Indonesian government devolved responsibility to provincial and local governments, ensuring compliance with the Ministry of Health's policy guidelines. Leimena mobilized rural communities to establish a *desa* [Bahasa Indonesia: village] hygiene service.[70] However, local governments' ability to implement delegated health programs was contingent on fiscal capacity. Financing the Bandung Plan proved contentious as most regencies were ill-equipped to integrate preventive and curative health services.

To address the Bandung Plan's limitations, Julie Sulianti Saroso (Technical Director of Maternal and Child Health Services) during the 1950 posited a comprehensive team approach. This involved liaising between central and provincial ministries of health in implementing health education across rural communities.[71] Saroso championed a nationwide school health program that integrated preventive and curative health services, promoted hygiene and nutrition education, vaccinated schoolchildren against infectious diseases, conducted dental screenings, and offered first aid training. She sought to embed maternal and child health into the broader architecture of rural health services. However, her attempts at coordination failed due to persistent health personnel shortages.[72]

Between 1957 and 1965, successive attempts to redress shortages of health personnel were unsuccessful. President Soekarno's authoritative tendencies, partly supported by the military and vested interests within the political elite, pushed Indonesia beyond the limits of its economic base, social structure, and political institutions.[73] In the name of continuing the revolution, Soekarno nationalized foreign enterprises in Indonesia and increased the power of the military. Then, to counterbalance the military, he supported the Partai Komunis Indonesia (PKI). In the words of historian Adrian Vickers, "The crash-through or crash approach led to the greatest disaster in the nation's history."[74]

Late in the evening of September 30, 1965, army units led by Col. General Untung launched a limited military coup in Jakarta to remove a council of generals alleged to be plotting to remove Soekarno with the aid of UK and US. The dramatic murder of six military generals, allegedly by the PKI, provided a fillip to General Soeharto to move to the center of Indonesian political life.[75] Between 1966 and 1968, Soeharto consolidated his power and in 1968 was proclaimed the President of Indonesia, heralding the New Order regime (1968–1998).

The health policy of the New Order bore the imprint of Siwabessy. After assuming office, suspended all employees suspected to harbor PKI sympathies and began the delicate task of rebuilding Indonesia's relations with the WHO that suffered considerable strain toward the late 1950s and early 1960s. In 1968, he convened a National Health Conference to expand healthcare across the Indonesian archipelago through a network of Puskesmas. Siwabessy's proposals were echoed in Indonesia's First Five-Year Plan (Repelita I, 1969–1974). During the Second Five-Year Plan (Repelita II, 1974–1979), Siwabessy proposed the integration of preventive and curative services and established a Puskesmas in each subdistrict to optimize the functioning of the Department of Health.[76]

The expansion of the Puskesmas across the Indonesian archipelago coincided with the emergence of the PHC paradigm. Indonesian delegates to the WHA, particularly Saroso and Nugroho, reported on current

PHC projects, strategically positioning their country as an active participant in the PHC discourse.[77]

Spearheaded by Nugroho, Community Health Development (CHD) evolved into a comprehensive social experiment in Central Java in 1963, amid Indonesia's political transition from the Old to the New Order. CHD recognized health's interdependence with all aspects of human life, championing initiatives to help people lead healthier lives.[78] By primarily mobilizing locally available resources—including money, people, and equipment—CHD moved beyond biomedicine's narrow confines to incorporate broader developmental efforts.

In 1963, the Indonesian Ministry of Health assigned Nugroho and his wife, a physician, to the Foundation for Christian Hospitals in Solo. The foundation had a small maternity clinic with 20 beds and served patients from Solo and neighboring villages. Nugroho conceptualized the maternity clinic as the nucleus of CHD.

To operationalize CHD, he improved staff conditions, created an esprit de corps, and raised their wages. Next, Nugroho upgraded the status of the maternity clinic to that of a maternity hospital. He envisioned the maternity hospital as a referral center for neighboring polyclinics. The enhancement of health services in the hospital was accomplished through simplification. In the words of Nugroho, "There was no expensive and complicated equipment. In place of an incubator, for example, a glass box heated with an electric light was used, because most of the auxiliary staff were untrained village girls."[79] To address the shortfall of skilled medical personnel, Nugroho's team hired paramedical personnel. However, Nugroho noted that the maternity hospital excluded underprivileged community members.

Mapping the constraints of clinic-based care, Nugroho reoriented his efforts toward broader rural challenges. In 1965, the Ministry of Health deputed Nugroho to Begajah, a village 20 kilometers to the south of Solo. There were two outpatient clinics in the village. Nugroho managed the clinic under the jurisdiction of the Solo maternity hospital. As Begajah was situated in a food-scarce region of Central Java, Nugroho frequently encountered several patients suffering from various degrees of malnutrition. Appalled by the continual confrontation with malnutrition in its various forms, Nugroho developed a strong desire to investigate the "roots of the misery."[80] To this end, he conducted a village survey to collect baseline data. However, due to political disturbances in Indonesia, associated with the September 30th Movement, the survey had to be suspended. Despite the challenges, Nugroho continued his community development work unperturbed. He converted the outpatient clinic into a health center, enabling him to respond to villagers' health and livelihood concerns.

During this period, Nugroho familiarized himself with rural infrastructure, decision-making process, and the socio-cultural background of villagers through personal observation. This was a particularly challenging time for him, as he was trained to diagnose and treat individual patients. However, he realized that to truly grasp villagers' problems, he had to be accepted as one of them. Loitering in the village, having tea in villagers' homes, sitting under a tree and observing women harvest paddy, and joking with the children, Nugroho learned about poverty.[81] His experience in Begajah enlightened Nugroho about the interconnectedness between socioeconomic well-being and good health:

> I learned to speak the same language of poverty, to see through the people's eyes the life they lived, almost a routine of shortcomings and hunger, without any hope of improvement. I understood their apathy and surrender and, worst of all, their loss of human dignity. This process of change in my way of thinking and feeling took place slowly.[82]

Without any preconceived design, Nugroho drew up a flexible program adapted to the baseline data collected from observation and personal contacts. He secured the support of the village headman and the *desa* administration to set up a local development committee, tasked with coordinating community initiatives. The committee would mobilize villagers in decision-making.

Recognizing the link between poor nutrition and agricultural underperformance, Nugroho piloted the enhancement of farm output as the central axis of intervention in Begajah's CHD. He assembled an interdisciplinary team led by a physician to operationalize this program. Using a demonstration plot provided by the village as a strategic lever, the team, in close cooperation with the government, introduced high-yielding rice that doubled output. In 1970, during an evaluation survey that included all children below the age of five, Nugroho's team recorded zero cases of malnutrition—a diagnostic milestone. Between 1966 and 1970, they offered health and nutrition courses to village women, triggering a marked decline in infant mortality.

Nugroho asserted that from the perspective of cost and benefit, health and nutrition education activities were exceedingly cheap. Yet, they produced disproportionately effective results:

> The model house that had been built as an example some years before was never thought to serve any useful purpose. The community had not been in the least interested, but now, after the standard of living had been raised and the community had reached the 'take-off level', bamboo walls were gradually replaced by brick walls, windows were put in the houses, glass tiles were used, and the gardens were well kept.[83]

Smiles, music in homes, children's laughter, and rippling paddyfields symbolized the village's recovery from structural deprivation.

In the second case, Nugroho pioneered a pilot community health insurance scheme (Bahasa Indonesia: *dana sehat*) in Solo, during the early 1970s. He organized groups of 15 households, where mothers contributed a fixed sum to a group fund that they could access whenever a sick family member wanted to see a doctor.[84] The elected leader would deposit group funds into a local bank account. Additionally, mothers were free to borrow from the fund to patch a leaky roof or buy a goat. Group pressure ensured that the loaned amount was promptly returned. A health visitor from Nugroho's team visited the groups once a month to encourage the mothers to discuss their problems freely. If a problem came up, the health visitor referred them to the nearest resource in town. For example, when a child had diarrhea, mothers were instructed how to manage symptoms, recording notes on the side of the house, which were then reviewed by Nugroho's team.[85]

What distinguished *dana sehat* from other community health insurance schemes was that within this framework, villagers were encouraged to contribute according to their capabilities.[86] The *dana sehat* health fund was created by collecting monthly subscriptions from the rural community valued at 0.5 percent of the family income, or approximately six US cents per month.[87] Since *dana sehat* was rooted in the Javanese principle of *gotong royong* [mutual self-help], wealthier individuals were expected to contribute more. If the monthly bill for healthcare exceeded the available subscription pool, the deficit was covered by credit cooperative funds. If the health bill was less than the subscription fees, the surplus was added to the cooperative's revolving fund.[88] A continuing monthly deficit prompted families to reexamine possible causes for high incidence of disease. With guidance from the Nugroho team, villagers soon learnt to conduct simple health surveys and address environmental sanitation. In addition to successful grassroots mobilization in rural Java, the *dana sehat* gained international visibility as it was congruent with the Basic Needs Approach—emphasizing nutrition, sanitation, and access to healthcare.

Interestingly, the formative period of Nugroho's CHD (1963–1970) coincided with the establishment of the Christian Medical Commission (CMC) in 1968. The CMC, a semiautonomous body, assisted the WCC in evaluating church-related medical programs in the developing world. Nugroho's Central Java experiment, launched in 1963, revealed that church-run hospitals prioritized curative care but failed to address basic community needs.[89] James C. McGilvray, the CMC's first director, was disturbed to find that the Church's curative services conflicted with the Christian emphasis on wholeness. McGilvray discovered Nugroho's project during a 1967 survey in Indonesia.[90] Nugroho presented his project to the CMC in 1971. In 1973, Joe de Wray—then with the Rockefeller Foundation in Bangkok—encountered Newell in a remote corner of India and apprised him of Nugroho's initiative. At the time, Newell was seeking innovative rural health care models.[91] Nugroho's *dana sehat*—a network of self-funded mothers' groups operating without external aid—attracted the WHO's attention in 1974. Newell subsequently invited Nugroho to contribute a chapter to *Health by the People*.

India

The origins of the Jamkhed Comprehensive Rural Health Project (CRHP) can be traced to the 1944 Bombay Plan, which emphasized increased production and equitable resource distribution as poverty alleviation strategies.[92] The Bhore Committee Report (1946) extended this developmental vision to health, arguing that unemployment and poverty undermined well-being through inadequate housing.[93] The Committee recommendations served as a prototype for health planning in post-independence India.

In 1952, the Government of India implemented some of the Bhore Committee recommendations. The country was divided into development blocks. Each block, serving 80,000 to 100,000 people, was assigned a primary health center, linked to sub-centers, each covering approximately 10,000 individuals.[94] In addition to establishing health centers, the Government of India instituted campaigns against malaria and tuberculosis. Although nearly 80 percent of state government budgets were allocated to medical colleges, primary health centers in rural areas suffered chronic infrastructural neglect and equipment shortages. These chronic imbalances in the distribution of public health resources underscored the urgency of alternate models—particularly those that championed community-based care.

Amid entrenched budgetary asymmetry and institutional inertia, efforts to recast rural health delivery were piloted through experiments such as at Narangwal in Punjab (1960–1975). The Narangwal initiative was spearheaded by Carl Taylor, in collaboration with the Indian Council of Medical Research and the Ministry of Health. Taylor was the founding chair of International Health at Johns Hopkins and a co-drafter of the Alma-Ata Declaration. The initiative demonstrated that village-level health services—spanning family planning, nutrition, and basic healthcare—could be delivered affordably.[95] The Jamkhed CRHP drew inspiration from Carl Taylor's experiment with the Auxiliary Nurse Midwife (ANM) to provide basic care to rural areas.[96]

The son of a schoolteacher, Rajanikant Arole (1934–2011) developed an early interest in medicine. After earning a science degree, he pursued medical education at Christian Medical College, Vellore, where he met Mabelle, his future wife.[97] United by a shared commitment to India's rural poor, the two physicians trained at Johns Hopkins under Taylor, whose Narangwal experiment demonstrated how university-based health projects could transform health outcomes in underserved areas. The Aroles formative exposure to interdisciplinary pedagogy and community-based care at Johns Hopkins shaped the strategic contours of the Jamkhed CRHP.

Shifting focus from treatment to addressing the structural determinants of care, the Aroles demonstrated that health could be an entering wedge into socioeconomic development.[98] Jamkhed, a poor village in Maharashtra, close to Rajanikant Arole's birthplace, became their focus. The Aroles targeted diseases caused by malnutrition, contaminated water, and inadequate sanitation—problems deeply entrenched in traditions, taboos, and social injustices affecting marginalized communities.[99]

When the Aroles launched the Jamkhed CRHP (1970), health indicators in the project area were among the worst in the world—an infant mortality rate of 176 per 1000, and a 40 percent malnutrition rate among children under five.[100] Additionally, one-third of the village population was migrating to sugarcane plantations in neighboring areas for short-term employment due to severe drought and ensuing starvation. Such intersecting crises—economic, nutritional, ecological, and migratory—prompted the Aroles to reconsider the demerits of hospital-based care.

In his address to the Annual Meeting of the CMC in June 1972, Rajanikant Arole reflected on his four years of work in a rural hospital. He admitted that both he and his wife had come to realize that their efforts were largely confined to providing curative care to hospitalized patients.[101] Seventy percent of the patients whom the Aroles treated suffered from preventable diseases. Most patients "cured" returned to the same insanitary conditions that caused their illness. In sum, the rural hospital offered an interim solution to health problems. Driven by this realization, the Aroles immersed themselves in the impoverished countryside near Jamkhed, trying to understand villagers' felt needs.

In talking to the villagers, the Aroles were amazed that healthcare was accorded a low priority. The greatest concerns were basic survival needs—food, water, schooling for children, and adequate roads for taking surplus crops to market.[102] During the drought, villagers mobilized resources to finance the digging of deep tubewells and recruited mobile health teams. These teams, composed of trained personnel and local representatives, promoted maternal and child health, responded to natural disasters, and treated leprosy and TB cases, while actively campaigning to reduce social stigma.

Having addressed villagers' immediate health needs, the Aroles realized a long-term solution required the recruitment of a village health worker for every community. However, young ANMs were reluctant to live in villages. The Aroles noted that nurturing mutual trust between health workers and rural communities was more effective than relying solely on formal education.[103] As one member of the CRHP team put it, "I can teach a chimpanzee how to give an injection but I need human beings to go to the villages and change attitudes towards health."[104] To operationalize this insight, the Aroles asked the village councils to appoint trusted middle-aged women from the community who would receive training in Jamkhed, work with families, and liaise with mobile health teams periodically.

The Jamkhed CRHP recognized the niche of Ayurvedic practitioners in furthering community health. To this end, the Aroles integrated them into child nutrition initiatives and the treatment of leprosy and tuberculosis patients.[105] Furthermore, they engaged the wives of Ayurvedic practitioners in antenatal outreach and maternal care.

The CRHP marked an epistemic shift in engaging with rural health. Moving away from treating illnesses in isolation, the Jamkhed program addressed the structural determinants that shaped community well-being. The Aroles recognized that poor conditions stemmed from unsafe water, caste-based social exclusion, low hygiene and nutrition awareness, and marginal farming conditions. This recognition led to a community-driven strategy that addressed the etiology of disease at its roots.

Jamkhed was one of the first projects of its kind to demonstrate the effectiveness of mobilizing illiterate female Community Health Workers (CHWs).[106] CHWs provided basic health care, and supported the poorest villagers. The CHWs maintained a basic health information system in each village that recorded births, deaths, family planning usage, and information from other sectors such as agriculture and the environment, often using indicators chosen by the locals. The aggregated data—displayed on a public village blackboard—mobilized the community in identifying issues and tracking health progress. Broadening its participatory ethos beyond clinical care, the Jamkhed CRHP built a demonstration and training farm where it introduced new crops appropriate to local conditions.[107]

The comprehensive approach to health, pioneered by the Aroles at Jamkhed, led to conspicuous achievements but also revealed a few limitations. Farmers' clubs improved land for agricultural production and watershed development, and learned to use appropriate technologies such as biogas and vermiculture.[108] Jamkhed's CHW model prompted the Indian government to initiate the world's second largest CHW program, following China. The government provided three-month training for 500,000 CHWs. Unfortunately, the program proved difficult to replicate across India due to poor selection of CHWs—often based on political connections—and insufficient support systems. Government planners prioritized training but neglected integration and long-term support.[109]

Thailand

Since 1975, Thailand has prioritized investment in decentralized health delivery while simultaneously strengthening its medical workforce. Over the decades, insurance schemes tailored to demographic segments improved financial access to care. This incremental strategy culminated in the introduction of Universal Health Coverage (UHC) in 2002.[110] The trajectory toward UHC was shaped by broader sociopolitical forces dating back to the late 1960s when the Vietnam War heightened fears of communist contagion. In response, Thai authorities targeted poverty: the perceived root of ideological unrest. Health—alongside education and agriculture—was reframed as a cornerstone of rural development and poverty alleviation, embedding care within a broader matrix of national stabilization.

In parallel with Thailand's push for rural health investment, the Rural Doctors' Movement emerged—a phalanx of progressive physicians committed to reducing health disparities in the underserved north and northeast. Despite operating under a military dictatorship, these physicians chose community health hospitals over emigration or private medical practice.[111] Their vision led to the creation of the Rural Doctor Society in 1978, which institutionalized equity-focused reforms. During the 1990s, following democratization, Society members assumed influential roles within the Ministry of Public Health, helping catalyze the introduction of UHC.

During the mid-1970s, 84 percent of Thailand's poor lived in rural areas, nearly two-thirds in the under-resourced northern and northeastern provinces.[112] Physicians, primarily drawn from the urban elite, emigrated abroad. The Vietnam War and military rule further obscured the structural realities confronting Thailand's peripheral communities.

During the democratic interregnum between 1973 and 1976, previously banned socialist ideas circulated among students and farmers. The Peasants Federation of Thailand, founded in 1974, mobilized impoverished villagers, while the National Student Center of Thailand evolved into a hub for student activism. Amid the surge of grassroots mobilization, a cadre of politically engaged doctors and students confronted systemic rural health infrastructure neglect. Sanguan Nitayarumphong, then a medical student at Mahidol University, spearheaded efforts to reorient the medical curriculum toward rural health and nurtured political engagement among aspiring physicians.[113]

In 1974, the Equality Action Group—a student-led collective—raised health awareness among secondary school pupils. Over 4000 student volunteers joined what became known as Return to the Countryside Campaign, spending a month in rural communities to understand local health challenges.[114] The campaign aligned with the Public Health for the Masses initiative, foregrounding the medical and infrastructural inequities facing Thailand's northern and northeastern provinces.

Sociologist Joseph Harris observes that medical activism in Thailand coincided with the global ascendance of the PHC paradigm, emphasizing health promotion, disease prevention, the strategic use of health volunteers, and community participation.[115] While the WHO-UNICEF Conference on PHC at Alma-Ata is acknowledged as a watershed moment in the dissemination of PHC ideals, Thailand's PHC experiments predate this international endorsement. As early as the 1960s, community health volunteers were mobilized for malaria control in Saraphi, reflecting local participation in healthcare delivery.[116]

In response to constraints imposed by state-led health provision, Thai medical activists formed an organization known as Rural Medical Federation in 1976. The Federation published a journal, documenting physicians' experiences in the countryside.[117] The group aspired to visit the PRC to study the Barefoot Doctor model, which they viewed offered a community-based alternative to Thailand's Bangkok-centric health infrastructure. Some activists framed their views in socialist terms, while others identified as "concerned student activists" interested in rural welfare.[118] A third strand rejected ideological labels, instead emphasizing the benefits of PHC. During his student days, Sanguan expressed interest in visiting Sweden, where UHC aligned with his social democrat leanings.[119] What unified Rural Medical Federation's members was their concern for the impoverished countryside, regardless of ideological orientation.

However, the Rural Medical Federation was founded at an unpropitious moment in Thailand's history. On October 6, 1976, right-wing paramilitary groups opened fire on some Thammasat University students, while a few others were hanged from a tamarind tree and burned with tires.[120] Amid a thorny political conflict, a military coup was staged against the elected government with royal assent. The coup claimed to purge the communist insurgency. The liberated zones of the Communist Party of Thailand (CPT), especially in the mountainous areas of the north and northeast, absorbed a mass influx of left-leaning and liberal university students. Several medical students and practitioners fled to join the CPT. A few students such as Viroj Tangcharoensathien entered private practice to support colleagues affiliated with the CPT's jungle-based medical service.[121]

Conceived during a time of political turbulence in Thailand, the Rural Medical Federation abruptly collapsed within a few months of its inception. However, in 1978, the Federation was renamed the Rural Doctor Society, to avoid associations with radical labor and peasant organizations, targeted by right-wing groups. The society brought together medical professionals committed to addressing social and economic disparities, limited healthcare access, and the struggles of rural poor.[122] Members focused on strengthening camaraderie among physicians stationed in Thailand's northern and northeastern provinces by organizing management training programs, creating handbooks, initiating activities, and providing mentorship through senior physicians.

According to sociologist Joseph Harris, members reoriented their roles to address the social determinants of health—collaborating with villagers to develop community gardens, revolving funds, village banks, and drug cooperatives.[123] Their connections to the Thai Ministry of Health opened venues for professional advancement, enabling them to manage the development of Thailand's fledging health insurance programs in the early 1980s.

By the 1990s, although rural Thais' access to health services had improved, many indigent patients struggled to get hospitalized. UHC was the Rural Doctor Society's holy grail. The society conducted research, set the agenda, and devised policy advocacy strategies that interested the Thai-Rak-Thai party.[124] The Thai-Rak-Thais won the 2001 election on the UHC platform. The lasting legacy of the Rural Doctor Society was the enshrinement of a constitutional provision which mandates the state to provide free healthcare to low-income citizens and free services for the prevention and control of communicable diseases.[125] Despite repeated coups, this clause has been retained in all succeeding constitutions since 1978. In acknowledgment of its historical and continued contribution to people's health, the Rural Doctor Society was conferred the Ramon Magsaysay Award in 2024, a testament to the Society's enduring impact on underserved rural communities.

Sri Lanka

In his autobiography *A Voyage Toward Health*, V.T.H. Gunaratne, Regional Director of the WHO Regional Office for South-East Asia (SEARO), between 1968 and 1981, contended that while drugs do not enhance health directly, they were central to the region's PHC strategy.[126] He emphasized that a rational selection of essential drugs forms the cornerstone of state PHC systems. Based on Sri Lanka's experience, he urged each Southeast Asian member state to identify and prioritize essential pharmaceuticals as a preliminary step toward self-reliance.

Since gaining independence from the UK in 1948, Ceylon (Sri Lanka since 1972), prioritized state-sponsored industrialization but neglected the pharmaceutical sector. This was partly due to its well-established network of colonial era health units, which reduced the perceived urgency for pharmaceutical investment.[127] By the 1950s, Ceylon increasingly relied on the UK and other Western nations for a steady supply of pharmaceuticals, raising concerns about long-term accessibility and affordability. Recognizing this dependency, Bibile—founder of the first department of pharmacology on Ceylon—proposed a solution: a streamlined list of essential drugs, generically procured through competitive bidding for the public sector.[128] In 1959, he authored *Ceylon Hospitals Formulary*, urging state-run hospitals to limit drug use to those listed in the formulary.[129]

Bibile's formulary offered a structured approach to sourcing generic drugs. In 1962, Ceylon suffered a foreign exchange crisis, triggered by its dependence on tea exports—whose prices fell by 70 percent.[130] This downturn severely impacted drug imports. At one point, 23 brands of tetracycline capsules, 12 of chloramphenicol, and 12 of tetracycline syrup were imported.[131] This proliferation of brands frustrated cost rationalization. Between 1965 and 1970, the drug import budget was cut from 33 million to 24 million rupees.[132] As medical needs grew, the per capita supply of pharmaceuticals dwindled.

In 1970, the United Front coalition, led by Sirimavo Bandaranaike, won the parliamentary elections on a socialist platform. The Bandaranaike administration consulted Bibile and physician-parliamentarian S. Wickremasinghe on pharmaceutical rationalization. The following year, Bibile and Wickremasinghe co-authored *The Management of Pharmaceuticals in Ceylon*, advancing three recommendations: reduce private-sector pharmaceutical imports; amend patent laws governing drug distribution; and import drugs in bulk to ensure supply continuity.[133]

Building on its recommendation to modify Ceylon's patent laws, the Wickremasinghe-Bibile Report (1971) proposed enabling local pharmaceutical production, promoting generic naming in prescriptions, disseminating unbiased pharmaceutical information, and phasing out advertising. Furthermore, the report recommended instituting pharmaceutical quality control. In 1972, the government established the State Pharmaceuticals Corporation of Sri Lanka (SPC), which implemented Bibile's plan between 1972 and 1976.[134]

While Sri Lanka translated Bibile's vision into practice by the mid-1970s, similar efforts in Pakistan and Mozambique were thwarted by an adverse trade balance and political turmoil, respectively.[135] Pharmaceuticals became the cornerstone of international dialogues on economic cooperation. At the United Nations Conference on Trade and Development convened in Nairobi, Kenya (1976), and the Fifth Non-Aligned Conference, convened in Colombo (1976), the importance of pharmaceuticals was highlighted. This momentum carried into the Group of 77 Conference on Economic Cooperation Among Developing Countries held in Mexico City (September 1976). The Colombo NAM Summit adopted Resolution 25, urging developing countries to cooperate with international organizations to promote pharmaceutical production, procurement, and distribution.[136] These collaborative efforts highlighted the growing recognition of pharmaceuticals as a critical plank for fostering economic cooperation and self-reliance in the Global South—anchored in the principle of pharmaceutical sovereignty.

Bibile's initiatives proved successful in Sri Lanka. The SPC imported large volumes of drugs for the private sector at a fraction of previous prices.[137] Purchasing from non-traditional suppliers—Hungary, Poland, and Yugoslavia—yielded significant savings on widely used drugs such as diazepam. Predictably, transnational pharmaceutical corporations circulated unsubstantiated rumors about the poor quality of generics.[138]

In 1974, the Sri Lankan Minister of Finance N.M. Perera threatened to nationalize Pfizer, citing exorbitant raw material pricing and non-compliance with SPC's generic labeling requirements.[139] In response, the US Pharmaceutical Manufacturers Association enlisted the American government to oppose the move. Washington escalated diplomatic pressure by threatening to suspend food aid to Sri Lanka—a reaction disproportionate to the economic losses incurred, given Sri Lanka's negligible share of the global pharmaceutical market.[140] Transnational corporations interpreted Sri Lanka's policy of promoting generic drugs as a structural impediment to their global business model.

Within the Sri Lankan medical profession, there was no organized support for Bibile's efforts. Amid a deepening economic crisis in 1976, the government halted the final stages of the pharmaceutical program, prompting Bibile's resignation from the SPC. The 1977 parliamentary elections resulted in a landslide victory for the United National Party, led by J.R. Jayewardene. While his administration liberalized the economy, the SPC continued to retain its monopoly over drug procurement and distribution. Transferred from the Ministry of Commerce to the Ministry of Health, the SPC's administrative shift proved cosmetic—Sri Lanka' s pharmaceutical policy remained largely unchanged.

For instance, Gladys Jayawardena, a retired microbiologist and a sister-in-law of the Sri Lankan president, chaired the 1978 SEARO Regional Seminar on Drugs Policies and Management. The conclusions that emerged from the seminar were identical to those raised by Bibile: the problems of transfer pricing, over-invoicing, and fluctuations in the prices of raw materials.[141] Furthermore, pharmacologist N.D.W. Lionel—a colleague of Bibile and a contributor to the Wickremasinghe-Bibile Report—was rapporteur to the 1977 WHO Expert Committee on the Selection of Essential Drugs.[142] Despite abrupt political shifts and significant constraints, Sri Lanka's pharmaceutical policy—engineered by Bibile—left an indelible imprint on global health discussions concerning essential drugs and healthcare equity.

Coda: Alma-Ata and Its Discontents

The development of PHC in Southeast Asia reveals a synergistic interchange between Cold War ideologies and local adaptations. Geopolitical considerations influenced the trajectory of the global campaigns against malaria and smallpox and the export of the Barefoot Doctors model to the Global South. However, local health actors—in Indonesia, India, Thailand, and Sri Lanka—reconfigured PHC to suit domestic requirements—within, and sometimes in spite of, Cold War constraints. This reinforces the centrality of context for understanding the evolution of particular healthcare models across the region. Antedating Cold War interventions, the Kalutara health unit in Ceylon—established in 1926 through a Rockefeller-colonial partnership—subsequently provided the prototype for the postcolonial state's integrated PHC network.

The Alma-Ata Declaration (1978) was an inflection point in the evolution of global health, shifting the focus from a narrow biomedical framework to a holistic approach. The Declaration defined PHC as essential healthcare, founded on practical, scientifically sound, and socially acceptable methods and technologies. It emphasized universal accessibility, active community participation, and affordability—nurturing self-reliance and empowering communities to determine and address their own health needs.[143] However, while PHC emphasized equity and universal access, an alternative model—Selective Primary Healthcare (SPHC)—introduced in

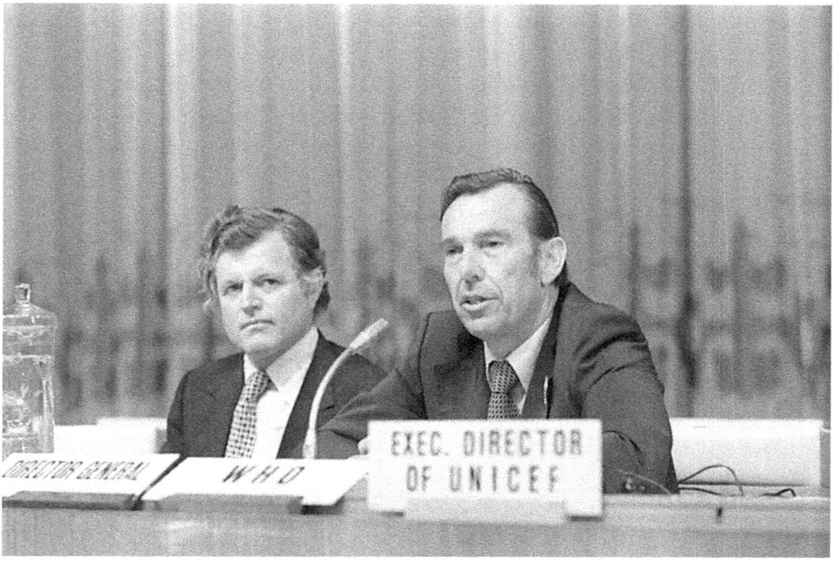

Image 7.3 U.S. Senator Edward Kennedy (left) made a surprise appearance at the 1978 Alma-Ata conference. At right is then WHO Director-General Halfdan Mahler. WHO Image Reference No: HQ 233206. With Permission from the WHO Photo Library

1979—prioritized cost-effective interventions to address the main health problems of developing countries (Image 7.3).[144]

The road from policy formulation to PHC implementation was circuitous. WHO member states embraced PHC as national policy, yet implementing "Health for All" within nation-state frameworks encountered three persistent challenges:

(1) Balancing vertical disease eradication campaigns with holistic health programs;
(2) Institutionalizing health equity and community participation;
(3) Securing sustainable funding for PHC.[145]

Despite the Alma-Ata Declaration's ambitious targets, its lack of an enforcement mechanism to uphold governments' compliance with human rights obligations for health highlighted the dichotomy between policy and implementation. In the two decades following Alma-Ata, neoliberalism permeated global development policy. In several developing nations such as India, structural adjustment programs sought to reduce budgetary deficits by restricting healthcare spending.[146] This led to underfunded health systems, a decline in the quality of health personnel, and worsening access to care for the poor. Conferences such as Bellagio (held in 1979) sought to tackle these deficiencies by emphasizing cost-effective health services.

The Bellagio Conference not only set the stage for the ascendance of SPHC but also revealed the gap between global health goals and actionable solutions. Seeking scalable and cost-effective health interventions, the Rockefeller Foundation sponsored a small but impactful conference entitled "Health and Population in Development" at Bellagio in 1979. This meeting aimed to enhance the integration of health and population initiatives at a time when global interest in reproductive health was waning, primarily due to a reaction against coercive and arbitrary population control measures in India.[147] The Bellagio discussions prioritized strategically targeted technical interventions aimed at addressing immediate public health problems of developing countries.

At Bellagio, Robert McNamara, the then president of the World Bank (1968–1981), defended the institution from critics alleging the Bank's neglect of social poverty and the fatigue of Global North donors working in developing nations.[148] Advocating modular solutions, he shifted the World Bank's focus from large-scale development projects to poverty reduction strategies, applying business management methods to international development.

McNamara adopted a conservative position on PHC—emphasizing economic realism over a rights-based approach:

> Given the obstacles they face, elimination of absolute poverty in the Low Income countries by the end of this century seems impossible. A more realistic target would be to reduce the proportion of their populations living in poverty to about 15 to 20 percent by the year 2000, which would still leave nearly 400 million people in absolute poverty. To realize even this gain will require massive efforts to raise the productivity and incomes of the poor.[149]

The quote reveals a strategic shift from utopian poverty elimination goals toward sustained reduction—acknowledging structural constraints—while advocating long-term policy interventions to raise living standards.

Julia Walsh and Kenneth S. Warren's 1979 paper, "Selective Primary Health Care: An Interim Strategy for Disease Control in Developing Countries," informed discussions at the Bellagio conference. They presented SPHC as "a rationally conceived, best-data-based, selective attack on the most severe public-health problems" in underdeveloped areas.[150] The SPHC approach focused on targeting malaria, tuberculosis, measles, or diarrheal diseases, for which proven interventions existed. The eradication of smallpox in 1980 illustrated the promise of targeted vaccination programs to reduce the burden of communicable diseases in developing countries.

In its original articulation in 1979, the contents of SPHC were vaguely delineated. Walsh and Warren outlined interventions such as measles and diphtheria-pertussis-tetanus vaccination (DPT), febrile malaria treatment, oral rehydration for infantile diarrhea, and promoting breastfeeding.[151] Over the following years, SPHC's focus narrowed to four key interventions: GOBI—growth monitoring, oral rehydration, breastfeeding, and immunization.

In 1983, under the leadership of UNICEF Executive Director James Grant (1980–1995), the agency announced GOBI as the main tool for a Child Survival and Development Revolution.[152] Several health ministries in developing countries emphasized aspects of GOBI to attract international aid under PHC banner—reframing these interventions as targeted intervention nodes into broader health system strengthening.

The only sphere where GOBI was unable to attain its full potential was growth monitoring of infants.[153] In 1980, the Tamil Nadu state government in southern India, with World Bank aid, implemented the Tamil Nadu Integrated Nutrition Project targeting infants in the 6–34 months age bracket, the critical group where most stunting occurred. The program's diagnostic criteria for supplementary feeding were epidemiologically targeted. Yet, national implementation faltered due to flaws in program design. Rolf Carrière—senior UNICEF consultant in 1980s Tamil Nadu—noted that the Indian government privileged easy-to-reach children between three and five, despite widespread malnutrition in the 6–34 months age group.[154] GOBI's selective traction in India revealed a trade-off between targeted interventions and inclusive health outcomes.

Between 1979 and 1981, SPHC's technocratic approach eclipsed Alma-Ata's idealism, revealing a fundamental tension between global health aspirations and actionable solutions. This dilemma highlighted difficult policy choices confronting Southeast Asian governments and international aid agencies. While SPHC recalibrated global health priorities to address resource deficits in developing countries through low-cost interventions such as GOBI, it sidestepped structural factors—access to potable water, sanitation, and health education. These elements—envisaged as quintessential in the Alma-Ata Declaration—were excluded from SPHC's reductionist logic.

Ultimately, the regional quest for PHC across Southeast Asia revealed normative dissonances of mapping lofty global health aspirations into deliverable outcomes at varying scales: local, national, regional, and international.

Notes

1. Draft of Dwight D. Eisenhower's Speech, "Security and Peace," 11/26/1957, 7th draft, White House Correspondence 1955 (2), Box 5, John Foster Dulles Papers: White House Memoranda Series, Dwight D. Eisenhower Presidential Library.
2. Marcos Cueto, *Cold War and Deadly Fevers: Malaria Eradication in Mexico, 1955–1975* (Baltimore, MD: Johns Hopkins University Press, 2007), 15.
3. WHA Resolution A 22/P&B/8, "Reexamination of the Global Strategy of Malaria Eradication," *Official Records of the World Health Organization: Twenty-Second World Health Assembly, part I*, no. 176, July 8–25, 1969 (Geneva: WHO, 1969), WHO Library and Historical Collections, Geneva (hereafter WHOL).
4. See Anne-Emanuelle Birn, "The Stages of International (Global) Health: Histories of Success or Successes of History?" *Global Public Health* 4, no. 1 (2009): 50–68.
5. Marcos Cueto, "The Origins of Primary Healthcare and SELECTIVE Primary Healthcare," *American Journal of Public Health* 94, no. 11 (2004): 1864–74, 1867.
6. Socrates Litsios, "The Long and Difficult Road to Alma-Ata: A Personal Reflection," *International Journal of Health Services* 32, no. 4 (2002): 709–32, 718.
7. Randall Packard, *A History of Global Health: Interventions into the Lives of Other Peoples* (Baltimore, Maryland: Johns Hopkins University Press, 2016).
8. Erez Manela, "A Pox on Your Narrative: Writing Disease Control into Cold War History," *Diplomatic History* 14, no. 2 (2010): 299–323, 306
9. Manela, "A Pox on Your Narrative," 307.

10. WHO, "Re- examination of the Global Strategy of Malaria Eradication," Resolution 22.39, *Twenty-Second World Health Assembly, Boston, Massachusetts (July 8 to July 25, 1968)*: *Part I, Resolutions and Decisions Annexes* (Geneva: WHO, 1969), WHOL.
11. Packard, *A History of Global Health.*
12. WHO, "Methodology of Planning an Integrated Health Programme for Rural Areas: Second Report of the Expert Committee on Public Health Administration," *WHO Technical Report Series* 83 (Geneva: WHO, 1954), WHOL.
13. Packard, *A History of Global Health.*
14. John Charnow and Sherwood C. Moe, "Henry Labouise: UNICEF Executive Director, 1965–1979," *Monograph X1 UNICEF History Series Monograph XI* (New York: UNICEF, 1988), Doc. CF/HST/MON/1988-011, UNICEF Archives.
15. Kathryn Sweet, "Women's Health in Laos: From Colonial Times to the Present," in *Translating the Body: Medical Education in Southeast Asia*, Hans Pols, C. Michele Thompson and John Harley Warner edited (Singapore: NUS Press, 2017), 116–45, 127.
16. Ibid., 127.
17. Vivek Neelakantan, "Mobilizing Applied Medical Knowledge in Indonesia: Soekarnoist Science and Asian-African Solidarity in the 1950s," in *Fighting for Health: Medicine in Southeast Asia*, C. Michele Thompson, Kathryn Sweet, and Michitake Aso edited (Singapore: NUS Press, 2024), 167–93, 176.
18. Nikita Chrusjtjov, *Uni Sovjet Sahabat Bagi Rakjat 2 jang Sedang Berdjoeang Untuk Kemerdekaanja* (Djakarta: Kedutaan Besar URSS, 1960), Perpustakaan Nasional Republik Indonesia or PNRI [Bahasa Indonesia].
19. D.D. Venediktov and V.I. Petrov, *Untuk Taraf Kesehatan jang Tertinggi* (Djakarta: Kedutaan Besar URSS, 1960), PNRI [Bahasa Indonesia].
20. Neelakantan, "Mobilizing Applied Medical Knowledge," 176.
21. Professor Dr Satrio and Mona Lohanda, "Perjuangan dan Pengabdian: Mosaik Kenangan Prof. Dr Satrio," *Penerbitan Sejarah Lisan Nomor 3* (Jakarta: Arsip Nasional Republik Indonesia, 1986), 206, The National Archives of Indonesia or ANRI [Bahasa Indonesia].
22. Neelakantan, "Mobilizing Applied Medical Knowledge," 176–77.
23. Neelakantan, "Mobilizing Applied Medical Knowledge," 177.
24. Jenna Grant, "'Cambodian Pathology': Imagining Modern Biomedicine in the Cambodian-Soviet Medical Journal, *Revue Médico-Chirurgicale de l' Hôpital de Amitié Khméro-Soviétique* (1961–71)," in *Translating the Body: Medical Education in Southeast Asia*, Hans Pols, C. Michele Thompson, and John Harley Warner edited (Singapore: NUS Press, 2017), 194–229.
25. Birn and Krementsov, "'Socialising' Primary Care?"

26. Niels Brimnes, "Negotiating Social Medicine in a Postcolonial Context: Halfdan Mahler in India, 1951–74," *Medical History* 67, no. 1 (2023): 5–22, 5.
27. Birn and Krementsov, "'Socialising' Primary Care?"
28. Ibid.
29. Ibid.
30. V. Djukanovic and E.P. Mach, *Alternative Approaches to Meeting Basic Needs in Developing Countries: A Joint WHO-UNICEF Study* (Geneva: WHO, 1975), WHOL.
31. Ibid.
32. Socrates Litsios, "Kenneth Newell: Primary Healthcare's Midwife," *Social Medicine* 14, no. 1 (2021): 28–36, 28.
33. Ibid., 28.
34. Kenneth Newell, "Health by the People," in *Health by the People*, Kenneth Newell edited (Geneva: WHO, 1975), 191–203, 192, WHOL.
35. Newell, "Health by the People," 199.
36. Victor Sidel, "The Barefoot Doctors of the People's Republic of China," *The New England Journal of Medicine* 286, no. 24 (June 15, 1972): 1292–1300.
37. Xiaoping Fang, "Communist Medicine: The Emergence of TCM and Barefoot Doctors, Leading to Contemporary Medical Markets," in *Routledge Handbook of Chinese Medicine*, Vivienne Lo, Michael Stanley-Baker and Dolly Yang (Abingdon, Oxon: Routledge, 2022), 638–48, 641.
38. Shirish Kavadi, "John B. Grant and Public Health in India," *Indian Journal of Medical Ethics* 4, no. 1 (2019), https://doi.org/10.20529/IJME.2019.010.
39. Sidel, "Barefoot Doctors," 1293.
40. Ibid., 1293.
41. Liping Bu, "Taking Our Own Road: Building the People's Health in Socialist China," in *Public Health and Cold War Politics in Asia*, Liping Bu edited (Abingdon, Oxon: Routledge, 2024), 32–56, 32.
42. Sidel, "Barefoot Doctors," 1294.
43. "WHO Visits China," *World Health: Magazine of the World Health Organization* (September 1974): 8–14, WHOL.
44. Ibid.
45. Ibid.
46. Ibid.
47. George T. Yu, "China and the Third World," *Asian Survey* 17, no. 11 (1977): 1036–48, 1037.
48. Yu, "China," 1043.
49. Jan Ovesen and Ing-Britt Trankell, *Cambodians and Their Doctors: A Medical Anthropology of Colonial and Post-Colonial Cambodia* (Copenhagen: NIAS Press, 2010), 91.
50. Ibid., 91.

51. Xun Zhou, "China's Barefoot Doctor to Alma Ata: The Primary Healthcare Movement in the Long 1970s," in *China, Hong Kong and the Long 1970s: Global Perspectives,* P. Roberts and O.A. Westad (Basingstoke, Oxon: Palgrave Macmillan, 2017), 135–57.
52. Birn and Krementsov, "'Socialising' Primary Care?"
53. Ibid.
54. Litsios, "The Long and Difficult Road to Alma-Ata," 715.
55. Birn and Krementsov, "'Socialising' Primary Care?"
56. Ibid.
57. Ibid.
58. Ibid.
59. Ibid.
60. Ibid.
61. Vivek Neelakantan, "Indonesian Health Policy between the Old and the New Orders," in *Public Health and Cold War Politics in Asia,* Liping Bu edited (Abingdon, Oxon: Routledge, 2024), 151–76, 154.
62. Johannes Leimena, "World Health and World Community," *The Ecumenical Review* 4 (1951):407–409, The World Council of Churches Archives, Geneva (hereafter WCC).
63. C.E.A. Winslow, *The Cost of Sickness and the Price of Health* (Geneva: WHO, 1951), WHOL.
64. Johannes Leimena, *Public Health in Indonesia: Problems and Planning* (Djakarta: G.C.T. van Dorp, 1956).
65. Liping Bu, "John B. Grant and Public Health in China," *Rockefeller Archive Center Research Reports* (2012), https://rockarch.issuelab.org/resources/27881/27881.pdf.
66. "Interviews: Charles Burton Fahs, Trip to the Far East (Djakarta)," Diary: Trip to the Far East, April 26 to June 23, 1954, Rockefeller Foundation Officers' Diaries RG 12, F-L, RAC; "Rockefeller," June 4, 1955, *Indische Courant*, June 4, 1955, 2, Koninklijke Bibliotheek (KB) [Dutch].
67. R.Z. Leirissa, *Kewarganegaraan Yang Bertanggung Jawab: Mengenang Dr. J. Leimena* (Jakarta: BPK Gunung Mulia, 1980), 21. [Bahasa Indonesia].
68. Vivek Neelakantan, *Science, Public Health and Nation-Building in Soekarno Era Indonesia* (Newcastle-upon-Tyne: Cambridge Scholars, 2017), 74.
69. Neelakantan, "Indonesian Health Policy," 155.
70. Neelakantan, "Indonesian Health Policy," 156.
71. Neelakantan, *Science, Public Health and Nation-Building*, 84.
72. Ibid., 84.
73. Neelakantan, "Indonesian Health Policy," 161.

74. Adrian Vickers, *A History of Modern Indonesia, Second Edition* (Cambridge: Cambridge University Press, 2013), 148.
75. Neelakantan, "Indonesian Health Policy," 162.
76. Neelakantan, "Indonesian Health Policy," 163.
77. Ibid., 163.
78. Gunawan Nugroho, Rufino Macagba, and George Dorros, *Building Community Health* (Health Development International and Visionary Healthcare Leadership Worldwide, 2001).
79. Gunawan Nugroho, "Starting from Scratch," *World Health* (1975): 26–29, 26, WHOL.
80. Gunawan Nugroho, "A Community Development Approach to Raising Health Standards in Central Java, Indonesia," in *Health by the People*, Kenneth Newell edited (Geneva: WHO, 1975), 91–111, 94, WHOL.
81. Nugroho, "A Community Development Approach," 95.
82. Ibid., 95.
83. Nugroho, "A Community Development Approach," 96.
84. Rufino Macagba, "Email Interview by Vivek Neelakantan," December 10, 2021.
85. Ibid.
86. Gunawan Nugroho and Katherine Elliott, "The Dana Sehat Programme in Solo, Indonesia," *Proceedings of the Royal Society B: Biological Sciences* 199 (1977): 145–50.
87. Nugroho and Elliott, "The Dana Sehat Programme," 148.
88. Nugroho and Elliott, "The Dana Sehat Programme," 149.
89. Socrates Litsios, "The Christian Medical Commission and the Development of the World Health Organization's Primary Healthcare Approach," *American Journal of Public Health* 94, no. 11 (2004): 1884–93, 1887.
90. James C. McGilvray, *The Quest for Health and Wholeness* (Tubingen: German Institute for Medical Missions Theology, 1981), 58.
91. Litsios, "The Christian Medical Commission," 1889.
92. Sir Purshottamdas Thakurdas, J.R.D. Tata, G.D. Birla et al., *A Plan of Economic Development for India, Part II: Role of the State* (Publisher Unknown: Bombay, 1944).
93. *Report of the Health Survey and Development Committee, Volume 1: Survey* (Delhi: Manager of Publications Government of India, 1946).
94. Drs. Mabelle and Rajanikant Arole, *A Comprehensive Rural Health Project: Jamkhed* (London: Macmillan, 1994), 41. Autobiography.
95. Carl Taylor, "The Doctor's Role in Rural Health Care," *International Journal of Health Services* 6, no. 2 (1976): 219–30.
96. Arole and Arole, *A Comprehensive Rural Health Project*, 40.
97. Stephen Pincock, "Obituary: Rajanikant Arole," *Lancet* 378, no. 9788 (July 2, 2011), 24.

98. Carl Taylor, "Foreword," in *A Comprehensive Rural Health Project: Jamkhed* (London: Macmillan, 1994), vi–vii.
99. Pincock, "Obituary," 24.
100. Henry Perry and Jon Rohde, "The Jamkhed Comprehensive Rural Health Project and the Alma-Ata Vision of PHC," *American Journal of Public Health* 109, no. 5 (2019): 699–704, 700.
101. Rajanikant S. Arole, "Comprehensive Rural Health Project Jamkhed, India: Address to the Christian Medical Commission at its Annual Meeting in June 1972," *Contact* 10 (1972): 1–9, WCC.
102. "Jamkhed, Maharashtra: A New Experience in Christian Medical Work in India," *Contact* 161/62 (1998): 10, WCC.
103. Ibid., 10.
104. Ibid., 10.
105. Arole, "Comprehensive Rural Health Project."
106. Perry and Rohde, "The Jamkhed Comprehensive Rural Health Project," 700.
107. Perry and Rohde, "The Jamkhed Comprehensive Rural Health Project," 701.
108. Ibid., 701.
109. Perry and Rohde, "The Jamkhed Comprehensive Rural Health Project," 703.
110. Viroj Tangcharoensathien, Waranan Wittayapiposakul, Warisa Panichkriangkrai, et al., "Health Systems Development in Thailand: A Solid Platform for Successful Implementation of Universal Health Coverage," *The Lancet* 391, no. 10126 (March 2018): https://doi.org/10.1016/S0140-6736(18)30198-3.
111. Joseph Harris, *Achieving Access: Professional Movements and the Politics of Health Universalism* (Ithaca: Cornell University Press, 2017), 36.
112. Harris, *Achieving Access*, 37.
113. Ibid., 37.
114. Harris, *Achieving Access*, 38.
115. Ibid., 38.
116. Sanguan Nityarumphong, "Evolution of Primary Health Care in Thailand: What Policies Worked?" *Health Policy and Planning* 9, no. 3 (1990): 246–54.
117. Harris, 38.
118. Harris, *Achieving Access*, 39.
119. Ibid., 39.
120. Davisakd Puaksom, "Thailand's Rural Doctor Society in the 1970s-80s and Its Struggles to Improve Health in the Countryside," in *The Geopolitics of Health in South and Southeast Asia: Perspectives from the Cold War to COVID-19, 1948–2021*, Vivek Neelakantan edited (Abingdon, Oxon: Routledge, 2023), 98–119, 102.

121. Puaksom, "Thailand's Rural Doctor Society," 103.
122. Harris, *Achieving Access*, 40.
123. Ibid., 40.
124. "Rural Doctors Movement," Ramon Magsaysay Award Foundation. Accessed March 14, 2025. https://rmaward.asia/rmawardees/rural-doctors-movement/?form=MG0AV3&form=MG0AV3.
125. Ibid.
126. V.T. Herat Gunaratne, *A Voyage Toward Health* (New Delhi: Tata MacGraw-Hill Publication Company, 1980), 115.
127. Soma Hewa, "Sri Lanka's Approach to Primary Health Care: A Success Story in South Asia," *Galle Medical Journal* 16, no. 2 (2011): 24–31. The Rockefeller Foundation inaugurated the Kalutara Health Unit in 1926. The unit conducted health surveys, compiled vital statistics, promoted health education, controlled infectious diseases, and developed maternal-child health and sanitation programs. Although health units improved public health across Ceylon, subsequent efforts by the colonial and postcolonial states were undermined by recurring malaria outbreaks. Following independence, Ceylon consolidated its early public health achievements by implementing a broad-based social welfare program. Free services—including maternity care, hospitalization, and essential drugs—helped fulfil basic needs.
128. Jeremy A. Greene, "Vital Objects: Essential Drugs and Their Critical Legacies," in *Reimagining (Bio) Medicalization, Pharmaceuticals and Genetics: Old Critiques and New Engagements*, Susan Bell and Anne Figert edited (Abingdon. Oxon: Routledge, 2015), 89–111, 93.
129. D.C. Jayasuriya, "Regulating the Drug Trade in the Third World," *World Health Forum* 2, no. 3 (1981): 423–26, WHOL.
130. Sirimavo R.D. Bandaranaike, "The Non-Aligned Movement and the United Nations," *The Black Scholar* 8, no. 3 (1976), 27–31, 34–38.
131. Sanjaya Lall and Senaka Bibile, "The Political Economy of Controlling Transnationals: The Pharmaceutical Industry in Sri Lanka, 1972–76," *International Journal of Health Services* 8, no. 2 (1978): 299–328, 302.
132. Ibid., 302.
133. S.A. Wickremasinghe and S. Bibile, "Pharmaceuticals Management in Ceylon," *The British Medical Journal* 3, no. 5777 (September 25, 1971): 757–58.
134. Greene, "Vital Objects," 93.
135. Jeremy A. Greene, "Making Medicines Essential: The Emergent Centrality of Pharmaceuticals in Global Health," *BioSocieties* 6, no. 1 (2011): 10–33, 17.
136. Greene, "Vital Objects," 94.

137. Krisantha Weerasuriya, "A Search for Balance: Pharmaceuticals in Sri Lanka: Pioneering Steps in a Receptive Environment and Subsequent Accommodations," *Development Dialogue* 1 (1995): 54–95, 62.
138. Ibid., 62.
139. Telegram From US Department of State to Secretary of State, "Minister Threatens Takeover of Pfizer in Sri Lanka," May 10, 1974, Wikileaks: Public Library of US Diplomacy. Accessed March 24, 2025. https://wikileaks.org/plusd/cables/1974COLOMB01305_b.html. Confidential.
140. Weerasuriya, "A Search for Balance," 62.
141. Weerasuriya, "A Search for Balance," 64.
142. Weerasuriya, "A Search for Balance," 70; WHO, "The Selection of Essential Drugs: Report of a WHO Expert Committee," *WHO Technical Report Series* 615 (Geneva: WHO, 1977), WHOL.
143. Cueto, "The Origins of Primary Healthcare," 1868.
144. Ibid., 1868.
145. Susan B. Rifkin, "Alma Ata after 40 years: Primary Health Care and Health for All—From Consensus to Complexity," *BMJ Global Health* 3 (2018): e001188, doi: 10.1136/ bmjgh-2018-001188.
146. Shailender Hooda, "Health System in Transition in India: Journey from State Provisioning to Privatization," *World Review of Political Economy* 11, no. 4 (2020): 506–32.
147. Cueto, "The Origins of Primary Healthcare," 1867; For details concerning the backlash against family planning in India during the political Emergency (1975), consult Rebecca Jane Williams, "Storming the Citadels of Poverty: Family Planning under the Emergency in India, 1975–1977," *The Journal of Asian Studies* 73, no. 2 (2014): 471–92.
148. Cueto, "The Origins of Primary Healthcare," 1868.
149. World Bank, *World Development Report 1978* (Washington D.C.: The World Bank, 1978), 33–34.
150. Julia Walsh and Kenneth S. Warren, "Selective Primary Health Care: An Interim Strategy for Disease Control in Developing Countries," *The New England Journal of Medicine* 301, no. 18 (1979): 967–74, 967.
151. Walsh and Warren, "Selective Primary Health Care," 972.
152. Marcos Cueto, "The WHO and Primary Healthcare during the 1980s," in *Health for All: The Journey of Universal Health Coverage*, in Sanjoy Bhattacharya and Alexander Medcalf edited (Hyderabad: Orient Blackswan, 2015).
153. Rolf Carrière, "Email Interview by Vivek Neelakantan," April 13, 2025.
154. Ibid.

CHAPTER 8

Conclusion

The Limits of International Technical Assistance in Health

While the remit of this monograph focuses on the emergence of international health in Southeast Asia, India, and Sri Lanka, the dialectic between internationalization and regionalization was not unique to this region. In Africa, donor support for public health programs was typically funneled through national and colonial governments, whereas in Asia, multilateral agencies were reluctant to direct resources through local governments, preferring instead to operate through regional agencies.[1] Between the 1950s and 1970s, there was a widespread apprehension across Southeast Asia, India, and Sri Lanka, that an overdependence on foreign aid would erode hard-won political independence. As a result, aid agencies preferred to work through regional initiatives. In doing so, they opened up a strategic intermediary space—a buffer zone that allowed decolonized Asian states to leverage international aid while insulating their domestic policies from donor overreach.

A distinctive feature of PHC evolution across Southeast Asia, India, and Sri Lanka between the 1950s and 1970s was the eradication model, exemplified by campaigns against malaria, tuberculosis, yaws, and smallpox. These initiatives relied on technical interventions, and coordinated by international aid agencies, but were countered by regional solidarity.

V. Neelakantan, *The Emergence of International Health Policy in Southeast Asia, India, and Sri Lanka, 1937–1978*,
https://doi.org/10.1007/978-3-032-21233-7_8

Eradication efforts also involved negotiating international health governance across scales: international organizations, national governments, and local programs. While framed in supposedly apolitical terms, eradication programs became enmeshed in Cold War politics. The mobilization of health resources often mirrored the mobilization of ideological alliances, transforming disease eradication into a proxy battlefield for competing visions of postwar development.[2]

Proximity to Cold War fault lines such as Vietnam, Korea, China, and the USSR, the salience of the population question, and the widespread perception of India as a prototype for international health initiatives in the developing world, gave Asia wider visibility in global debates on disease eradication and PHC. This visibility was amplified not only by proximity to geopolitical conflicts but also by the multiplicity of Cold Wars. These included the US-supported campaigns against Communist insurgents in Indonesia, Malaya, and the Philippines, the Indochina wars, and the non-aligned but assertive orientation of 1950s Indonesia and India.[3] Together, these dynamics transformed postcolonial Asian states into the primary crucible for Cold War health interventions. At the same time, the Asian trajectory toward PHC points to the imperative to reconcile international health norms with local realities, the need to explore alternative models of healthcare, and the process of double decolonization—against colonial powers and international aid agencies that succeeded them. In this sense, this monograph contributes not only to regional histories of health in Asia, but to the politics of international health.

The divergence between internationalization and regionalization in health governance is exemplified in the journey from Bandoeng to Alma-Ata between 1937 and 1978.

The journey from Bandoeng (1937) to Alma-Ata is not a teleological account documenting Southeast Asia's linear progress toward PHC. Rather, it exemplifies the region's persistent quest for autonomy—an ongoing struggle against foreign interventions in governance and health. Despite differing contexts, a fundamental thread connecting the Intergovernmental Conference of Far-Eastern Nations on Rural Hygiene at Bandoeng (1937), the Asian-African Conference (1955), and Alma-Ata (1978) was the urgency for locally driven solutions and raising living standards. The same critique of externally imposed technical solutions was highlighted by William Lederer and Eugene Burdick in *The Ugly American*.

Set in the fictional principality of Sarkhan, roughly corresponding to Laos in 1958, the novel critiqued international aid interventions that, divorced from lived experiences, escalated technological dependency. Although the novel expresses a great deal of frustration with the shortcomings of US Cold War diplomacy in Southeast Asia, it also presents solutions for course correction.[4] One of the exemplary Cold Warriors from the novel, retired American engineer Homer Atkins registers the need in rural Sarkhan for some kind of efficient pump to lift water from one terraced paddy to another. But what good is an imported technology if it cannot relate to the very people it aims to help? He could have easily imported such pumps from the US, but rejects such an alternative. Atkins asserts, "It's no good if I go spending a hundred thousand dollars bringing in something. It has to be something right here, something the natives understand."[5]

Working alongside a local mechanic Jeepo, Atkins designs a pump from bicycle parts but Jeepo comes up with crucial adjustments based on the observation of his neighbors' behavior.[6] Together they develop a locally appropriate technology, launching a company to market these low-cost yet effective pumps throughout Sarkhan. Atkin's character closely resonates with the personality of celebrated urban planner Albert Mayer who left his New York practice to work in India.[7] In 1948, Jawaharlal Nehru invited him to launch a pilot community development project in Etawah, northern India.

Like Atkins, Mayer rejected imported technologies and instead focused on villagers' felt needs. He mobilized rural communities around Etawah to construct schools, roads, and wells, using locally available materials. Etawah ultimately became the cornerstone of the nationwide community development program launched in India during the 1950s.

Nevertheless, the history of international health is replete with examples of well-intentioned interventions floundering for lack of local adaptation. The trajectory of the Global Malaria Eradication Program (1955–1969) illustrates how technical assistance—when disconnected from community engagement—can undermine the goal of eradication. Notably, in 1957, the Eisenhower administration's support for the WHO's global efforts to eradicate malaria was not driven by health considerations alone but was part of a wider geopolitical strategy to combat communism. However, the campaign relied exclusively on insecticide DDT and standardized treatment protocols—overlooking underlying socioeconomic factors, ecological dynamics, and behavioral heterogeneity among anopheline mosquito species. For instance, early malaria eradication efforts in Indonesia during the 1950s registered institutional optimism. However, the exclusion of rural communities, in conjunction with anopheline resistance to DDT, led to the recrudescence of the disease in localities previously deemed disease-free.[8]

The failure of malaria eradication—akin to the critiques of technical assistance echoed in *The Ugly American*—revealed that international health interventions must be locally embedded and enlist community participation. Only grassroots engagement ensures enduring impact.

Equilibrium Between International Health Goals and Actionable Solutions

The Bandoeng Conference was convened in 1937 when social medicine had reached a crescendo. Eleven years later, the Preamble of the WHO reinforced a broad vision of social medicine that underscored health as a fundamental human right guaranteed by the state. However, by the 1950s, the WHO abandoned its broad mandate in favor of technical interventions favoring targeted solutions against diseases such as malaria, tuberculosis, and yaws. While these interventions achieved discernible success, they marked a departure from the holistic ideals of social medicine, prioritizing efficiency over health reforms.

The mandate of social medicine finds a compelling narrative in Hindi novelist Phanishwar Nath Renu's *Maila Anchal* [Hindi: Soiled Border], published in 1954. Set on the eve of Indian independence in the district of Purnia in rural Bihar (eastern India), the chief protagonist of the novel is Prashant, a newly graduated physician. He embodies the aspirations of a newly independent nation, striving to bridge the gap between modern medicine and the entrenched social realities such as caste-based exclusion confronting rural communities. Instead of pursuing further studies abroad, he settles down in Maryganj village, Purnia, due to his commitment to serve the underprivileged. Prashant conducts research on malaria and kala azar, then endemic to the area, and connects these diseases to broader social and environmental determinants of health.[9] His deployment of sarcasm in the novel is subtle yet impactful, allowing him to assess how health education initiatives in post-independent India offered symbolic solutions rather than structural change. In the context of malaria eradication, he notes that persuading villagers to use DDT and mosquito nets is ineffective; even getting them to apply bitter-scented oils as mosquito repellents is a luxury.[10] His novel illustrates how even well-meaning health policies failed to redress entrenched rural inequalities.

Renu's novel resonates with Gunnar Myrdal's concerns in *Asian Drama*, where he explores the persistent gulf between aspirations and reality in social and economic development across the postcolonial state in Asia.[11] In this context, the recommendations of India's Health Survey and Development Committee (The Bhore Committee) become relevant, offering a blueprint for reflecting the need to harmonize aspirational goals and actionable solutions. The Committee emphasized adequate health protection to all, covering both curative and preventive aspects, irrespective of their ability to pay for it.[12] In addition, it linked public health to the improvement of nutritional standards, elimination of unemployment, the provision of a living wage to all workers, and improvement of agricultural and industrial production.

Despite its bold vision, the implementation of the Bhore Committee recommendations faced several challenges. Although India's postcolonial state sought to improve living standards, progress was impeded by the refractoriness of socioeconomic and political realities and administrative fractures. One key challenge was the devolution of public health to the provinces under the Government of India Act (1919), resulting in uneven regional implementation. For example, the 1949 Report of the Environmental Hygiene Committee noted that funds allocated for water supply at the provincial level frequently lapsed due to limitations of materials and manpower.[13] Furthermore, the Priorities Subcommittee of the National Planning Committee contended that the housing problem in India was not of the same urgency as food, reflecting the government's focus on fulfilling the population's immediate survival needs over long-term infrastructural development.[14]

As in independent India, public health efforts in postwar Indonesia were similarly enmeshed in the nation's broader economic and political struggles. In 1949, subsequent to the transfer of political sovereignty to the Indonesian republic, the country inherited a ruined health system, punctuated by the scars of warfare. With only 1200 physicians for a population of approximately 70 million—one physician per 70,000—the Ministry of Health launched emergency programs to control infectious diseases (smallpox, cholera, plague) and endemic conditions (malaria, tuberculosis, yaws, leprosy).[15] By the mid-1950s, these campaigns precipitated a decline in mortality, engendering optimism about Indonesia's public health gains despite a severe physician shortage. During this period, the

Ministry of Health had launched a number of bold initiatives, notably the ambitious Bandung Plan (1951), which envisioned the integration of preventive and curative care. Integration was impeded by Indonesia's decentralized governance, political deadlocks, financial instability, and corruption.

Amid Indonesia's efforts to leverage public health in postwar national reconstruction, celebrated writer Pramoedya Ananta Toer portrayed everyday hardships of Indonesians. In a sarcastic vein he wrote:

> A small guerrilla squad that is cautious is not likely to lose ten people in two years, yet in my peaceful kampung, with its stink and its condition, people die one after another. They die a cheap death, friend. Like this, at the back of my house, soon after I started living in Kebun Djahé Kober, one person died of a chronic venereal disease.[16]

The invisibility of death and disease in Toer's *kampung* [Bahasa Indonesia: informal urban settlement] reveals how entrenched socioeconomic realities shaped public health outcomes. His choice of a *kampung*—situated 500 meters from the presidential palace when the WHO-sponsored disease eradication campaigns were underway—illustrates the disconnect between Indonesia's aspirations for modernity and the invisible poor.

Renu and Toer's narratives mirror the challenges faced by the WHO and other international aid agencies: the disconnect between international health goals and the overlooked realities of the targeted population. A lingering question in Chaps. 4 and 5 is why the proverbial magic bullet eclipsed the comprehensive social medicine approach championed by Andrija Štampar and Ludwik Rajchman—figures foundational to the WHO and UNICEF.

While Štampar and Rajchman emphasized structural reforms in sanitation, nutrition, and healthcare access, by the 1950s, international health campaigns gravitated toward controlling endemic diseases, favoring targeted interventions such as vaccines and antibiotics.

Catalyzed by the Cold War, WHO's and UNICEF's reorientation toward disease eradication came at the risk of subordinating more holistic interventions—particularly maternal and child health—in order to align with American funding priorities.

Likewise, the ILO's advocacy for Universal Health Coverage (UHC) was congruent with the Preamble of the WHO which proclaims the human right to the highest attainable standard of health. However, the

WHO's response to the ILO's recommendations on UHC was lukewarm. Political resistance from donor countries, particularly the US, and recipient allies in Southeast Asia—such as the Philippines—complicated efforts to align the WHO's policies with ILO's UHC vision. The WHO's noncommittal approach to particular models of healthcare financing revealed its inclination toward the eradication model over broader structural reforms.

By 1969, the shortcomings of the WHO's single-disease approach became increasingly apparent. As a result, the agency reevaluated its flagship initiative—the malaria eradication program—and shifted its emphasis toward strengthening basic health services.[17]

In 1973, a joint WHO-UNICEF study concluded that international health interventions had marginal impact on health problems in developing countries. The study identified key factors that contributed to strengthening basic health services. These included immunization, maternal care, postnatal childcare, family planning, potable water supplies, sanitation and vector control, health and nutrition education, diagnosis and treatment of common diseases, emergency medical care, and referral services.[18]

Building on the WHO-UNICEF collaborative study, PHC emerged as a critique of the diffusion of technologically intensive healthcare from developed to developing countries. This critique was influenced by John Bryant's *Health and the Developing World*. Bryant argued that although the medical answers to malaria or typhoid were well-known, getting rid of mosquitos or providing clean water would consume significant resources in developing countries.[19] The persistence of malnutrition, gastroenteritis, and pneumonia in impoverished communities was not merely a reflection of disease prevalence, but of deeply rooted socioeconomic inequities. Confronting intractable and entrenched challenges, PHC had to transcend the biomedical model to address structural determinants—ensuring contextually appropriate, technically feasible solutions within constrained state capacity.

Beyond critiquing technologically oriented healthcare, PHC was a product of broader socio-political movements, particularly the decolonization of Africa and the rise of leftist ideologies in the Global South. These movements demanded the redistribution of resources that recognized sovereignty of postcolonial states vis-à-vis global powers, rather than uncritically adapting Western biomedical models to local contexts. Radical agrarian reforms, expanded access to education, employment, and housing were fundamental to addressing socioeconomic inequities underpinning disease.[20]

In 1974, the UN General Assembly adopted a resolution on the Establishment of a New International Economic Order (NIEO) to uplift less-developed countries. Meanwhile, as embedded liberalism and planned modernization were in deep crisis and communism weakened in its traditional Eastern European and Asian strongholds, conditions emerged for the pluralization of political ideologies.[21] Détente had terminated the binary geopolitical logic of the early Cold War. The collapse of the Bretton Woods exchange system in 1971 had revealed the tenuousness of global governance institutions. The Vietnam War upended Cold War hierarchies.

The paradigmatic shift from the Old Order—focused on efficiency, growth, and profit maximization—to the NIEO, called for equitable access to resources, markets, and technology for developing countries. The quest for rational and equitable pharmaceutical policies constituted part of Third World efforts to establish a NIEO. NIEO's emphasis on strengthening technical cooperation in the Global South and economic self-sufficiency provided an impetus to developing countries such as Sri Lanka to establish centralized procurement of essential medicines. This shift in economic philosophy directly influenced the Alma-Ata Declaration, reinforcing the inseparability between health and socioeconomic development.[22]

Amid this global reorientation of approaches toward international development, aid agencies such as the UN and the WHO began to recalibrate their institutional priorities and operational strategies. Three key ideas that permeated the Alma-Ata Declaration included appropriate technologies, opposition to medical elitism, and health as a tool for socioeconomic development.[23] At Alma-Ata, WHO Regional Director for South-East Asia (SEARO), V.T.H. Gunaratne, forcefully articulated these concerns, highlighting their significance in shaping PHC.

Gunaratne observed that South-East Asia's health infrastructure prioritized hospitals, clinics, and training personnel in Western institutions. However, these approaches proved incongruous to local needs.[24] Between the 1950s and 1970s—as regional states grappled with fragile health systems—aid agencies such as the WHO and UNICEF focused on vertical programs targeting malaria, tuberculosis, and yaws. While these initiatives helped reduce disease-related morbidity, they diverted scarce resources from basic health services.

Gunaratne argued that weak health infrastructures not only deepened socioeconomic challenges but also reinforced the cyclical relationship between poverty and health outcomes.[25] This argument aligns with Gunnar Myrdal's cumulative causation theory, which highlights how structural inequities self-perpetuate over time.[26] Gunaratne further substantiates this perspective by demonstrating how nutritional deficiencies eroded productivity and work capacity—fueling a vicious cycle of malnutrition and diminished output that reproduced structural poverty.

Attempts to break the cyclical relationship between poverty and ill health were undermined by unfavorable doctor-to-population and hospital-bed-to-population ratios, as well as the limited number of rural health centers. In rural areas, low agricultural productivity and weak purchasing power of most families were exacerbated by systemic factors such as inequitable land tenure, limited water for irrigation, intensifying pressure of population on land, and access to timely credit. Some of these inequities were embedded within the traditional social structures of SEARO member states. In urban slums, poverty and poor health were exacerbated by rapid rural migration to cities, outpacing the ability of industry to generate meaningful employment.[27] Emphasizing the interconnectedness between health and socioeconomic development, Gunaratne asserted that "Better Health for All" cannot be viewed in isolation from a more rational and just socioeconomic configuration, as it both influences and contributes to broader development efforts. He explained that health operates both as a cause and consequence of such development. Toward the end of his Alma-Ata address, Gunaratne highlighted a paradox: despite advances in medical technology, their impact on rural health remained minimal.[28] Several factors contributed to the limited basic health services across the SEARO region including a lack of political will, the low priority accorded to health in development plans, inadequate community participation, low per capita health expenditure, and an uneven distribution of medical personnel between rural and urban areas. Gunaratne lamented the slow integration of PHC into rural development across South-East Asia.

While SEARO member states faced significant challenges in integrating PHC as a key pillar of rural development, the Western Pacific region encountered similar logistical challenges. In response, the WHO Regional Office for the Western Pacific (WPRO) engineered a strategy that sought to strike a balance between international health goals and tangible outcomes. Francisco Dy, the WPRO Regional Director from the Philippines

(1966–1979), drew inspiration from China's Barefoot Doctors' model, advocating for the training of villagers as frontline medical providers in inaccessible regions.[29] Dy's endorsement embedded PHC within WPRO's rural health strategy.

While SEARO and WPRO sought to recalibrate international health goals to member state priorities, Southeast Asia's vast epidemiological, socioeconomic, and political diversity posed structural impediments to the implementation of a cohesive regional health strategy. Both agencies operated within financial constraints and donor-imposed conditionalities. In the aftermath of Alma-Ata, the shift from holistic, community-based interventions to technical disease-specific strategies prioritizing cost-effectiveness further diluted PHC's implementation.

The Alma-Ata Declaration (1978) reaffirmed that "health, which is a state of complete physical, mental and social wellbeing, and not merely the absence of disease or infirmity, is a fundamental human right."[30] The Declaration imbued the WHO definition of health with normative depth and an actionable framework. However, since 1980, international health interventions have tended to focus on atomized priorities such as disease eradication and improving health service delivery—resulting in siloed interventions that obscure the broader structural determinants of health.

This monograph challenges mainstream international health narratives which privilege WHO-led initiatives.[31] These narratives have overlooked how local actors recalibrated PHC to national priorities—resisting international prescriptions, diverting resources toward community health, or selectively appropriating elements from PHC, SPHC, and Basic Needs. Furthermore, the overemphasis on the WHO-driven policy framework has obscured alternative models to international health governance, such as the Basic Needs Approach introduced by the ILO and Selective Primary Health Care (SPHC) developed by UNICEF. Rather than being at odds with PHC, these approaches embodied divergent operational logics. PHC sought to integrate health within broader socioeconomic frameworks; the Basic Needs Approach prioritized the production of what was essential to meeting human needs; and SPHC emphasized targeted cost-effective interventions. The WHO Director General Halfdan Mahler was reticent to incorporate Basic Needs into his articulation of PHC, fearing backlash from developing countries over perceived WHO interference in domestic affairs.[32]

The Legacy of Southeast Asia's Public Health Initiatives

Southeast Asia pioneered international health initiatives long before the PHC paradigm gained international currency. Rural hygiene initiatives—such as the Rockefeller Foundation's anti-hookworm campaigns across Ceylon, the Philippine Islands, the Netherlands Indies, and British India—revealed a complex interplay of colonial governance, nationalist thinking, and medical philanthropy. Foundational efforts between 1915 and 1939, along with the Bhore Committee's advocacy for a publicly funded health system in India in 1946, prefigured the region's subsequent engagement with PHC. Far from being a passive recipient of US and WHO-led frameworks, Southeast Asia's trajectory toward Alma-Ata demonstrates how regional governance, political imperatives, and localized adaptations shaped the PHC paradigm.

Southeast Asia's PHC trajectory illustrates persistent tensions between national sovereignty, international priorities, and the agenda of donors, revealing the fractured nature of international health governance. The four case studies in Chap. 7—drawn from Indonesia, India, Thailand, and Sri Lanka—illustrate that PHC was not a top-down WHO imposition, but evolved through geopolitical rivalries, local adaptations, and negotiations between governments and international aid agencies.

While the WHO championed PHC as a transformative strategy, Southeast Asian states navigated its implementation by reconciling decentralized health governance with national oversight. In Indonesia, the Puskesmas network integrated PHC into rural health services.[33] Sri Lanka's system, shaped by its welfare-state legacy, incorporated elements of decentralized health delivery. Sri Lanka's current concern is sustaining the country's momentum in maternal and child health and infectious disease prevention, while confronting emerging challenges—non-communicable diseases and rising out-of-pocket expenditures. To manage these transitions, the government plans to link peripheral health centers to referral institutions, promoting resource-sharing and accountability within demarcated catchment areas.[34]

Southeast Asia's approach to PHC reflects a deep-rooted commitment to equity and community participation. While policy intent is congruent with Alma-Ata principles, implementation has varied across sub-national and national levels due to political, economic, and social constraints. By contrast,[35] the successes of these provinces contrast with hurdles faced by other parts of Southeast Asia where fragmented health systems, inequitable resource distribution, and donor-driven priorities have eroded the translation of Alma-Ata principles into actionable goals. By contrast, in South Asia, particularly India, the southern states of Kerala and Tamil Nadu have been acclaimed as models of public sector financing and of achieving good health outcomes at a relatively low cost.[36] Yet, these successes were not easily replicable elsewhere across India and Southeast Asia, since implementation was contingent on distinctive political cultures (particularly Kerala's leftist politics, and Tamil Nadu's welfare populism), high levels of community mobilization, and enduring institutional legacies.[37]

The contrast becomes stark when set against South Asia, where fragmented health systems, inequitable distribution of medical personnel, and donor-imposed priorities frequently impeded the translation of Alma-Ata principles into tangible outcomes.

For instance, in Indonesia, the Ministry of Health sets national standards for medical education, service provision, and guidelines for treatment. Previously epidemiological data flowed systematically between the center, the provinces, and the districts. However, with the implementation of administrative decentralization since 2001, district administrations directly receive funds from Jakarta, bypassing provincial reporting mechanisms. This shift compromised supervisory provincial insights that once facilitated coordinated health planning, affecting rational resource distribution.[38] The Indonesian Ministry of Health controls disease eradication programs which focus on single disease issues: malaria, TB, and HIV/AIDS are current favorites. Many of these programs reflect the priorities of institutional donors and current global health trends rather than Indonesia's needs. Similarly in Cambodia, aid fragmentation in the health sector—with an inclination toward prevention and treatment of communicable diseases that pose an international security risk—has undermined PHC.[39]

Systemic failures continue to impact health systems across Southeast Asia, overshadowing meaningful progress and highlighting the necessity to address the social determinants of health. The persistent disregard for human rights undermines health outcomes. While high population densities and close human-animal proximity amplify the region's vulnerability to zoonotic diseases, governments prioritize containment over addressing poor living conditions. Tensions between biological risk and state sovereignty escalated during the 2006–2007 avian influenza outbreak, when Indonesian Health Minister Siti Fadilah Supari asserted viral sovereignty.

She declared domestic viral samples destined for global research as national patrimony—fueling vaccine equity debates that resurfaced during the COVID-19 pandemic.

Reclaiming Southeast Asia's agency in international health policy would imply revisiting historical lessons, not with the purpose to critique policy failures, but to reimagine alternate health models. COVID-19 exposed structural fault lines in the region's health systems, particularly in India and Malaysia, reinforcing the shortcomings of centralized health interventions and the efficacy of civil society responses. In the Indian context, while the Second Wave of the pandemic (2021) exposed institutional fragilities undergirding the country's health infrastructure, it also galvanized community participation. NGOs arranged for supplies of oxygen and helped people register for vaccination. Accredited Social Health Activists established community trust regarding the safety and efficacy of vaccination.[40] In Southeast Asia, the pandemic served as a stark reminder that the region's socioeconomic growth was distributed inequitably. In Malaysia, civil society groups made the Malay hashtag "MigranJugaManusia," which translates to Migrants are Human Too, to highlight the plight of migrant workers.[41]

Southeast Asia's health activism has a long genealogy that traces back to the early 1930s—around the same time social medicine reached its zenith in Europe. In British India and the Netherlands Indies, international agencies—such as the Rockefeller Foundation—along with missionaries, nurses, and nationalist physicians, trained local populations in rural hygiene. Medical nationalism in colonial Southeast Asia laid the groundwork for the emergence of social medicine. Yet despite its diverse lineages, social medicine remains obscured beneath flagship government schemes—malaria eradication, community development, and family planning.

In Indonesia, India, Thailand, and Sri Lanka, PHC draws on enduring traditions of community participation. The future of PHC in the region depends on the resilience of such grassroots initiatives. However, health activists are marginalized under neoliberal economic regimes that favor privatized healthcare. As Pratik Chakrabarti asserts, "Health activism cannot by itself compensate for inadequate state investment in health care, but it can be a foundation for future investment by the state in public health."[42] Recognizing the critical role of local health activists who have linked PHC to social determinants of health is not merely an act of acknowledgment—it is a necessary step toward forging policies that secure long-term investment in health infrastructure, enabling equitable health access for future generations.

Notes

1. See, for example, James L.A. Webb, and Tamara Giles-Vernick, "Introduction," in *Global Health in Africa: Historical Perspectives on Disease Control*, Tamara Giles-Vernick, and James L.A. Webb edited (Athens, Ohio: Ohio University Press, 2013), 1–24, 6.
2. For the Soviet perspective on disease eradication refer Marek Eby, "Cold War Form: International Content?: The Martsinovskii Institute, the World Health Organization, and the Wider Networks of International Malariology," in *International Organizations and the Cold War: Competition, Cooperation, and Convergence*, Sandrine Kott, Eva-Maria Muschik, and Elisabeth Roehrlich edited (London: Bloomsbury Academic, 2025), 145–62.
3. Odd Arne Westad, *The Global Cold War* (Cambridge: Cambridge University Press, 2007).
4. Daniel Immerwahr, "The Ugly American: Peeling the Onion of an Iconic Cold War Text," *Journal of American-East Asian Relations* 26 (2019): 7–20, 9.
5. William Lederer and Eugene Burdick, *The Ugly American* (New York: W.W. Norton and Co., 1958), 216.
6. Lederer and Burdick, *The Ugly American*, 225.
7. Immerwahr, *The Ugly American*, 11.
8. Vivek Neelakantan, "The Campaign Against the Big Four Endemic Diseases and Indonesia's Engagement with the WHO During the Cold War 1950s," in *Public Health and National Reconstruction in Post-War Asia: International Influences, Local Transformations*, Liping Bu and Ka-che Yip edited (Abingdon, Oxon: Routledge, 2014), 154–74.
9. Phanishwar Nath Renu, *Maila Anchal* (Allahabad: Rajkamal Publication, 1954).
10. Ibid.
11. Gunnar Myrdal, *Asian Drama: An Inquiry into the Poverty of Nations*, volume 1 (New York: Pantheon, 1968), 34.
12. *Report of the Health Survey and Development Committee Summary*, volume 2 (New Delhi: Government of India Press, 1946).
13. Government of India Ministry of Health, *Report of the Environmental Hygiene Committee*, October 1949 (New Delhi: Government of India Press, 1949), 9.
14. Ibid.

15. Vivek Neelakantan, *Science, Public Health and Nation-Building in Soekarno-Era Indonesia* (Newcastle-upon-Tyne: Cambridge Scholars, 2017), 1.
16. Pramoedya Ananta Toer, “My Kampung,” Djakarta, July 1952, in *Tales from Djakarta: Caricatures of Human Beings and their Circumstances*, trans. Sumit Mandal (Ithaca: Southeast Asia Program, Cornell University Press, 1999), 54–59, 54.
17. WHA Resolution A 22/P&B/8, “Reexamination of the Global Strategy of Malaria Eradication,” *Official Records of the World Health Organization: Twenty-Second World Health Assembly, part I*, no. 176, July 8–25, 1969 (Geneva: WHO, 1969), WHO Library and Historical Collections, Geneva (hereafter WHOL).
18. V. Djukanovic and E.P. Mach, *Alternative Approaches to Meeting Basic Health Needs in Developing Countries: A Joint WHO-UNICEF Study* (Geneva: WHO, 1975), WHOL.
19. John Byrant, *Health and the Developing World* (Ithaca: Cornell University Press, 1972).
20. Marcos Cueto, Theodore Brown, and Elizabeth Fee, *The World Health Organization: A History* (Cambridge: Cambridge University Press, 2019), 172.
21. Nils Gilman, “The New International Economic Order: A Reintroduction,” *Humanity* 6, no. 1 (Spring 2015). Accessed April 29, 2025. https://humanityjournal.org/issue6-1/the-new-international-economic-order-a-reintroduction/
22. World Health Organization, *Declaration of Alma-Ata*, International Conference on Primary Health Care, Alma-Ata, USSR, September 6–12, 1978, WHOL, https://iris.who.int/handle/10665/347879, accessed May 10, 2025.
23. Cueto, Brown, and Fee, *The World Health Organization*, 177.
24. *WHO Report of the Regional Director for South-East Asia to the International Conference on Primary Health Care, Alma-Ata, USSR*, September 6–12, 1978, Jacket 6, Document No. P-21-87-5, *The International Conference on Primary Health Care*, Registry Files, The WHO Archives, Geneva (hereafter WHOA).
25. Ibid.
26. Gunnar Myrdal, *An American Dilemma: The Negro Problem and Modern Democracy,* volume 1 (New York: Harper and Brothers, 1944), 101.
27. *WHO Report of the Regional Director for South-East Asia.*
28. Ibid.
29. Paul Majendie, “WHO Plan for Rural Medicine,” *New Nation,* July 26, 1978, 8, National Library Board, Singapore (NLB).

30. *Primary Health Care; Report of the International Conference on Primary Health Care, Alma-Ata, USSR*, September 6–12, 1978 (Geneva: WHO, 1978), WHOL.
31. Randall Packard, *A History of Global Health: Interventions into the Lives of Other Peoples* (Baltimore, MD: Johns Hopkins University Press, 2016); see also Anne-Emanuelle Birn and Nikolai Krementsov, "'Socialising' Primary Care? The Soviet Union, WHO and the 1978 Alma-Ata Conference," *BMJ Global Health* 3 (2018): e000992. Doi: 10.1136/bmjgh-2018-000992.
32. Fernando Antônio Pires-Alves and Marcos Cueto, "The Alma-Ata Decade: The Crisis of Development and International Health," *Ciência & Saúde Coletiva* 22 (2017): 2035–44.
33. Vivek Neelakantan, "Indonesian Health Policy Between the Old and the New Orders," in *Public Health and Cold War Politics in Asia*, Liping Bu edited (Abingdon, Oxon: Routledge, 2024), 151–76, 163.
34. Susie Perera, Sudha Ramani, Taufique Jaarder, et al., "Reorienting Health Systems Towards Primary Health Care in South Asia," *The Lancet Regional Health–Southeast Asia* 28 (2024): 100466.
35. Ibid.
36. Ibid.
37. Andrew Wyatt, "Populism and Politics in Contemporary Tamil Nadu," *Contemporary South Asia* 21 (2013): 365–81.
38. Elizabeth Pisani, "Medicine for a Sick System," *Inside Indonesia* 113 (January 26, 2013). Accessed May 3, 2025. https://www.insideindonesia.org/editions/edition-111-jan-mar-2013/medicine-for-a-sick-system
39. Suyeon Lee and Funcie Y. Park, "Examining Aid Fragmentation and Collaboration Opportunities in Cambodia's Health Sector," *Global Health* 20, no. 62 (2024), https://doi.org/10.1186/s12992-024-01063-7
40. Pratik Chakrabarti, "Health as Activism: Rethinking Social Medicine in India," *The Lancet* 399 (June 4, 2022): 2096–97, 2096.
41. Khoo Ying Hooi, "Southeast Asia's Pandemic Politics and Human Rights: Trends and Lessons," *LSE Blogs*, October 1, 2020. Accessed May 5, 2025. https://blogs.lse.ac.uk/seac/2020/10/01/southeast-asias-pandemic-politics-and-human-rights-trends-and-lessons/#comments
42. Chakrabarti, "Health as Activism," 2097.

Bibliography

Primary Sources

A. Archives and Special Collections

Archives of the League of Nations, Geneva

League of Nations Secretariat

R19/12B/32210	Dossier concerning the Fifth Congress of the Far Eastern Association of Tropical Medicine, 1924
R839/12B/21836	Collaboration between the Health Organization of the League of Nations and the International Health Board of the Rockefeller Foundation, 1922
R843/12B/23230/25592	Commission d' Enquête en Extrême Orient, 1922
R903/12B/30818/35026	Far Eastern Sanitary Convention, 1925

V. Neelakantan, *The Emergence of International Health Policy in Southeast Asia, India, and Sri Lanka, 1937–1978*,
https://doi.org/10.1007/978-3-032-21233-7

C/167M/43/1924/III	Report presented to the Health Committee of the League of Nations, 1924
R925/12B/34275/45102	Far East Epidemiological Intelligence Bureau: Organisation of the Work of the Bureau, 1925
R983/12B/52362	Conference on Health Problems in the Pacific Islands, Melbourne (1926)
R925/12B/34275/42212	Epidemiological Intelligence Bureau in the Far East: Proceedings of the Singapore Conference, February 1925
R6093/8A/25509/8855	Rural Hygiene Conference in the Far East: Correspondence Exchanged during Pampana's Mission, April to August 1936
R6017/8A/37715/8855	Rural Hygiene Conference in the Far East, August 1937: Speeches by Delegates, Rapporteurs, etc.
R6107/8A/37714/8855	Rural Government Conference in the Far East, August 1937: Reports of Commissions
R6096/8A/26763/8855	Intergovernmental Conference of Far-Eastern Countries on Rural Hygiene, Item V, Hygiène Rural Conférence en Extrême-Orient: Rapports des Gouvernements, 1937
R 6094/8A/26055/8855	Rural Hygiene: Study of the Fly Problem in the Far East, 1936–39
R6150/8A/42169/47155	Postwar Health Problems: International Health Organization, 1943
6199/8D/43551/347	Eastern Bureau Singapore: Reopening of the Bureau, Transfer of Assets to the World Health Organization, 1947

Rockefeller Archive Center, Tarrytown, New York

Field Offices Series 2	Rockefeller Sanitary Commission for the Eradication of Hookworm
	Disease Records; Philippines
Record Group 2	General Correspondence
	Indonesia HYD-2
Record Group 5	International Health Board Records
	Project Correspondence
	Sub Group 2, India
Record Group 12	Officers' Diaries
	Fahs, Charles Burton
	Heiser, Victor G.
	Sawyer, Wilbur

Rockefeller Foundation Annual Reports (various years)

University of Auckland Libraries and Learning Services

Western Pacific Health Services, *Fourth Annual Report (1931)*

United Nations Archives, New York City

S-1271-0000-0066-00001	UNRRA and San Francisco Conference, 1943–49
S-1241-10000-10047-100001	Committee for the Far East, 1943–49
S-11560-10000-10014-100001	Report of the Activities of the Interim Commission of the WHO, 1947–50

UN Digital Library, New York City

E/H/PC/17	Technical Preparatory Committee for the International Health Conference: Summary Record of the Seventh Meeting (1946)
A/RES/57/I	56th Plenary Meeting: UN Assembly First Session, 1946

National Archives of India, New Delhi

Identifier PR_000003001391	Department of Education and Health
Identifier PR_000005014082	Reports and Memoranda Circulation: Health Survey and Development Committee (1943)
Identifier: PR_000001593212	Inter Asian Relations Conference (New Delhi) in March (1947)
Identifier PR_000005014113	Ministry of External Affairs
Identifier PR_ 000005014106	Ministry of External Affairs

National Archives of Singapore

Oral History Collection

Chellapah, Wilfred. Oral History Interview conducted by the National Archives of Singapore. Accession No. 000353. Reel 9 of 19. Singapore: National Archives of Singapore, November 7, 1983.

UTS Library Special Collections, Sydney

PRS Mani Collection

Yale University Archives

Henry Ernst Sigerist Papers

University of Pittsburgh Digital Collections

Szeming Sze Papers

Sze, Szeming. *The Origins of the World Health Organization: A Personal Memoir*. Boca Raton: IISZ Publications, 1982.

Archives of the World Health Organization, Geneva

I. Oral History Collections

Siegel, Milton P. *Transcripts of an Oral Interview by Gino Levy and Norman Howard Jones*, November 15–19, 1982. World Health Organization Archives.

II. WHO Archives on Microform

WHO First Generation Files (WHO. I)	1945–50
WHO Second Generation Files (WHO. II)	1950–55
WHO Project Files	1945–86

III. Registry Files

Document P-21-87-5, Jacket 2	The International Conference on Primary Health Care

IV. WHO Library and Historical Collections

Official Records of the WHO (various years)
Minutes of the Technical Preparatory Committee
Summary of Resolutions and Decisions adopted at the World Health Assembly
Verbatim Records of Plenary Sessions
Annual Reports of SEARO Regional Director to the Regional Committee (various years)
Annual Reports of the WPRO Regional Director to the Regional Committee (various years)

V. WHO Publications

Djukanovic, V., and E. P. Mach. *Alternative Approaches to Meeting Basic Needsin Developing Countries.* Geneva: World Health Organization, 1975.

Newell, Kenneth. "Health by the People." In *Health by the People*, Kenneth Newell edited, 191–203. Geneva: WHO, 1975.

Nugroho, Gunawan. "A Community Approach to Raising Health Standards in Central Java, Indonesia." In *Health by the People*, Kenneth Newell edited, 91–111. Geneva: WHO, 1975.

Winslow, C. E. A. *The Cost of Sickness and the Price of Health.* World Health Organization Monograph Series, no. 7. Geneva: World Health Organization, 1951.

World Health Organization. *Constitution of the World Health Organization.* In *Basic Documents*, 49th edition. Geneva: WHO, 2020

World Health Organization and United Nations Children's Fund. *Primary Health Care: A Joint Report by the Director-General of the World Health Organization and the Executive Director of the United Nations Children's Fund.* Geneva: World Health Organization, 1978.

World Health Organization. *The World Health Organization: Twenty Years in South-East Asia, 1948–67.* New Delhi: SEARO, 1967.

World Health Organization, Regional Office for the Western Pacific. *Fifty Years of the World Health Organization in the Western Pacific Region.* Manila: WPRO, 1998.

VI. WHO Technical Reports

World Health Organization. *Methodology of Planning an Integrated Health Programme for Rural Areas: Second Report of the Expert Committee on Public Health Administration.* WHO Technical Report Series 83. Geneva: World Health Organization, 1954.

World Health Organization. *The Selection of Essential Drugs: Report of a WHO Expert Committee.* WHO Technical Report Series, No. 615. Geneva: World Health Organization, 1977.

Harry S. Truman Presidential Museum and Library

Oral History Collections

Hyde, Henry van Zile. Oral History Interview by Richard D. McKinzie, July 16, 1975. Harry S. Truman Presidential Museum and Library.
Morse, David. "Oral History Interview by James R. Fuchs." August 3, 1977. Harry S. Truman Presidential Museum and Library.

Harvard University Libraries

Tozzer Library

Cora Dubois Papers

Schlesinger Library

Martha May Elliot Papers

Seeley G. Mudd Library, Princeton

Maurice Pate Papers

UNICEF Archives and Historical Collections, New York City

I. UNICEF Archives

CF/HST/034/anx.02/05	UNICEF Goals in Maternal and Child Welfare: Statement by Maurice Pate at the Annual Meeting of the American Public Health Association, October 22, 1959
CF/NYH/USAA/DB01/ HS/1996–0067	Excerpts of Interview with Milton Siegel by John Charnow, Interviewed May 11, 1984
CF/HST/1985–044	Reflections on Dr Ludwik Rajchman's Contribution to UNICEF: A Personal Memoir, September 3, 1985
CF/HST/INT/ HEY–001/M	Interview with E.J.R. Heyward Conducted by Mrs. Margaret Catley-Clarkson, July 14, 1983
CF/RAI/USAA/DPP/ RAM/2010/00091	Interview with Lord Noel-Baker Concerning Ludwig Rajchman, Considered as Founder of UNICEF, July 1, 1982
CF/HST/INT/ KEE–009/M	Interview with Spurgeon Milton Keeny Conducted by Peter Jessup, November 27, 1980

II. UNICEF Historical Collections

Black, Maggie. *The Children and the Nations: A Story of UNICEF* (New York: UNICEF, 1986).
Charnow, John, and Sherwood C. Moe. "Henry Labouisse: UNICEF Executive Director, 1965–1979." Monograph XI, UNICEF History Series. New York: UNICEF, 1988. New York: UNICEF Archives.
Wong, Wah. "UNICEF in Asia: A Historical Perspective." UNICEF History Series Monograph X. New York: UNICEF, 1988.

University of Minnesota Libraries

Elmer L. Anderson Library

University of Minnesota Libraries. *YMCA Biographical Files: S.M. Keeny; Kautz Family Papers.* Kautz Family YMCA Archives.

Tamil Nadu State Archives, Chennai

GO 1313	Health Department MS Series
GO 3069	MS Series
GO 2682	MS Series

Parliament of India Digital Collections

Lok Sabha Debates

Senate of the Philippine Legislative Digital Resources

Republic Act No. 747. *Official Gazette* 48(7), 1952: 2582.

Archives of the International Labour Organization, Geneva

I. ILO Archives

File No. 1110–1, File Series WHO, Registry 177769	WHO International Conference on Primary Healthcare, Alma Ata, USSR, September 6 to 11, 1978
File No. 177, Jacket 1, Registry 159775	The Etawah Pilot Development Project, September 1951 to December 1958
File No. 177, Jacket 2, File Series MI	Mission: Surendra Kumar Jain (August 1976 to November 1986)
WHO File 1119–1, Registry 177769	WHO International Conference on Primary Healthcare

II. ILO Library

Hopkins, M.J.D. "Basic Needs Approach to Development Planning: A View." *World Employment Program Research Papers*, Doc. WEP-32/WP3. Geneva: International Labour Organization, 1977.

International Labour Conferences Proceedings (various years).

ILO. *Preparatory Asian Regional Conference of the International Labour Organisation: Record of Proceedings, October to November 1947*. Geneva: ILO, 1948.

International Labour Office. Report of a Joint WHO-ILO Committee on Personal Health and Social Security," November 10 to 16, 1970. Doc. D.2.1971. Geneva: ILO,

———. "Expanded Program of Technical Assistance: Report to the Government of Burma on Social Security," Doc. ILO/TAP/Burma/R. l. Geneva: ILO, 1952.

International Labour Organization. "The Economic Background of Social Policy

Including Problems of Industrialization." Report IV. *Preparatory Asian Regional Conference of the International Labour Conference of the International Labour Organization*. New Delhi: ILO, 1947.

———. "Problems of Social Security: First Item on the Agenda." Report I. *Preparatory Asian Regional Conference of the International Labour Organization*. New Delhi: ILO, 1947.

Report of the Director-General. *Preparatory Asiatic Regional Conference of the International Labour Organisation, New Delhi, 1947*. New Delhi: ILO, 1947.

Ron, Aviva, Brian, Abel Smith, and Giovanni Tambouri. *Health Insurance in Developing Countries: The Social Security Approach.* Geneva: International Labour Organization, 1990.

Szal, Richard J. *Health, Employment and Development.* Paper presented at the WHO International Conference on Primary Health Care, Alma-Ata, USSR, September 6–12, 1978. Geneva: International Labour Organization, 1978.

III. <u>ILO Centenary Project</u>

Rodgers, Gerry. "Surendra Kumar Jain: Interview for the ILO Century Project." March 2008. ILO Century Project.

Dwight D. Eisenhower Presidential Museum and Library

John Foster Dulles Papers: White House Memoranda Series

Arsip Nasional Republik Indonesia, Jakarta

<u>Oral History Collection</u>

Professor Dr Satrio and Mona Lohanda. "Perjuangan dan Pengabdian: Mosaik Kenangan Prof. Dr Satrio." *Penerbitan Sejarah Lisan Nomor 3.* Jakarta: Arsip Nasional, 1986. In Bahasa Indonesia.

B. Official Publications, Pamphlets, and Medical Literature

Asian Relations Conference. *Being Report of the Proceedings of the First Asian Relations Conference: New Delhi, March to April 1947.* New Delhi, 1948.

Bandaranaike, Sirimavo R.D. "The Non-Aligned Movement and the United Nations." *The Black Scholar* 8, no. 3 (1976): 26–31.

Borkar, G. *Health in Independent India: A Decade of Progress.* New Delhi: Ministry of Health, 1958.

Burckel, Christian, edited. *Who's Who in the United Nations.* New York: Christian Burckel and Associates, 1951.

Byrant, John. *Health and the Developing World.* Ithaca: Cornell University Press, 1972.

Calderwood, Howard. "The World Health Organization and its Regional Organizations." *Temple Law Quarterly* 37, no. 1 (1963): 15–27.

"Communiqué of the Bandung Conference." *Current Science* 26, no. 166 (1955): 371–75.

Curtin, P.W.E. "Effect of the Colombo Plan." *Pakistan Horizon* 7, no. 2 (1954): 76–79.

Darling, A.T., M.A. Barber and H.P. Hacker, *Hookworm and Malaria Research in Malaya, Java and the Fiji Islands: Report of the Uncinariasis Commission to the Orient, 1915–17*. New York: The Rockefeller Foundation International Health Board, 1920.

Dole, Lionel. "French Doctors Doubt Efficacy of BCG." *People's Health* 4, no 4 (1950).

"Far Eastern Association of Tropical Medicine." *The British Medical Journal* 1, no. 2470 (May 2, 1908): 1061–62.

"Far Eastern Rural Hygiene Conference." *Current Science* 6, no. 2 (1937): 70–72.

Fifield, Russell H. "The Hukbalahap Today." *Far Eastern Survey* 20, no. 2 (1951): 13–18.

Goodman, Neville. "The World Health Organisation and its Interim Commission." *The Lancet* (September 1946): 358–59.

Government of India Ministry of Health. *Report of the Environmental Hygiene Committee*, October 1949. New Delhi: Government of India Press, 1949.

Government of India Planning Commission. *The First Five-Year Plan: Draft Outline*. New Delhi: Government of India, 1951.

Greene, Katrine R.C. "UNRRA's Record in China." *Far Eastern Survey* 20, no. 10 (1951): 100–105.

"Health of India." *The British Medical Journal* no. 4444 (March 16, 1946): 395–96.

Heiser, Victor. "Practical Experiences with Beriberi and Unpolished Rice in the Philippines." *Journal of the American Medical Association* LVI, no. 17 (1911): 1237–38.

Hoadley, Stephen J. "The Rise and Fall of the Basic Needs Approach." *Cooperation and Conflict* 16, no. 3 (1981): 149–64.

Hydrick, John Lee. *Intensive Hygiene Work in the Netherlands East Indies*. New York City: Rockefeller Foundation, Netherlands Information Bureau, 1944.

Jeyasuria, L.W. *A Review of the Rural Health Services in West Malaysia*. Kuala Lumpur: Ministry of Health, 1967.

Kroef, Justus van der. "Point Four in Southeast Asia." *Current History* 22, no. 128 (1952): 193–99.

Lall, Sanjaya and Senaka Bibile. "The Political Economy of Controlling Transnationals: The Pharmaceutical Industry in Sri Lanka, 1972–76." *International Journal of Health Services* 8, no. 2 (1978): 299–328.

Leimena, Johannes. *Public Health in Indonesia: Problems and Planning*. Djakarta: G.C.T. van Dorp, 1956.

Leonard, Larry L. "UNRRA and the Concept of Regional International Organization." *Iowa Law Review* 30 no. 4 (1945): 489–514.

League of Nations Health Organisation. *Report of the Intergovernmental Conference of Far-Eastern Nations on Rural Hygiene Held at Bandoeng (Java), August 3rd–13th, 1937*. Geneva: League of Nations Health Organisation, 1937.

Majid, Abdul. *Public Health Activities in Afghanistan*. New Delhi: Asian Relations Conference, 1947.

Maung, Mya. "The Burmese Way to Socialism beyond the Welfare State," *Asian Survey* 10, no. 6 (1970): 533–51.

McCarrison, Robert. "Rice in Relation to Beri-Beri in India." *The British Medical Journal* 1, no. 3297 (1924): 414–20.

McGilvray, James C. *The Quest for Health and Wholeness*. Tubingen: German Institute for Medical Missions Theology, 1981.

Mehta, Usha. "The Working of the Employees' State Insurance Scheme in India: An Aspect of Centre-State Relations." *Indian Journal of Political Science* 22, no. 3 (1961): 205–13.

Monteiro, E.S. "International Cooperation in Postgraduate Medical Education in Malaya." *The British Medical Journal* 2, no. 5148 (1959): 330–32.

Myrdal, Gunnar. *Asian Drama: An Inquiry into the Poverty of Nations*, Volume 1. New York: Pantheon, 1968.

———. *Asian Drama: An Inquiry into the Poverty of Nations*, Volume 2. New York: Pantheon, 1968.

———. *An American Dilemma: The Negro Problem and Modern Democracy*, Volume 1. New York: Harper and Brothers, 1944.

Nicholls, William. "Accommodating Economic Change in Underdeveloped Countries." *The American Economic Review* 49, no. 2 (1959): 156–68.

Nityarumphong, Sanguan. "Evolution of Primary Health Care in Thailand: What Policies Worked?" *Health Policy and Planning* 6, no. 3 (1990): 254–62.

Nugroho, Gunawan and Katherine Elliott. "The Dana Sehat Programme in Solo, Indonesia." *Proceedings of the Royal Society B: Biological Sciences* 199 (1977): 145–50.

Nugroho, Gunawan, Rufino Macagba, and George Dorros. *Building Community* Health. Health Development International and Visionary Healthcare Leadership Worldwide, 2001 [Place of publication not identified].
Pardee, Ruth E. "First Aid for China." *Pacific Affairs* 19, no. 1 (1946): 75–89.
Philippine Government. "President's Month in Review: February 1949." *Messages of the President Elpidio Quirino*, Proclamations Book 6, Volume 3. Manila: Bureau of Printing, 1949.
Polson, Robert A. "Community Development in the Philippines: Observations and Comments." *Philippine Sociological Review* 4, no. 4 (1956): 7–14.
Raja, K.C.K.E. *Health Problems of India*. New Delhi: Indian Council of World Affairs, 1947.
Rajagopalachari, C. *B.C.G. Vaccination: Why I Oppose It*. Madras: K.J. Ramanujam, 1955.
Raman, A.V. "American Citizens' View on BCG." *People's Health* 4, no. 4 (1950).
———." Editorial." *People's Health* 4, no. 4 (1950).
———, "BCG: What About It?" *People's Health* 3, no. 3 (1949).
Report of the Health Survey and Development Committee, Volume II. New Delhi: Government of India, 1946.
———. *Report of the Health Survey and Development Committee*, Volume I. New Delhi: Government of India, 1946.
Ryle, John A. "Social Medicine: Its Meaning and Its Scope." *The Milbank Memorial Fund Quarterly* 22, no. 1 (1944): 58–71.
Sawyer, Wilbur A. "Achievements of UNRRA as an International Organization." *American Journal of Public Health* 37 (1947): 41–58.
———. *Advantages of Nation-Wide and International Organization of Disease Control, with Special Reference to Hookworm Disease and Beri-Beri*. Singapore: Government Printing Office, 1923.
Sein, Maung. *Health Problems of Burma*. New Delhi: Indian Council of World Affairs, 1947.
Sharp, Walter. "The New World Health Organization." *American Journal of International* Law 41, no. 3 (1947): 409–30.
Sidel, Victor. "The Barefoot Doctors of the People's Republic of China." *The New England Journal of Medicine* 286, no. 24 (June 15, 1972): 1292–1300.

Sigerist, Henry. *Medicine and Health in the Soviet Union*. New York: Citadel Press, 1937.

Soetopo, M, R. Wasito, H., Soedarsono, and D. Tjokrodipo. "The Indonesian Treponematoses Control Project." *Bulletin of the World Health Organization* 15, no.6 (1956): 937–58.

Soetopo, M, and R. Wasito. "Experience with Yaws Control in Indonesia: Preliminary Results with a Simplified Approach," *Bulletin of the World Health Organization* 8 (1953): 275–91.

Sukanto, Julie. "Education and Welfare in Indonesia." *Pakistan Horizon* 1, no. 2 (1948): 131–36.

Taylor, Carl. "The Doctor's Role in Rural Health Care." *International Journal of Health Services* 6, no. 2 (1976): 219–30.

Thakurdas, Sir Purshottamdas, J.R.D. Tata, G.D. Birla et al. *A Plan of Economic Development for India, Part II: Role of the State*. Bombay: [Publisher unknown], 1944.

Thompson, Virginia and Richard Adloff. "Social Welfare in Southeast Asia." *Far Eastern Survey* 18, no. 2 (1949): 136–40.

Walsh, Julia and Kenneth S. Warren. "Selective Primary Health Care: An Interim Strategy for Disease Control in Developing Countries." *The New England Journal of Medicine* 301, no. 18 (1979): 967–74.

Weerasuriya, Krisantha. "A Search for Balance: Pharmaceuticals in Sri Lanka: Pioneering Steps in a Receptive Environment and Subsequent Accommodations." *Development Dialogue* 1 (1995): 54–95.

Weintraub, Philip. "UNRRA: An Experiment in International Welfare Planning." *The Journal of Politics* 7, no. 1 (1945): 1–24.

Wickremasinghe, S.A. and S. Bibile. "Pharmaceuticals Management in Ceylon." *The British Medical Journal* 3, no. 5777 (September 25, 1971): 757–58.

Woodbridge, George. *UNRRA: A History of the United Nations Relief and Rehabilitation Administration*, volume I. New York: Columbia University Press, 1950.

World Bank. *World Development Report 1993: Investing in Health*. New York: Oxford University Press, 1993.

———. *World Development Report 1978*. Washington D.C.: The World Bank, 1978.

Yu, George T. "China and the Third World." *Asian Survey* 17, no. 11 (1977): 103648.

Dutch Publications: Koninklijke Bibliotheek (KB), National Library of the Netherlands, The Hague

Redevoeringen van de Leden van den Volksraad: Abdul Firman Gelar Maharadja Soangkoepon en Abdul Rasjid Gelar Maharadja Mahkota Soangkoepon over het Zittingsjaar, 1936–37. Buitenzorg: Buitenzorgsche Drukkerij, 1938.

Bahasa Indonesia Pamphlets: Perpustakaan Nasional Republik Indonesia, Jakarta

Chrusjtjov, Nikita. *Uni Sovjet Sahabat Bagi Rakjat 2 jang Sedang Berdjoeang Untuk Kemerdekaanja.* Djakarta: Kedutaan Besar URSS, 1960.

Venediktov, D.D. and V.I. Petrov. *Untuk Taraf Kesehatan jang Tertinggi.* Djakarta: Kedutaan Besar URSS, 1960.

Office of the Historian (Foreign Relations of the United States Series)

Raether, Karl, and Harriet Schwar, edited. Foreign Relations of the United States, 1952–1954, East Asia and the Pacific. Vol. 12, pt. 2. Washington, DC: U.S. Government Printing Office, 1987. Department of State, Office of the Historian.

C. Memoirs, Biographies, Political Writings, and Fiction

Arole, Mabelle and Rajanikant Arole. *A Comprehensive Rural Health Project: Jamkhed.* London: Macmillan, 1994.

Balińska, Marta A. *For the Good of Humanity: Ludwik Rajchman, Medical Statesman,* trans. Rebecca Howell. Budapest: Central European University Press, 1998.

Brown, Arthur. "Personal Experiences in the Malaria Eradication Campaign, 1955–1962." *Journal of the Royal Society of Medicine* 95 (March 2002): 154–56.

Bowles, Chester. *Ambassador's Report.* New York: Harper and Brothers, 1954.

Gullick, M. "Recollections of My Time in Malaya (1945–1956), Part 2." *Journal of the Malaysian Branch of the Royal Asiatic Society* 87, no. 1 (2014): 53–81.

Gunaratne, V.T. H. *A Voyage Toward Health.* New Delhi: Tata McGraw-Hill Publication Company, 1980.

Heiser, Victor. *An American Doctor's Odyssey: Adventures in Forty-Five Countries.* New York: W.W. Norton, 1936.

Keeney, S.M. *Half of the World's Children: A Diary of UNICEF at Work in Asia.* Association Press: New York, 1957.

———. "Two Cooperative Projects of WHO and UNICEF," *Public Health Reports* 68, no. 6 (1953): 607–608.

Lederer, William and Eugene Burdick. *The Ugly American.* New York: W.W. Norton and Co., 1958.

Leirissa, R.Z. *Kewarganegaraan Yang Bertanggung Jawab: Mengenang Dr. J. Leimena.* Jakarta: BPK Gunung Mulia, 1980. In Bahasa Indonesia.

Mayer, Albert. *The Story of Rural Development at Etawah, Uttar Pradesh: Pilot Project, India.* Berkeley: University of California Press, 1958.

Nehru, Jawaharlal. "The Development of the Nation," September 14, 1952. In *Selected Works of Jawaharlal Nehru* 19 (July 19, 1952 to October 18, 1952), Second Series. New Delhi: Jawaharlal Nehru Memorial Fund, 1996.

———. "Speech at the Closing Plenary Session of the Asian Relations Conference: Asian Relations Organization." April 2, 1947. In *Selected Works of Jawaharlal Nehru,* vol. 2. New Delhi: Jawaharlal Nehru Memorial Fund, 1984, 247–51.

Pincock, Stephen. "Obituary: Rajanikant Arole." *Lancet* 378, no. 9788 (July 2, 2011): 24.

Renu, Phanishwar Nath. *Maila Anchal.* Allahabad: Rajkamal Publication, 1954. In Hindi.

Thurman, Ernestine S. "Asia: A Challenge to Scientists." *AIBS Bulletin* 12, no. 1 (1962): 24–27.

Toer, Pramoedya Ananta. "My Kampung." *Djakarta*, July 1952. In *Tales from Djakarta: Caricatures of Human Beings and Their Circumstances*, translated by Sumit Mandal, 54–59. Ithaca: Southeast Asia Program, Cornell University Press, 1999.

D. Newspapers and Periodicals

Koninklijke Bibliotheek (KB), National Library of the Netherlands, The Hague

Dutch Newspapers

De Sumatera Post
Het Nieuws van den Dag voor Nederlandsch-Indië
Indische Courant

Gandhi Bhavan Collection, Bangalore

Harijan

Leiden University Library

Digital Collection: Malay Newspapers

Asia Raya

KITLV Collection: Malay Medical Periodicals

Berita Ketabiban

National Library of Australia, Canberra

Warwick Daily News

JSTOR South Asia Open Archives

Amrita Bazar Patrika

The National Library Board, Singapore

Indian Daily Mail
Morning Tribune
National Straits Times Reporter
New Nation
The Singapore Free Press
Singapore Standard
The Straits Times

New York Times Archives

The New York Times

Tamil Nadu State Archives Library Annex, Chennai

The *Miscellany: Monthly Journal of the South Indian Branch of the Indian Medical Association*

WHO Library and Historical Collections, Geneva

Chronicle of the World Health Organization
World Health Forum
World Health: Magazine of the World Health Organization

ILO Library, Geneva

International Labour Review

The World Council of Churches, Geneva

Contact
The Ecumenical Review

University of Michigan Library

The Michigan Daily

Secondary Sources: Monographs, Edited Volumes, Peer-Reviewed Articles, PhD Theses, Research Reports, and Academic Blogs

Abeyasekare, Susan. "Health as a Nationalist Issue in Colonial Indonesia." In *Nineteenth and Twentieth Century Indonesia: Essays in Honour of Professor J.D. Legge*, edited by C.D. Cowan and O.W. Wolters, 1–9. Clayton, Victoria: Monash University Press, 1986.

Acharya, Amitav. "Asia is Not One." *The Journal of Asian Studies* 69, no. 4 (2010): 1001–13.

Acuin, Jose. Rebecca Firestone, Thein Thein Htay, et al. "Southeast Asia: An Emerging Focus for Global Health." *The Lancet* 377, no. 9765 (February 2011): 534–35.

Akami, Tomoko. "The League of Nations Health Organization." *Oxford Biographies in the History of Medicine*, Jacalyn Duffin edited. Oxford: Oxford University Press, 2025.

———. "Imperial Polities, Intercolonialism, and the Shaping of Global Governing Norms: Public Health Expert Networks in Asia and the League of Nations Health Organization, 1908–37." *Journal of Global History* 12, no.1 (2017): 4–25.

Aloni, Omer. *The League of Nations and the Protection of the Environment.* Cambridge: Cambridge University Press, 2022.

Amrith, Sunil, and Glenda Sluga. "New Histories of the United Nations." *Journal of World History* 19, no. 3 (2008):251–74.

———. *Decolonizing International Health: India and Southeast Asia, 1930–65.* Basingstoke: Palgrave Macmillan, 2006.

Anderson, Benedict, *The Spectre of Comparisons: Nationalism, Southeast Asia and the World.* London: Verso, 1998.

———. *Java in a Time of Revolution: Occupation and Resistance, 1944–46.* Ithaca: Cornell University Press, 1972.

Anderson, Mark, Kristin Becknell, and Joanna Taliano. "History of Humanitarian Emergencies." In *Health in Humanitarian Emergencies: Principles and Practices for Public Health and Healthcare Practitioners,* edited by David Townes, 9–24. Cambridge: Cambridge University Press, 2018.

Anderson, Warwick. *Colonial Pathologies: American Tropical Medicine, Race and Hygiene in the Philippines.* Durham, NC: Duke University Press, 2006.

———. Anderson, Warwick. "Going through the Motions: American Public Health and Colonial Mimicry.'" *American Literary History* 14, no. 4 (2002): 686–719.

Arnold, David. "Death and the Modern Empire: The 1918–19 Influenza Epidemic in India." *Transactions of the Royal Historical Society* 29 (2019): 181–200.

———. "British India and the Beriberi Problem, 1798–1942." *Medical History* 54, no. 3 (2010): 295–314.

———. "Nehruvian Science and Postcolonial India." *ISIS* 104, no. 2 (2013): 360–70.

———. "Tropical Governance: Managing Health in Monsoon Asia, 1908–1938." *Asia Research Institute Working Paper* Series 116 (2009). Accessed April 10, 2025. https://papers.ssrn.com/sol3/papers.cfm?abstract_id=1645149.

Aso, Michitake. "Patriotic Hygiene: Tracing New Places of Knowledge Production about Malaria in Vietnam, 1919–75." *Journal of Southeast Asian Studies* 44, no. 3 (2013): 423–43.

Baru, Rama V. "Changing Avatars of Social Medicine in the Indian Subcontinent." In *Medicine on a Larger Scale: Global Histories of Social Medicine*, edited by Anne Kveim Lie, Jeremy Greene, and Warwick Anderson, 278–96. Cambridge: Cambridge University Press, 2025.

———. "The Bhore Committee and Recent Debates." *Seminar* 714 (2019). Accessed July 14, 2024. https //www.india-seminar.com/2019/714/714_rama_v_baru.htm.

Bayly, Christopher, and Tim Harper. *Forgotten Wars: The End of Britain's Asian Empire*. London: Penguin, 2007.

Benzian, Habib, and Manu Raj Mathur. "Indonesia Leaves SEARO: What it Means for Regional Health and WHO. *The Lancet Regional Health–Southeast Asia* 43 (2025): 10031, https://doi.org/10.1016/j.lansea.2025.100660.

Bhattacharya, Sanjoy, and Carlos Eduardo D' Avila Pereira Campani. "Re-assessing the Foundations: Worldwide Smallpox Eradication, 1957–67," *Medical History* 64, no. 1 (2020): 71–93.

———. "International Health and the Limits of its Global Influence: Bhutan and the Worldwide Smallpox Eradication Programme," *Medical History* 57, no. 4 (2013): 461–86.

———. *Expunging Variola: The Control and Eradication of Smallpox in India*. Hyderabad: Orient Longman, 2006.

Birn, Anne-Emanuelle, and Nikolai Krementsov. "'Socialising' Primary Care? The Soviet Union, WHO and the 1978 Alma-Ata Conference." *BMJ Global Health* 3 (2018): e000992.

———. "Philanthrocapitalism, Past and Present: The Rockefeller Foundation, the Gates Foundation, and the Setting(s) of the International/ Global Health Agenda." *Hypothesis* 12, no. 1 (2014): e8. doi:10.5779/hypothesis. v12i1.229.

———. With Elizabeth Fee. "The Art of Medicine: The Rockefeller Foundation and the International Health Agenda." *The Lancet* 381, no. 9878 (September 2013): 1618–19.

———. "The Stages of International (Global) Health: Histories of Success or Successes of History?" *Global Public Health* 4, no. 1 (2009): 50–68.

Brimnes, Niels. "Rallying around the Magic Wand: Visions of Social Medicine, Public Health and Disease Control in India." In *Yearbook for the History of Global Development: Health and Development*, edited by Iris Borowy, and Bernard Harris, 175–91. Oldenburg: de Gruyter, 2023.

———. "Negotiating Social Medicine in a Postcolonial Context: Halfdan Mahler in India, 1951–74." *Medical History* 67, no. 1 (2023): 5–22.

———. *Languished Hopes: Tuberculosis, the State and International Assistance in Twentieth Century India.* Hyderabad: Orient Blackswan, 2015.
Borowy, Iris. *Coming to Terms with World Health: The League of Nations Health Organisation, 1921–46.* Frankfurt: Peter Lang, 2009.
Brown, Theodore, and Elizabeth Fee. "The Bandoeng Conference of 1937: A Milestone in Health and Development." *American Journal of Public Health* 98, no. 1 (2008): 42–43.
———. "Andrija Štampar: Charismatic Leader of Social Medicine and Public Health." *American Journal of Public Health* 96, no. 2 (2006): 1382–85.
Bu, Liping. "Taking Our Own Road: Building the People's Health in Socialist China." In *Public Health and Cold War Politics in Asia*, edited by Liping Bu, 32–56. Abingdon, Oxon: Routledge, 2024.
———. "John B. Grant and Public Health in China." *Rockefeller Archive Center Research Reports.* Sleepy Hollow, NY: Rockefeller Archive Center, 2012. https://rockarch.issuelab.org/resources/27881/27881.pdf.
———. "Beijing First Health Station: Innovative Public Health Education and Influence on China's Health Profession." In *Science, Public Health and the State in Modern Asia*, edited by Liping Bu, Darwin H. Stapleton and Ka-che Yip, 129–43. Abingdon, Oxon: Routledge, 2012.
Buchwald, Henry. *Healthcare Upside Down: A Critical Examination of Policy and Practice.* Cham: Springer Nature, 2022.
Chakrabarti, Pratik. "Health as Activism: Rethinking Social Medicine in India." *The Lancet* 399 (June 4, 2022): 2096–97.
Cho, Ho Hee. *Imperial Health: Centralisation of Medical Institutions in the South Pacific.* PhD diss., Oxford University, 2022.
Clarke, Philip, and Guido Erreygers. "Edgar Sydenstricker: A Pioneer of Health Economics." The *European Journal of the History of Economic Thought* 29, no. 6 (2022): 1066–88.
Cueto, Marcos. "The History of International Health: Medicine, Health and Two Socio-Medical Perspectives, 1851–2000." In *The Oxford Handbook of Global Health Politics*, edited by Colin McInnes, Kelley Lee and Jeremy Youde. New York: Oxford University Press, 2020.
———. With Theodore Brown, and Elizabeth Fee. *The World Health Organization: A History.* Cambridge: Cambridge University Press, 2019.
———. "The WHO and Primary Healthcare during the 1980s." In *Health for All: The Journey of Universal Health Coverage*, edited by

Sanjoy Bhattacharya and Alexander Medcalf. Hyderabad: Orient Blackswan, 2015.
———. *Cold War and Deadly Fevers: Malaria Eradication in Mexico, 1955–1975*. Baltimore, MD: Johns Hopkins University Press, 2007.
———. *The Value of Health: A History of the Pan American Health Organization*. Washington DC: PAHO, 2006.
———. "The Origins of Primary Healthcare and SELECTIVE Primary Healthcare." *American Journal of Public Health* 94, no. 11 (2004): 1864–74.
Cui, Ziqi, Jing Li, Ling Meng, et al. "Nipah Virus: a Re-emerging Public Health Concern." *Lancet Microbe* 5, no. 3 (March 2024): e212.
Davies, Sara. *Containing Contagion: The Politics of Disease Outbreaks in Southeast Asia*. Baltimore, MD: Johns Hopkins University Press, 2019.
Dutta, Binayak. "Challenging Times, Challenged Body: Decolonization, Displacement and Disease among East Pakistani Refugees in South Assam, 1947–54." In *Playing with Nature: History and Politics in North-East India*, edited by Sajal Nag, 255–72. Abingdon, Oxon: Routledge, 2018.
Duus, Peter. "Diplomacy and Statecraft: The Vision of a Greater East Asia Co-Prosperity Sphere." *Diplomacy and Statecraft* 7, no. 1 (2007): 54–72.
Eby, Marek. "Cold War Form: International Content?: The Martsinovskii Institute, the World Health Organization, and the Wider Networks of International Malariology." In *International Organizations and the Cold War: Competition, Cooperation, and Convergence*, edited by Sandrine Kott, Eva-Maria Muschik, and Elisabeth Roehrlich, 145–61. London: Bloomsbury Academic, 2025.
Emmerson, Donald K. "Southeast Asia: What is in a Name." *Journal of Southeast Asian Studies* 15, no. 1 (1984): 1–21.
Fang, Xiaoping. "Communist Medicine: The Emergence of TCM and Barefoot Doctors, Leading to Contemporary Medical Markets." In *Routledge Handbook of Chinese Medicine*, edited by Vivienne Lo, Michael Stanley-Baker, and Dolly Yang, 638–48. Abingdon, Oxon: Routledge, 2022.
Fee, Elizabeth, Marcos Cueto, and Theodore Brown. "At the Roots of the World Health Organization's Challenges: Politics and Regionalization." *American Journal of Public Health* 106, no. 11 (2016): 11–16.
Frankel, Francine. *India's Political Economy: The Gradual Revolution, 1947–1977*. Princeton: Princeton University Press, 1977.

Gillespie, James A. "Social Medicine, Social Security and International Health, 1940–60." In *The Politics of Healthy Life: An International Perspective*, edited by Esteban Rodrìguez Ocaña, 219–40. Manchester: Manchester University Press, 2002.

Gilman, Nils. "The New International Economic Order: A Reintroduction." *Humanity* 6, no. 1 (Spring 2015). Accessed April 29, 2025. https://humanityjournal.org/issue6-1/the-new-international-economic-order-a-reintroduction/.

Gorsky, Martin, and Christopher Sirrs. "The Rise and Fall of 'Universal Health Coverage' as a Goal of International Politics, 1925–52." *American Journal of Public Health* 108, no. 3 (2018): 334–42.

Grant, Jenna. "'Cambodian Pathology': Imagining Modern Biomedicine in the Cambodian-Soviet Medical Journal, *Revue Médico-Chirurgicale de l' Hôpital de Amitié Khméro-Soviétique* (1961–71)." In *Translating the Body: Medical Education in Southeast Asia*, edited by Hans Pols, C. Michele Thompson, and John Harley Warner, 194–229. Singapore: NUS Press, 2017.

Greene, Jeremy A. "Vital Objects: Essential Drugs and Their Critical Legacies." In *Reimagining (Bio) Medicalization, Pharmaceuticals and Genetics: Old Critiques and New Engagements*, edited by Susan Bell, and Anne Figert, 89–111. Abingdon. Oxon: Routledge, 2015.

———. "Making Medicines Essential: The Emergent Centrality of Pharmaceuticals in Global Health." *BioSocieties* 6, no. 1 (2011): 10–33.

Greenough, Paul. "Indian Famines and Peasant Victims: The Case of Bengal in 1943–1944." *Modern Asian Studies* 14, no. 2 (1980): 205–35.

Grundy-Warr, Carl, and Shaun Lin. "COVID-19 Geopolitics: Silence and Erasure in Cambodia and Myanmar in Times of Pandemic." *Eurasian Geography and Economics* 61, nos. 4–5 (2020): 493–510.

Guénel, Annick. "The 1937 Bandung Conference on Hygiene: Towards a New Vision of Healthcare?" In *Global Movements, Local Concerns: Medicine and Health in Southeast Asia*, edited by Laurence Monnais and Harold Cook, 62–80. Singapore: NUS Press, 2012.

Haas, Ernst. Functionalism *and International Organization*. Stanford, CA: Stanford University Press, 1964.

Hall, D.G.E. *A History of South-East Asia*. New York: St. Martin's Press, 1955.

Harder, Andrew. "The Politics of Impartiality: The United Nations Relief and Rehabilitation in the Soviet Union, 1946–47." *Journal of Contemporary History* 47, no. 2 (2012): 347–67.

Harris, Joseph. *Achieving Access: Professional Movements and the Politics of Health Universalism*. Ithaca: Cornell University Press, 2017.

Harrison, Mark. "A Global Perspective: Reframing the History of Health, Medicine, and Disease." *Bulletin of the History of Medicine* 89, no. 4 (2015): 639–89.

Henderson, William. "The Development of Regionalism in Southeast Asia." *International Organization* 9, no. 4 (1955): 463–76.

Hewa, Soma. "Tropical Disease and Imperial Medicine in Colonial Sri Lanka." *Galle Medical Journal* 24, no. 2 (2019): 25–32.

———. "The Alma-Ata Declaration, Rockefeller Foundation and the Development of Primary Health Care in Sri Lanka: A Model for Health Prevention." In *Science, Public Health and the State in Modern Asia*, edited by Liping Bu, Darwin Stapleton and Ka-che Yip, 71–92. Abingdon, Oxon: Routledge, 2012.

———. "Sri Lanka's Approach to Primary Health Care: A Success Story in South Asia." *Galle Medical Journal* 16, no. 2 (2011): 24–31.

———. "The Hookworm Epidemic on the Plantations in Sri Lanka." *Medical History* 38 no.1 (1994): 73–90.

Heydon, Susan. *Modern Medicine and International Aid: Khunde Hospital, Nepal, 1966–1998*. Hyderabad: Orient Blackswan, 2009.

Hooda, Shailender. "Health System in Transition in India: Journey from State Provisioning to Privatization." *World Review of Political Economy* 11, no. 4 (2020): 506–32.

Huff, Gregg. *World War II and Southeast Asia: Economy and Society Under Japanese Occupation*. Cambridge: Cambridge University Press, 2020.

———. "The Second World War Vietnam and Java Famines." *Modern Asian Studies* 53, no. 6 (2019): 1–36.

Hull, Terence. "Conflict and Collaboration in Public Health: The Rockefeller Foundation and the Dutch Colonial Government in Indonesia." In *Public Health in Asia and the Pacific: Historical and Comparative Perspectives*, edited by Milton J. Lewis and Kerrie L. Macpherson, 139–52. Abingdon, Oxon: Routledge, 2008.

Immerwahr, Daniel. "The Ugly American: Peeling the Onion of an Iconic Cold War Text." *Journal of American-East Asian Relations* 26 (2019): 7–20.

———. Immerwahr, Daniel. *Thinking Small: United States and the Lure of Community Development*. Cambridge, MA: Harvard University Press, 2015.

Jagtiani, Sharinee. "'Foreign Armies are Functioning on Indian Soil': India, Indonesian Decolonization and Onset of the Cold War (1945–49)." *Cold War History* 22, no. 3 (2022): 305–24.

Johnston, G.A. *International Social Progress: The Work of the International Labour Organization*. London: George Allen and Unwin Ltd., 1924.

Jolly, Richard. *UNICEF (United Nations Children's Fund): Global Governance that Works*. Abingdon, Oxon: Routledge, 2014.

Jones, Norman Howard. *The Scientific Background of the International Sanitary Conferences*. Geneva: WHO, 1975.

Jose, Ricardo Trota. "Food Production and Food Distribution Programmes in the Philippines during the Japanese Occupation." In *Food Supplies and the Japanese Occupation in South-East Asia,* edited by Paul Kratoska, 67–100. Basingstoke, Oxon: Macmillan, 1998.

Kahin, G.M. *Nationalism and Revolution in Indonesia*. Ithaca: Cornell University Press, 2003.

Kavadi, Shirish. "John B. Grant and Public Health in India," *Indian Journal of Medical Ethics* 4, no.1 (2019). https://doi.org/10.20529/IJME.2019.010.

———. Kavadi, Shirish. "'Parasites Lost and Parasites Regained': Rockefeller Foundation's Anti-Hookworm Campaign in Madras Presidency." *Economic and Political Weekly* 42, no. 2 (2007): 130–37.

———. "'Wolves Come to Take Care of the Lamb': The Rockefeller Foundation's Hookworm Campaign in Madras Presidency." In *The Politics of the Healthy Life: An International Perspective*, edited by Esteban Rodrìguez-Ocaña, 89–111. Sheffield: European Society for the History of Medicine, 2002.

Khan, Shamshad. "Systems of Medicine and Nationalist Discourse in India: Towards 'New Horizons' in Medical Anthropology and History." *Social Science and Medicine* no. 62 no.11 (2006): 2786–97.

Khoo, Ying Hooi. "Southeast Asia's Pandemic Politics and Human Rights: Trends and Lessons." *LSE Blogs*, October 1, 2020. Accessed May 5, 2025. https://blogs.lse.ac.uk/seac/2020/10/01/southeast-asias-pandemic-politics-and-human-rights-trends-and-lessons/#comments.

Knapton, Samantha and Katherine Rossy. "Introduction." In *Relief and Rehabilitation in a Post-War World*, edited by Samantha Knapton, and Katherine Rossy. London: Bloomsbury, 2024.

Knoll, Eva-Maria. "Malaria Eradication and Modernization in Maldives and Sri Lanka." In *The Geopolitics of Health in South and Southeast Asia:*

Perspectives from the Cold War to COVID-19, edited by Vivek Neelakantan, 77–98. Abingdon, Oxon: Routledge, 2023.

Kott, Sandrine, and Joëlle Droux. "Introduction," in *Global Social Rights: The International Labour Organization and Beyond*, edited by Sandrine Kott, and Joëlle Droux, 1–16. Basingstoke: Palgrave Macmillan, 2013.

Lachenal, Guillaume. "A Genealogy of Treatment as Prevention (TasP): Prevention Therapy, and the Tensions of Public Health in African History." In *Global Health in Africa: Historical Perspectives on Disease Control*, edited by Tamara Giles-Vernick, and James L.A. Webb Jr, 70–91. Athens: Ohio University Press, 2013.

Lee, Kelley. *The World Health Organization*. Abingdon, Oxon: Routledge, 2009.

Lee, Suyeon and Funcie Y. Park. "Examining Aid Fragmentation and Collaboration Opportunities in Cambodia's Health Sector." *Global Health* 20, no. 62 (2024). https://doi.org/10.1186/s12992-024-01063-7.

Legge, J.D. "The Writing of Southeast Asian History." In *The Cambridge History of Southeast Asia: Volume 1, From Early Times to 1800*, edited by Nicholas Tarling, 1–50. Cambridge: Cambridge University Press, 1992.

Lin, Yi-Tang. *Statistics and the Language of Global Health: Institutions and Experts in China, Taiwan and the World, 1917–60*. Cambridge: Cambridge University Press, 2022.

Litsios, Socrates. "Kenneth Newell: Primary Healthcare's Midwife." *Social Medicine* 14, no. 1 (2021): 28–36.

———. "Cora Du Bois Brief Stint with the World Health Organization, 1950–51: Right Time, Wrong Place." *International Journal for Health Services* 48, no. 4 (2018): 716–34.

———. Rural Hygiene in the Early Years of the World Health Organization: Another Casualty of the Cold War?" *Anais do Instituto de Higiene e Medicina Tropical* 15 (August 2016): 125–32.

———. "Revisiting Bandoeng." *Social Medicine* 8, no. 3 (2014): 113–19.

———. "Bandoeng Conference of 1937." *American Journal of Public Health* 98, no. 5 (2008): 777.

———. Litsios, Socrates. "The Christian Medical Commission and the Development of the World Health Organization's Primary Healthcare Approach." *American Journal of Public Health* 94, no. 11 (2004): 1884–93.

———. "The Long and Difficult Road to Alma-Ata: A Personal Reflection." *International Journal of Health Services* 32, no. 4 (2002): 709–32.

Lowe, Celia. "Viral Sovereignty: Security and Mistrust as Measures of Future Health in the Indonesian H5N1 Outbreak." *Medical Anthropology Quarterly* 6, no. 3 (2019): 109–32.

Lynn-Pearson, Jessica. *The Colonial Politics of Global Health: France and the United Nations in Postwar Africa.* Harvard: Harvard University Press, 2018.

Maday, André de. *Le Charte International du Travail.* Neuchâtel: F. Ridier et cie, 1921. In French.

Magden, Kirsta K. "'The First Line of Defense': British Quarantine and the Port Sanitary Authorities in the Nineteenth Century." *Social History of Medicine* 15, no. 3 (2002): 413–28.

Manderson, Lenore. "Wireless Wars in the Eastern Arena: Epidemiological Surveillance, Disease Prevention and the Work of the Eastern Bureau of the League of Nations Health Organisation, 1925–1942." In *International Health Organisations and Movements*, edited by Paul Weindling, 109–33. Cambridge: Cambridge University Press, 1995.

Manela, Erez. "Smallpox and the Globalization of Development." In *The Development Century: A Global Perspective*, edited by Stephen J. Macekura and Erez Manela, 83–104. Cambridge: Cambridge University Press, 2018.

———. "A Pox on Your Narrative: Writing Disease Control into Cold War History." *Diplomatic History* 14, no. 2 (2010): 299–323.

Mark, Ethan. Japan's *Occupation of Indonesia during the Second World War: A Transnational History.* London: Bloomsbury, 2018.

Maul, Daniel. "The ILO in Asia and the Beginnings of Technical Assistance." In *The ILO from Geneva to the Pacific Rim: East Meets West*, edited by Jill M. Jensen, and Nelson Lichtenstein, 110–34. Basingstoke: Palgrave Macmillan, 2016.

———. *Human Rights, Development and Decolonization: The International Labour Organisation, 1940–70.* Basingstoke: Palgrave Macmillan, 2012.

Moni, Michele, and Klaus Peterson. "Cold War and Social Security in Burma and Malaysia." In *From Colonialism to International Aid: External Actors and Social Protection in the Global South*, edited by Carina Smith, 45–78. Basingstoke: Palgrave Macmillan, 2020.

Monnais, Laurence, and Hans Pols. "Imperial Social Medicine in Southeast Asia: The Bandung Intergovernmental Conference on Rural Hygiene."

In *Medicine on a Larger Scale: Global Histories of Social Medicine*, edited by Ann Kveim Lie, Jeremy Alan Greene and Warwick Anderson, 81–105. Cambridge: Cambridge University Press, 2025.

———. With C. Michele Thompson, and Ayo Wahlberg, edited. *Southern Medicine for Southern People: Vietnamese Medicine in the Making*. Newcastle-upon-Tyne: Cambridge Scholars, 2012.

Naono, Atsuko. "Rural Health in Modern Southeast Asia." In *Histories of Health in Southeast Asia; Perspectives on the Long Twentieth Century*, edited by Tim Harper, and Sunil Amrith, 99–117. Bloomington: Indiana University Press, 2014.

Neelakantan, Vivek. "Mobilizing Applied Medical Knowledge in Indonesia: Soekarnoist Science and Asian-African Solidarity in the 1950s." In *Fighting for Health: Medicine in Southeast Asia*, edited by C. Michele Thompson, Kathryn Sweet, and Michitake Aso, 167–93. Singapore: NUS Press, 2024.

———. "History of Pandemics in Southeast Asia: A Return of National Anxieties?" *ISIS* 114, S1 (2023): S419–46.

———. "Introduction." In *The Geopolitics of Health in South and Southeast Asia: Perspectives from the Cold War to COVID-19*, edited by Vivek Neelakantan, 1–26. Abingdon, Oxon: Routledge, 2023.

———. "The Monsoon Asia of Geographers: The Cold War Beginnings of the WHO Regional Office for Southeast Asia (SEARO), 1948–60." In *The Geopolitics of Health in South and Southeast Asia: Perspectives from the Cold War to COVID-19*, edited by Vivek Neelakantan, 27–53. Abingdon, Oxon.: Routledge, 2023.

———. "Indonesian Health Policy between the Old and the New Orders." In *Public Health and Cold War Politics in Asia*, edited by Liping Bu, 151–76. Abingdon, Oxon: Routledge, 2023.

———. "'No Nation Can Go Forward When it is Crippled by Disease': Philippine Science and the Cold War, 1946–65." *Southeast Asian Studies* 10, no. 1 (2021): 53–88.

———. "Tuberculosis Control in Postcolonial South India and Southeast Asia: Fractured Sovereignties in International Health, 1948–60." *Wellcome Open Research* 2 (4). https://doi.org/10.12688/wellcomeopenres.10544.2.

——— *Science, Public Health and Nation-Building in Soekarno-Era Indonesia*. Newcastle-upon-Tyne: Cambridge Scholars, 2017.

———. “The Campaign Against Yaws in Postcolonial Indonesia: Forgotten Disease, Unfinished Victories.” *IIAS Newsletter* 61, no. 4 (2014): 10–11.

———. “The Campaign Against the Big Four Endemic Diseases and Indonesia’s Engagement with the WHO during the Cold War 1950s.” In *Public Health and National Reconstruction in Post-War Asia: International Influences, Local Transformations*, edited by Liping Bu, and Ka-che Yip, 154–74. Abingdon, Oxon: Routledge, 2014.

———. “Eradicating Smallpox in Indonesia: The Archipelagic Challenge.” *Health and History* 12, no. 1 (2010): 61–87.

Nguyen, Thuy Linh. “French Educated Midwives and the Medicalization of Childbirth in Colonial Vietnam.” *Journal of Vietnamese Studies* 5, no. 2 (2010): 133–82.

O’ Shaughnessy, Patrick. “Parachuting Cats and Crushed Eggs: The Controversy Over the Use of DDT to Control Malaria.” *American Journal of Public Health* 98, no. 11 (2008): 1940–48.

Ovesen, Jan and Ing-Britt Trankell. *Cambodians and their Doctors: A Medical Anthropology of Colonial and Post-Colonial Cambodia.* Copenhagen: NIAS Press, 2010.

Packard, Randall. *A History of Global Health: Interventions into the Lives of Other Peoples.* Baltimore, MD: Johns Hopkins University Press, 2016.

———. *The Making of a Tropical Disease: A Short History of Malaria.* Baltimore, MD: Johns Hopkins University Press, 2007.

Perera Susie, Sudha Ramani, Taufique Jaarder, et al. “Reorienting Health Systems Towards Primary Health Care in South Asia.” *The Lancet Regional Health- Southeast Asia* 28 (2024): 100466.

Perry, Henry, and Jon Rohde. “The Jamkhed Comprehensive Rural Health Project and the Alma-Ata Vision of PHC.” *American Journal of Public Health* 109, no. 5 (2019): 699–704.

Pires-Alves, Fernando Antônio, and Marcos Cueto. “The Alma-Ata Decade: The Crisis of Development and International Health.” *Ciência & Saúde Coletiva* 22 (2017): 2035–44.

Pisani, Elizabeth. “Medicine for a Sick System.” *Inside Indonesia* 113 (January 26, 2013). Accessed May 3, 2025. https://www.insideindonesia.org/editions/edition-111-jan-mar-2013/medicine-for-a-sick-system.

Por, Heong Hong. “Tool of Domination and Act of Benevolence: Medicine and Healthcare during the Malayan Emergency, 1948–60.” In *Fighting for Health: Medicine in Cold War Southeast Asia*, edited by

C. Michele Thompson, Kathryn Sweet, and Michitake Aso, 53–83. Singapore: NUS Press, 2024.

Pols, Hans. *Nurturing Indonesia: Medicine and Decolonisation in the Dutch East Indies.* Cambridge: Cambridge University Press, 2018.

Puaksom, Davisakd. "Thailand's Rural Doctor Society in the 1970s-80s and Its Struggles to Improve Health in the Countryside." In *The Geopolitics of Health in South and Southeast Asia: Perspectives from the Cold War to COVID-19, 1948–2021*, edited by Vivek Neelakantan, 98–119. Abingdon, Oxon: Routledge, 2023.

———. "A Promise of Desire: On the Politics of Health and Moral Discourse in Thailand, 1950–2010." In Public Health and National Reconstruction in Post-War Asia: International Influences, Local Transformations, edited by Liping Bu and Ka-che Yip, 175–96. London: Routledge, 2015.

Ramanna, Mridula. *Bombay Presidency, 1850–1920: Disease, Sanitation and Public Health Personalities.* New Delhi: Primus, 2024.

Reinisch, Jessica. "Auntie UNRRA at the Crossroads." *Past and Present* 218, supplement 8 (2013): 70–97.

Ridlo, Ilham A. "Indonesia Just Left WHO's Southeast Asia Region: Here's Why It Matters for Global Health." *Science Watchdog.id,* May 26, 2025.Accessed May 28, 2025. https://sciencewatchdog.id/2025/05/26/indonesia-just-left-whos-southeast-asia-region-heres-why-that-matters-for-global-health/.

Rifkin, Susan B. "Alma Ata after 40 years: Primary Health Care and Health for All—From Consensus to Complexity." *BMJ Global Health* 3, no.3 (2018): e001188. doi:10.1136/ bmjgh-2018-001188.

Saavedra, Monica. "Politics and Health in the WHO Regional Office for South East Asia: The Case of Portuguese India, 1949–61." *Medical History* 61, no. 3 (2017): 380–400.

Sabharwal, Gopa. "In Search of an Asian Vision: The Asian Relations Conference of 1947." In *Imagining Asia(s): Networks, Actors, Sites,* edited by Andrea Acri, Kashshaf Ghani, Murari Jha and Sraman Mukherjee, 60–90. Singapore: ISEAS, 2019.

Sato, Shigeru. "Oppression and Romanticism: The Food Supply in Japan during the Japanese Occupation." In *Food Supplies and Japanese Occupation in Southeast Asia*, edited by Paul Kratoska, 167–86 Basingstoke: Macmillan, 1998.

Sen, Amartya. "Famines as Failures of Exchange Entitlements." *Economic and Political Weekly* 11, no. 31/33 (1976): 1273–80.

Siddiqui, Javed. *World Health and World Politics: The World Health Organization and the UN System*. London: Hurst and Company, 1995.

Silverstein, Sara. "Man with an Impossible Mission? Andrija Štampar's Separation of Politics and Healthcare in Yugoslavia and the World Health Organization." *Rockefeller Archive Center Research Reports*. Sleepy Hollow, NY: Rockefeller Archive Center, 2013. https://rockarch.issuelab.org/resources/27898/27898.pdf.

Sinha, Subir. "Lineages of the Developmentalist State: Transnationality and Village India, 1900–1965." *Comparative Studies in Society and History* (2008): 57–90.

Sirrs, Christopher. "Promoting Health Protection Worldwide: The International Labour Organisation and Health Systems Financing, 1952–2012." *International History Review* 42, no. 2 (2020): 371–90.

Smith, Alexander Cameron. "Australian Imperialism and International Health in the Pacific Islands," *Australian Historical Studies* 41, no. 1 (2010): 57–74.

Standing, Guy. "The ILO: An Agency for Globalization?" *Development and Change* 39, no. 8 (2008): 355–84.

Stapleton, Darwin H. "A Lost Chapter in the Early History of DDT: The Development of Anti-Typhus Technologies by the Rockefeller Foundation's Louse Laboratory, 1942–44." *Technology and Culture* 46, no. 3 (2005): 513–40.

Stein, Eric A. "Hygiene and Decolonization: The Rockefeller Foundation and Indonesian Nationalism, 1933–58." In *Science, Public Health and the State in Modern Asia*, edited by Liping Bu, Darwin Stapleton and Ka-che Yip, 51–70. Abingdon, Oxon: Routledge, 2012.

Stevenson, Michael A. and Andrew F. Cooper. "Overcoming Constraints of State Sovereignty: Global Health Governance in Asia." *Third World Quarterly* 30, no. 7 (2009): 1379–94.

Stoler, Ann Laura. *Along the Archival Grain: Epistemic Anxieties and Colonial Common Sense*. Princeton: Princeton University Press, 2009.

Subrahmanyam, Arjun, and Michael Sturma. "Asian Labourers, the Thai Government and the Thai-Burma Railway." *Journal of Contemporary History* 56, no. 2 (2020): 364–85.

Sweet, Kathryn. "Women's Health in Laos: From Colonial Times to the Present." In *Translating the Body: Medical Education in Southeast Asia*, edited by Hans Pols, C. Michele Thompson, and John Harley Warner, 116–45. Singapore: NUS Press, 2017.

Tagliacozzo, Eric. "Pilgrim Ships and the Frontiers of Contagion: Quarantine Regimes from Southeast Asia to the Red Sea." In *Histories of Health in Southeast Asia: Perspectives on the Long Twentieth Century*, edited by Tim Harper, 47–60. Bloomington, Indiana: Indiana University Press, 2014.

Takuma, Kayo. "The Far Eastern Bureau of the League of Nations: Linking the Regional and International Orders Through Health Work." In *East Asians in the League of Nations: Actors, Empires, and Regions in Early Global Politics*, edited by Christopher Hughes, and Hatsue Shinahora, 61–80. Basingstoke: Palgrave Macmillan, 2023.

Tangcharoensathien, Viroj, Waranan Wittayapiposakul, Warisa Panichkriangkrai, et al. "Health Systems Development in Thailand: A Solid Platform for Successful Implementation of Universal Health Coverage." *The Lancet* 391, no. 10126 (March 2018). https://doi.org/10.1016/S0140-6736(18)30198-3.

Tappan, Jennifer. "The True Fiasco: The Treatment and Prevention of Severe Acute Malnutrition in Uganda, 1950–74." In *Global Health in Africa: Historical Perspectives on Disease Control*, edited by Tamara Giles Vernick, and James L.A. Webb Jr, 92–116. Athens: Ohio University Press, 2013.

Tarling, Nicholas. "The United Kingdom and the Origins of the Colombo Plan." *The Journal of Commonwealth and Comparative Politics* 24, no. 1 (2008): 3–36.

Thakur, Vineet. "An Asian Drama: The Asian Relations Conference, 1947." *International History Review* 41, no. 3 (2019): 673–95.

Than, Tharaphi. "The Languages of Pyidawtha and the Burmese Approach to National Development." *Southeast Asia Research* 21, no. 4 (2013): 639–54.

Van Daele, Jasmiene. "The International Labor Organization (ILO) in Past and Present Research." *International Review of Social History* 53, no. 3 (December 2008): 485–511.

Vandenbosch, Amry, and Richard Butwell. *The Changing Face of Southeast* Asia. Lexington, Kentucky: Kentucky University Press, 1966.

Vickers, Adrian. *A History of Modern Indonesia, Second Edition*. Cambridge: Cambridge University Press, 2013.

Villani, Angela. "Children in the Development Debate: The Role of UNICEF from 1947 to the First UN Development Decade." *Journal of World History* 32, no. 3 (2021): 405–38.

———. "Planning the Needs of Children in the Global South: UNICEF's Contribution to the Development Debate during the 1960s." *Histoire Politique* no. 41 (2020). Accessed November 27, 2024. https://journals.openedition.org/histoirepolitique/356

Webb, James L.A., and Tamara-Giles Vernick. "Introduction." In *Global Health in Africa: Historical Perspectives on Disease Control*, edited by Tamara Giles-Vernick, and James L.A. Webb, 1–24. Athens, Ohio: Ohio University Press, 2013.

Westad, Odd Arne. *The Global Cold War: Third World Interventions and the Making of Our Times.* Cambridge: Cambridge University Press, 2007.

Webster, David. "Development Advisors in a Time of Cold War and Decolonization: The United Nations Technical Assistance Administration, 1950–59." *Journal of Global History* 6, no. 2 (2011): 249–72.

Williams, Rebecca Jane. "Storming the Citadels of Poverty: Family Planning under the Emergency in India, 1975–1977." *Journal of Asian Studies* 73, no. 2 (2014): 471–92.

Weindling, Paul. "Philanthropy and World Health: The Rockefeller Foundation and the League of Nations Health Organization." *Minerva* 35 (1997): 269–81.

Whiteside, Noel. "The Beveridge Report and its Implementation: A Revolutionary Project?" *Dans Histoire et Politique* 3 (2014): 24–37.

Wyatt, Andrew. "Populism and Politics in Contemporary Tamil Nadu." *Contemporary South Asia* 21 (2013): 265–81.

Zhou, Xun. "China's Barefoot Doctor to Alma Ata: The Primary Healthcare Movement in the Long 1970s." In *China, Hong Kong and the Long 1970s: Global Perspectives,* edited by P. Roberts, and O.A. Westad, 135–57. Basingstoke, Oxon: Palgrave Macmillan, 2017.

Index[1]

[1] Note: Page numbers followed by 'n' refer to notes.

V. Neelakantan, *The Emergence of International Health Policy in Southeast Asia, India, and Sri Lanka, 1937-1978*,
https://doi.org/10.1007/978-3-032-21233-7

GPSR Compliance
The European Union's (EU) General Product Safety Regulation (GPSR) is a set of rules that requires consumer products to be safe and our obligations to ensure this.

If you have any concerns about our products, you can contact us on

ProductSafety@springernature.com

In case Publisher is established outside the EU, the EU authorized representative is:

Springer Nature Customer Service Center GmbH
Europaplatz 3
69115 Heidelberg, Germany

www.ingramcontent.com/pod-product-compliance
Ingram Content Group UK Ltd.
Pitfield, Milton Keynes, MK11 3LW, UK
UKHW020937180926
475692UK00004B/81

* 9 7 8 3 0 3 2 2 1 2 3 2 0 *